WOMEN IN STRESS

Women in Stress
A Nursing Perspective

Edited by
DIANE K. KJERVIK, R.N., M.S.
Assistant Professor, School of Nursing
University of Minnesota
Minneapolis, Minnesota

IDA M. MARTINSON, R.N., Ph.D., F.A.A.N.
Professor of Nursing, School of Nursing
Lecturer in Physiology, School of Medicine
University of Minnesota
Minneapolis, Minnesota

Appleton-Century-Crofts/New York

Dedicated to Women and Those Who Care

Prentice-Hall International, Inc., London
Prentice-Hall of Australia, Pty. Ltd., Sydney
Prentice-Hall of India Private Limited, New Delhi
Prentice-Hall of Japan, Inc. Tokyo
Prentice-Hall of Southeast Asia (Pte.) Ltd., Singapore

Design: Judith C. Allan

Illustration Credits:
Opener for Part I: THE GRANGER COLLECTION
Opener for Parts II, III, and IV: PHOTOGRAPHS BY KEN HEYMAN

Main entry under title:

Women in stress.

   Includes index.
   1. Nursing--psychological aspects. 2. Women--
Psychology. 3. Stress (Psychology) 4. Gynecologic
nursing--Psychological aspects. I. Kjervik, Diane K.,
1945-   II. Martinson, Ida Marie, 1936-
RT86.W58   610.73'678'01   78-22077
ISBN 0-8385-9829-3

PRINTED IN THE UNITED STATES OF AMERICA

CONTRIBUTORS

ANDERSON, STEVEN
Graduate Student
Department of Physiology
School of Medicine
University of Minnesota
Minneapolis, Minnesota

ALBRECHT, MARIE, R.N. M.S.
Assistant Professor
University of Minnesota
School of Nursing
Minneapolis, Minnesota

BRAND, KAREN PAULSEN, R.N., M.S.
Instructor
University of Minnesota
School of Nursing
Minneapolis, Minnesota

BRANCH, HOLLY, R.N., M.S.
Partner in Private Practice
Health Counseling Services
Minneapolis, Minnesota

BUSH, MARY ANN, R.N., M.S.
Clinician, Consultant, and Coordinator
Carver County Community
Health Program
Waconia, Minnesota

CANEDY, BRENDA HARAM, R.N., M.S.
Instructor
University of Minnesota
School of Nursing
Minneapolis, Minnesota

DYER, RUTH, R.N., M.S.
Instructor
University of Michigan
School of Nursing
Ann Arbor, Michigan

FINCK, KAREN, R.N., M.S.
Partner in Private Practice
Health Counseling Services
Minneapolis, Minnesota

GLASS, LAURIE K., R.N., M.S.
Assistant Professor
University of Wisconsin-Milwaukee
School of Nursing
Milwaukee, Wisconsin

GORDON, VERONA C., R.N., M.S.
Associate Professor
University of Minnesota
School of Nursing
Minneapolis, Minnesota

GRONSETH, EVANGELINE, R.N., Ph.D.
Research Associate
University of Minnesota
School of Nursing
Minneapolis, Minnesota
School of Nursing

JOSTEN, LA VOHN, M.N.
Maternal and Child Health Consultant
Minneapolis Health Department
Minneapolis, Minnesota

JUAREZ, MAUREEN, R.N., M.S.
Instructor
University of Minnesota
School of Nursing
Minneapolis, Minnesota

KIRESUK, TOM, Ph.D.
Chief Clinical Pathologist
Hennepin County Medical Center;
Director
Program Evaluation Resource Center
Minneapolis, Minnesota

KJERVIK, DIANE K., R.N., M.S.
Assistant Professor
University of Minnesota
School of Nursing
Minneapolis, Minnesota

LeDRAY, LINDA, R.N., M.S.
Clinical Nursing Coordinator for Psychiatry
Hennepin County Medical Center;
Director
Sexual Assault Research Service
Minneapolis, Minnesota

LUND, SANDER, B.A.
Associate Director
Program Evaluation Research Center
Hennepin County Medical Center
Minneapolis, Minnesota

MARTINSON, IDA M., R.N.,
Ph.D., F.A.A.N.
University of Minnesota
School of Nursing;
Lecturer
Department of Physiology
School of Medicine
University of Minnesota
Minneapolis, Minnesota

McELMURRY, BEVERLY LaBELLE,
R.N., Ph.D.
Associate Professor
Department of Nursing
Northern University
DeKalb, Illinois

MENIKHEIM, MARIE, R.N., M.S.
Nursing Curriculum Coordinator
Metropolitan State University
St. Paul, Minnesota

VALENTI, CAROL, R.N., B.S.N., M.S.W.
Department of Mental Health
St. Louis Park Medical Center
Minnetonka, Minnesota

WEISENSEE, MARY G., R.N., M.S.
Assistant Professor
University of Minnesota
School of Nursing
Minneapolis, Minnesota

Contents

Preface

This book was developed from the editors' long-term interest in stress and its effect on women. As this book approached completion, an editorial appeared in the September 15, 1977 *American Nurse* by Mary Reres with the title, "Coping With Stress in Nursing". She writes, "Stress has become the companion of this generation more than for any other age." We agree and hope that this book will serve as a text for an elective course in undergraduate nursing programs and a source book for graduate nursing students. Women's Studies Departments would also find the material appropriate regarding women in nursing as the largest group of professionals in the health care system.

Part I: These four chapters begin with a detailed discussion of the leadership role of Florence Nightingale as this continues to be felt today, followed by an historical view of women and nursing. The damage to nurses' opinions of themselves as a result of historical factors will be described and assertiveness as a means of raising an individual nurse's self-esteem will be discussed. This section will close with a look at challenges which await nurses as they move into the future.

Part II: This part starts with discussion of some basic differences in the male and female response to stress, followed by a more in-depth discussion of female sexuality. The next two chapters speak to the more social aspects of stress in communication patterns as well as in sexism. The final two chapters broaden the viewpoint to include the cultural dimension of Mexican-American aspects in illness as well as the stressful effect of poverty.

Part III: This section begins with the acute and chronic aspects of the battering and rape experiences of women. The woman's role in child abuse is then considered. The section closes with an introduction to the whole area of women and pain.

Part IV: The last part opens with a discussion of the loss of the childbearing capacity first through hysterectomy—one of the most common surgical procedures performed today—followed by the more natural loss through menopause. A more subtle loss with resulting stress will be covered by a discussion of the effects of divorce. This section closes with the more personal and ultimate loss of first a spouse through death, and then a child.

In the preparation of a manuscript of this nature (i.e., one involving values relating to intimate matters such as sex role identity) support, encouragement and critical evaluation of the concepts presented are essential. The editors wish to thank Geoffrey Abbott and Paul Martinson as "men behind the scenes" who provided these necessitities. Their ability to view the feminist message as a challenge and an opportunity rather than a threat was an asset in this process.

Also, numerous colleagues, friends, relatives and nursing students provided valuable comments regarding these topics. These persons have included, among others, Marcea Doremus, Andrea Thomson, and Charlotte Striebel. Special appreciation is expressed to Betty Lockhart for her assistance in coordinating the book.

Part I
Evolutionary Stress in the Development of Nursing's Professional Role

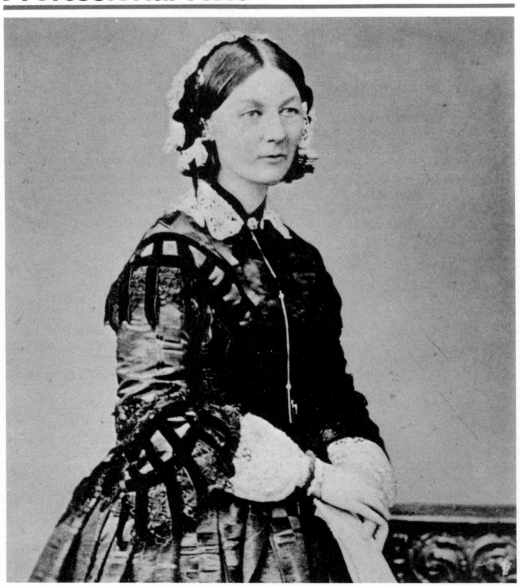

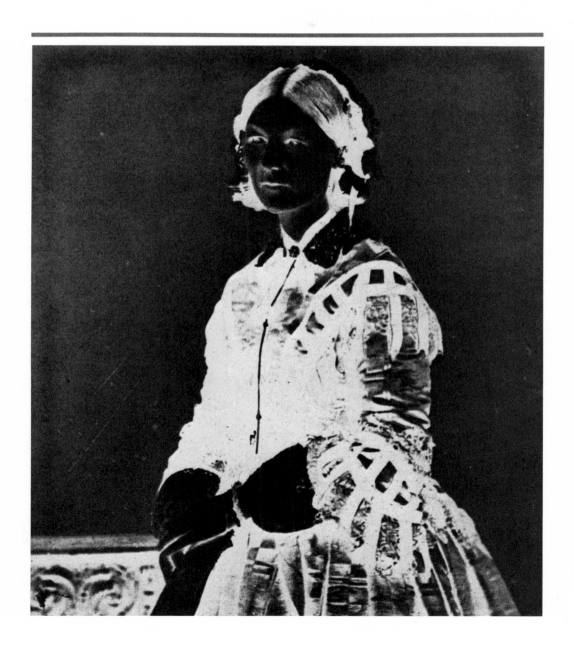

1
Florence Nightingale

Woman with a Vision

BRENDA HARAM CANEDY

To be on the leading edge of innovation is to court exhilaration, probably frustration, and surely stress. Innovation is seldom heralded as an unmixed blessing. Change suggests the insecurity of the unknown, and this can seem less appealing than even the possible discomfort of the known. It can be frankly unappealing from a position of established privilege.

To be a woman who innovates, and particularly one who innovates on a grand scale, is to face challenge from two directions. Women in Western culture have been regarded in great part as preservers of values approved for them by men; to innovate is antithetical with such societal norms. Furthermore, the innovator causes unrest, confusion, and upheaval and is thus likely to be relatively unwelcomed by those in power.

So a woman committed to a vision requiring innovation must be willing to undergo stress and to deal with it in ways that enhance her personal mental, emotional, and physical resources if her dream is to prosper. One who was committed and dealt successfully with the problems of the stresses visited upon her was Florence Nightingale. It is her environment, the mission she chose to pursue, and the ways she elected to respond to the stresses caused by the dichotomies between these two that will concern us here.

THE SETTING

Victoria came to Britain's throne in 1837 to begin a reign of 64 years, a period that has become synonymous with the apogee of British world influence. The Victorians themselves conceived of their period as "an age of transition," which is in itself peculiarly Victorian, "for although all ages are ages of transition, never before had men thought of their own time as an era of change *from* the past *to* the future."[1] And the transition to which they were referring was not out of the immediate past but out of the Middle Ages: "the medieval tradition from which they had irrevocably broken—Christian orthodoxy under the rule of king and nobility; the social structure of fixed classes, each with its recognized rights and duties; and the economic organization of village agriculture and town guilds."[2] This idea of the period as a time of the demise of feudalism was not an abstraction. Victorians who had come to adulthood as the period was beginning felt they had lived in two quite different words:

> It was only yesterday; but what a gulf between now and then! *Then* was the old world. Stage-coaches, more or less swift, riding-horses, pack-horses, highway-men, knights in armour, Norman invaders, Roman legions, Druids, Ancient Britons painted blue, and so forth—all these belong to the old period. I will concede a halt in the midst of it, and allow that gunpowder and printing tended to modernise the world. But your railroad starts the new era, and we

of a certain age belong to the new time and the old one. We are of the time of chivalry as well as the Black Prince or Sir Walter Manny. We are of the age of steam.[3]

When a transition comes swiftly and distinctly, it has aspects of destruction and reconstruction: As formulas of the old order are attacked, changed, or dispensed with, here and there emerge beginnings of the new. By 1830 both trends could be seen. Twenty years later, in the heart of the period, what new had emerged? What was "the state of society and of the human mind"?[4]

The State of Society: Industrial and Democratic

By the end of the century an industrial and democratic society replacing the agrarian and feudal order of the past had clearly emerged.[5] With the advent of a democracy, political power moved from the aristocracy to the people, primarily through the Reform Bills of 1832, 1867, and 1884, and at the same time there arrived what often is called a democratic society. John Stuart Mill wrote of this innovation, "Human beings are no longer born to their place in life ... but are free to employ their faculties, and such favourable chances as offer, to achieve the lot which may appear to them most desirable."[6] But the primary cause of this dissolution of the old conception of status was economic—the drawing of men off the land through commerce and the opening of new and independent careers to talent.[7] The Industrial Revolution underlay the new order in politics as well, and "once the middle class attained political as well as financial eminence, their social influence became decisive. The Victorian frame of mind is largely composed of their characteristic modes of thought and feeling."[8]

Striking though the impact of democracy was, far more so was the astounding industrial development that came with the use of new machinery and processes of manufacturing, locomotion, and communication.[9] This development changed fundamentally Britain's economic life. The old order of fixed regulation and its parallel of fixed social status were gone, replaced by the new principle of laissez-faire: "To live in this dynamic, freewheeling society was to feel the enormous pressure of work, far beyond anything known before."[10] Employers worked almost as long hours as those they employed, and even the professions felt the pressure,[11] all of which was due as much to the social system as to business conditions. The boundaries of class had given way, and it had become possible as never before to rise in the world through one's own effort; so the struggle for success was joined by the struggle for rank.[12] Personal ambition aside, material goods once unknown or available only to those of wealth were suddenly available on a broad scale; to possess the "paraphernalia of gentility,"[13] one increased his work load.[14] And as the wealth of the wealthy grew, it advanced the style of living in the middle and upper classes until the Victorian scrambled for things his father had been able to ignore.[15]

As the tempo of work increased, so did the tempo of life, and with striking impact. "The most salient characteristic of life in this latter portion of the 19th century is its SPEED," commented one observer.[16] Suddenly instead of horses and sailing vessels there were railroads and steamships, and they brought in their wake a new speed of living:

Faster locomotion, of goods and letters and people, simply increased the number of things one crowded into a day, and the rush from one to another. Once upon a time "people did not run about the town or the land as we do." They traveled less often, did not hurry to catch trains, wrote one letter a morning instead of ten. Now "we are whirled about, and hooted around, and rung up as if we were all parcels, booking clerks, or office boys."[17]

If the speed of life has increased in the twentieth century, the impression of speed has declined, for what today is commonplace was then astonishing innovation. The Victorians may have had more leisure than we do, but it didn't seem so. They felt they lived lives "without leisure and without pause—a life of *haste*—above all a life of excitement, such as haste inevitably involves—a life filled so full . . . that we have no time to reflect where we have been and whither we intend to go . . . still less what is of value, and the purpose, and *the price* of what we have seen, and done, and visited."[18]

There was as well an intellectual basis for this sense of fast-paced, teeming life, for education had spread and was accompanied by vast increases in knowledge and in the amount of publication: "Even idleness is eager now,—eager for amusement; prone to excursion-trains, art-museums, periodical literature, and exciting novels; prone even to scientific theorizing, and cursory peeps through microscopes."[19]

"That constant sense of being driven—not precisely like 'dumb' cattle, but cattle who must read, write, and talk more in twenty-four hours than twenty-four hours will permit, can never have been known to them,"[20] wrote Frances Cobbe in the 1860s as she compared her own generation with that of the first 30 years of the century, words that could as well describe the gulf between her day and ours.

The State of Mind: Doubt

The transition in the human mind was at first less apparent than that in society, but there were signs to sensitive observers that the traditional framework of thought was breaking down. Thomas Arnold noted in 1838 an "atmosphere of unrest and paradox hanging around many of our ablest young men of the present day." He spoke of "questions as to great points in moral and intellectual matters; where things which have been settled for centuries seem to be again brought into discussion."[21] That was where it began. Thus Houghton[21a]:

In 1850 the age is still one of "fusion and transition. . . . Old formula, old opinions, hoary systems are being thrown into the smelting-pan; they are fusing—they must be cast anew; who can tell under what new shapes . . . they will come forth from the moulds?"[22] In the seventies men are still searching— "amid that break-up of traditional and conventional notions respecting our life, its conduct, and its sanctions, which are undeniably befalling our age,— for some clear light and some sure stay."[23] By the eighties "the disintegration of opinion is so rapid that wise men and foolish are equally ignorant where the close of this waning century will find us."[24] Though the Victorians never ceased to look forward to a new period of firm convictions and established beliefs, they had to live in the meantime between two worlds, one dead or dying, one struggling but powerless to be born, in an age of doubt.

What John Morley had said of the 1850s and 1860s was true of the entire period, although the intensity and repercussions were greater as the years passed: "It was the age of science, new knowledge, searching criticism, followed by multiplied doubts and shaken beliefs."[25] The very effort to resolve the situation made it worse; new solutions bred new controversies that raised new questions. It was not only in religion that one faced a series of alternatives, but in ethical theory and the conception of man. Even the political-economic order of bourgeois capitalism, if an established fact in the outer environment of 1850, was not above question in the world of ideas. But it was not simply the presence of competing philosophies that called all into doubt; it was also the atmosphere of the time. As communication burgeoned, both scientific and historical knowledge increased, so that the Victorians were virtually engulfed yet left to deal with the perplexing implications of it all. John Stuart Mill's diary entry for January 13, 1854, gives the flavor of this confusion and doubt:

> Scarcely any one, in the more educated classes, seems to have any opinions, or to place any real faith in those which he professes to have. . . . It requires in these times much more intellect to marshall so much greater a stock of ideas and observations. This has not yet been done, or has been done only by very few: and hence the multitude of thoughts only breeds increase of uncertainty. Those who should be guides of the rest, see too many sides to every question. They hear so much said, or find that so much can be said, about everything, that they feel no assurance of the truth of anything.[26]

In all this turmoil, however, doubt never reached the point of positive skepticism nor was there ever a denial of the mind as a valid instrument of truth. The seeds of that radical doubt were planted by the 1870s, but they didn't grow until modern sociology, anthropology, and psychology had had their impact, with the implications of rationalization and relativism.[27] Uncertain though they might be as to which theory to accept or which faculty of the mind to rely on, it never occurred to the Victorians to doubt their capacity to arrive at truth. And it was faith in the existence of ultimate truths—in religion and ethics, politics, economics, aesthetics, and even the natural sciences—and in the ability of man's mind to discover them that united the contenders of every persuasion. That, it might be said, was the one intellectual certitude in Victorian Britain; with such a foundation, the world remained a rational place. But after 1870 the concepts of the relativity of knowledge and the subjectivity of thought began to gain foothold.[28]

Skepticism, doubt, and uncertainty in the 1860s became a settled state of baffled judgment, and a mind without beliefs began to surface.[29] Most Victorians were probably aptly described by John Stuart Mill in his comment, "The men of the present day rather incline to an opinion than embrace it; few . . . have full confidence in their own convictions"; or, in a variant phrase, people "have no strong or deep-rooted convictions at all."[30] And how could it have been otherwise in a period of dissolving creeds and clashing theories?

The impact of the two salient features of this "age of transition"—bourgeois industrial society and widespread doubt about the nature of man, society, and the universe—was felt to some degree by everyone in all classes, but what were the implications for the upper- and middle-class women of the period?

The family and its rituals were at the center of Victorian life. Usually women have been concerned with home and family, so the family-centeredness of Victorian life would seem to reflect a change of the masculine attitude. In the eighteenth century the coffee shop was often the center of men's social life, for there they "smoked, dined, wrote letters, discussed politics and literature, and got drunk."[31] With the next century came a radical change, recorded and in part explained in 1869 by John Stuart Mill:

> The association of men with women in daily life is much closer and more complete than it ever was before. Men's life is more domestic. Formerly, their pleasures and chosen occupations were among men, and in men's company: their wives had but a fragment of their lives. At the present time, the progress of civilization, and the turn of opinion against the rough amusements and convivial excesses which formerly occupied most men in their hours of relaxation—together with (it must be said) the improved tone of modern feeling as to the reciprocity of duty which binds the husband towards the wife—have thrown the man very much more upon home and its inmates, for his personal and social pleasures: while the kind and degree of improvement which has been made in women's education, has made them in some degree capable of being his companions in ideas and mental tastes.[32]

Improved education for women was hardly a factor before the middle of the century, but the Evangelical revival had a sobering impact on convivial excesses and did much to engender a greater sense of duty. Moreover, work was no longer simply a means of supporting a family, but also a means of helping it up the social ladder. Ambitious middle-class fathers were preoccupied with seeing their sons into the most prestigious Oxford and Cambridge colleges or into a good profession and with marrying their daughters to gentlemen of good birth. However,

> . . . the greater *amount* of family life and thought would not in itself have created "that peculiar sense of solemnity" with which, in the eyes of a typical Victorian like Thomas Arnold, "the very *idea* of family life was invested."[33] That idea was the conception of the home as a source of virtues and emotions which were nowhere else to be found, least of all in business and society.[34]
> . . . This is the true nature of home—it is a place of Peace; the shelter, not only from all injury, but from all terror, doubt, and division. In so far as it is not this, it is not home; so far as the anxieties of the outer life penetrate into it, and the inconsistently-minded unknown, unloved, or hostile society of the outer world is allowed by either husband or wife to cross the threshold, it ceases to be home; it is then only a part of the outer world which you have roofed over, and lighted a fire in. But so far as it is a sacred place, a vestal temple, a temple of the hearth watched over by Household Gods . . . so far as it is this, and roof and fir types only of a nobler shade and light,—shade as of a rock in a weary land, and light as of the Pharos in the stormy sea;—so far it vindicates the name and fulfills the praise, of Home.[35]

It was a place, then, of shelter from the anxieties and incursions of the outside world. It was also a shelter for the moral and spiritual values that the critical and commercial spirits of the time seemed bent on obliterating; and it was therefore a sacred place as well, a temple. Upon the priestess of the temple, the wife and mother, rested the task of maintaining these moral and spiritual values against the drift of industrialism and doubt.[36]

Society: A Haven of Stability

There was also a linking factor between home and family and the political and economic world outside, "an extremely flexible mechanism, useful to social groups faced with the consequences of increased population and urban growth, industrial development and political realignment which were the characteristics of the first half of the century."[37] That factor was the system of organizing social and domestic life that began to be codified in the 1820s under the rubric Society. The system had existed after a fashion before that time, centering around the Court, but in the second quarter of the nineteenth century it became greatly expanded and infused with a new authority, which set it flourishing into ever wider geographic and social circles for the next century. This system of quasi-kinship relationships was used as a means of "placing" mobile individuals during the period of upheaval brought on by industrialization and urbanization within a group that based membership on common claims to status honour which were in turn based on a particular life style. Such claims were in this case defined as the attributes of English "ladies" and "gentlemen."

Like any status group, the traditional aristocratic elite were obsessively concerned with the matter of access to their number, and with industrialization new forms of wealth as well as newly wealthy groups produced such a torrent of applicants to those ranks that the life style itself was threatened with inundation. Thus arose the strictly structured access rituals of nineteenth century Society and etiquette. Those who maintained the fabric of Society were middle- and upper-class women who acted as leaders but also as arbiters of social acceptance or rejection.

> By effectively preventing upper- and middle-class women from playing . . . any part in public life whatsoever, the Victorians believed that one section of the population would be able to provide a haven of stability, of exact social classification in the threatening anonymity of the surrounding economic and political upheaval. . . .
> . . . the shift from a society where patronage and familial or client relationship were the norm to a system where individual achievement was rewarded with great wealth and power, was bewildering to those living through the change. Increased geographical mobility through better transport also disrupted received notions of social placing. In contradistinction to these chaotic new developments, the rules of Society and the confining of social life to private homes made possible the minute regulation of personal daily life. It also made possible the evaluation and placing of newcomers in the social landscape. It legitimated the break with kin and the neglect of kinship interaction when these became incompatible with social mobility and in some cases even provided a network of pseudo-kin as replacements. Finally, the filtering of personnel through the sieve of Society regulated access to political power, economic position and the accumulation of capital.[38]

At a time when men were learning to perform new, more professional tasks in a vastly expanded outside world, women were being forced to operate in a more narrowly personal and private sphere. Their "career" line consisted of using every personal attraction that could be mustered to reinforce status inherited through family and thereby maneuver marriage, thus gaining the first rung on Society's ladder. A girl's education was aimed at accomplishments useful in Society and took place at home, a setting that helped to mold suitable attitudes and behavior patterns for her anticipated role. Attention in Society went to married women, and power and influence within this sphere tended to come late in life. The supreme authority of the dowagers, the arbiters, made it difficult indeed for any girl to deviate from the approved path. There was vigilant attention to her every move, and the fact that social pressure was often brought to bear on her mother and other relatives as much as on the girl herself promoted a heavy psychological burden.

Because economic position no less than social status was a function of home affiliations, girls and women were particularly vulnerable to sudden financial shifts brought on by changes within the family. And if the woman or girl were suddenly faced with loss of income, there was no viable economic alternative; the chronic underemployment and exploitation of governesses and lady companions were recognized by the Victorians themselves.[39]

> Married women, too, had no legal right to what income of their own they might possess and even after the passing of the Married Women's Property Acts [1870, 1882], little customary right. All these factors taken together weave a pattern which offered very limited scope for control over their own life chances, despite, in some cases, considerable material wealth.[40]

In the 1840s the sanctions laid upon girls or women who really were not fitted for or refused to accept the strictures determined by Society were severe indeed. At that period it could require the forces of a religious call and near insanity to break the bonds. Yet several generations later, as the century was nearing its close, for many girls the demands of Society still appeared to be in direct conflict with the nascent women's professions.[41] Such situations created genuine conflicts of loyalty which have often been dismissed as examples of feminine instability when in fact it could be argued that the very existence of alternative activities or even occupations made the girl's position even more uneasy: when there are no opportunities, there are no choices to be confronted.

> Most men could choose whether or not to enter Society. In any case, those who had other occupations to perform could use their wives (or sisters, daughters) to represent them. The great majority of women had no choice. The results were, as expected, a "failure of nerve" on the part of most women even when given the opportunity for achievement. . . .
> The insistence on women remaining private, or at least amateur figures, explains some of the contradictions in the nineteenth-century record. . . . Those whose private resources were great . . . were able to operate in a wider sphere. . . . It was middle-class women without resources and barred from public positions who were at the greatest disadvantage.[42]

And so it remained well into the twentieth century.

THE WOMAN

To understand Florence Nightingale is to comprehend that the young woman in search of a mission that would challenge all her talents returned from the experience of the Crimean War with insight into military administration and such a grasp of the subject that Queen Victoria was led to "wish we had her at the War Office."[43] The chief desire of her life was to raise nursing to the rank of a trained calling, but her first duty, as she saw it, was to use her experience, in so far as possible, to improve the medical administration of the army. To accomplish this mission she set out systematically to bury her public image, to disappear from public view, and this she did with the intensity and single-mindedness that she brought to bear on all important matters in her life.

After her return from the Crimea she refused all invitations, public and private, even a reception given in her honor at Chatsworth, the Seat of the Duke of Devonshire, to which she was invited by the Duke himself. She refused to make public statements or appearances, refused even to have her portrait painted. It was expected by those in power that she would, on her return, make revelations; but there was no attack, no revelation, and no justification. Rather she set forth with incredible patience and self-effacement to win over to her side those in authority. In taking this course she was refusing to use a potent weapon, for at that point adoration of her had grown to a phenomenal level. "She may truly be called the voice of the people at present," wrote a civilian physician, Dr. Pincoffs, who had been an eyewitness to her work in the Crimea to Mrs. Nightingale, her mother. "The publicity and the talk there have been about this work [improving the medical administration of the army] have injured it more than anything else," she wrote in August 1856 in a private note, "and in no way, I am determined, will I contribute by making a show of myself."[44]

The Private Years: The Personality Forms

This intensity and a shy, self-absorbed introspection marked her from childhood, as did her acute powers of observation and the methodical noting of what she saw. Of her early years she later reminisced:

My greatest ambition . . . was not to be remarked. I was always in mortal fear of doing something unlike other people, and I said, "If I were sure that nobody would remark me I should be quite happy." I had a morbid terror of not using my knives and forks like other people when I should come out. I was afraid of speaking to children because I was sure I should not please them.[45]

By the time she was seven, she was keeping a journal, recording all manner of things about her world, such as in the entry made on August 26, 1827:

On Wednesday Aunt Mai [Mr. Nightingale's sister Mary Shore] was married to Uncle Sam [Mrs. Nightingale's brother Samuel Smith]. I, Papa, Uncle Sam, Pop [Florence's sister Parthenope] and Mr. Bagshaw (the clergyman) went first. Mama and Aunt Mai in the bride's carriage. Aunt Julia [Mrs. Nightingale's sister Julia Smith] and Miss Bagshaw came last. When they were married we were all kneeling on our knees except Mr. Bagshaw. Papa took Aunt Mai's hand and gave it to Uncle Sam. We all cried except Uncle Sam, Mr. Bagshaw and Papa.[46]

Or on Sunday, November 15, 1829:

I, obliged to sit still by Miss Christie [the governess], till I had the spirit of obedience. Carters and Blanche [her cousins] here, not allowed to be with them. Mama at Fair-Oaks ill. Myself unhappy, bad eyes, shade and cold.[47]

Florence was a writer of letters. At the age of ten during a visit with her Uncle Octavius Smith at "Thames Bank," a house which then adjoined his distillery at Millbank, she wrote to Parthenope:

Give my love to Clémence [the girls' maid], and tell her, if you please, that I am not in the room where she established me, but in a very small one; instead of the beautiful view of the Thames, a most dismal one of the black distillery, and, whenever I open my window, the nasty smell rushes in like a torrent. But I like it pretty well notwithstanding. . . . I went up into the distillery to the very tip-top by ladders with Uncle Oc and Fred [her cousin] Saturday night. We walked along a great pipe. We have had a good deal of boating which I like very much. We see three steam-boats pass every day, the *Diana*, the *Fly*, and the *Endeavour*. My love to all of them except Miss W——. Give my love particularly to Hilary [her cousin Hilary Bonham Carter]. Your affecte and only sister. Dear Pop, I think of you, pray let us love one another more than we have done. Mama wishes it particularly, it is the will of God, and it will comfort us in our trials through life. Goodbye.[48]

Possessed of a keen intellect, she, with her sister, was educated by their father (himself a well-educated and well-informed man) in Latin, Greek, modern languages, constitutional history, composition, and mathematics, a range of studies far outside the usual curriculum for women of the period. To her father's guidance she was indebted for the mental grasp and powers of intellectual concentration that were to distinguish her work in life.

There was also the stimulation of a large circle of friends both within and outside the family. Had the family not been so close and so large, Florence might have negotiated her independence more easily. But as often happens in such families, there was one woman to whom they all turned when trouble came or help was needed—Florence—and she responded. In 1845 while nursing her father's mother, she wrote to Hilary Bonham Carter: "I am very glad sometimes to walk in the valley of the shadow of death as I do here; there is something in the stillness and silence of it which levels all earthly troubles. God tempers our wings in the waters of that valley, and I have not been so happy or so thankful for a long time. . . ."[49]

To be of service in this way filled a need in her. There was social life in London as well and travel on the Continent and later in Greece and Egypt. In the summer of 1839, when the family had returned from an extended European trip, the girls were presented at Court and family life resumed its appointed social round; but Florence had had an experience that marked her deeply, "a call from God."

In her private diary she wrote: "On 7 February 1837, God spoke to me and called me to His service."[50] This was not an inward revelation; it came, as to Joan of Arc, as an objective voice outside herself, which spoke in human words. She was not yet 17 when the voices first spoke to her, but they were not a phenomenon of adolescence. In a private note of 1874—nearly 40 years later—she wrote of the times when she had heard these voices: in 1837 when she received her call; in 1853 before she went to Harley Street to the Institution for the Care of Sick Gentlewomen; once in 1854 before she went to the Crimea; and once in 1861 after Sidney Herbert's death.

Although she sometimes enjoyed social pleasures and intellectual society, she reproached herself for doing so, feeling that the life of society was a distraction into the wrong path, away from the service she was to perform. Even housekeeping brought questions for her, which she could pose with her incisive wit:

> (Letter to an old family friend, Mary Clarke Mohl, then in Paris, July 1847): I am fed up to my chin in linen and glass, and I am very fond of housekeeping. In this too-highly-educated, too-little-active age it, at least, is a practical application of our theories of something—and yet, in the middle of my lists, my green lists, brown lists, red lists, of all my instruments of the ornamental in culinary accomplishments which I cannot even divine the use of, I cannot help asking in my head, Can reasonable people want all this? Is all this china, linen, glass necessary to make man a Progressive animal? Is it even good Political Economy (query, for "good," read "atheistical" Pol. Econ?) to invent wants in order to supply employment? Or ought not, in these times, all expenditure to be reproductive? "And a proper stupid answer you'll get," says the best Versailles [china] service; "so go and do your accounts; there is one of us cracked."[51]

Yet she was an affectionate and dutiful daughter who obeyed and yielded to family expectation for many years. She strived to think that her duty lay at home and that the social round and household tasks were all she had the right to expect, but they became increasingly distasteful to her. In her diary entry of July 7, 1846, she wrote: "What is my business in this world and what have I done this last fortnight? I have read the *Daughter at Home* to Father and two chapters of Mackintosh; a volume of *Sybil* to Mama. Learnt seven tunes by heart. Written various letters. Ridden with Papa. Paid eight visits. Done company. And that is all."[52] And as she later reflected on the Victorian family pastime of reading aloud:

> To be read aloud to is the most miserable exercise of the human intellect. Or rather, is it any exercise at all? It is like lying on one's back, with one's hands tied, and having liquor poured down one's throat. Worse than that, because suffocation would immediately ensue, and put a stop to this operation. But no suffocation would stop the other.[53]

Still the sense of vocation elsewhere strengthened and deepened in her, and she struggled with it.

One can learn a great deal about the inner life of the woman through her habit of writing what she called "private notes." She poured herself out on paper—her frustrations, her desires, her secrets, her questions, her unhappiness—and she wrote on anything at hand—letter margins, blotting paper, odd scraps of paper—sometimes dating her thoughts, sometimes not. There are those notes which are simply a sentence or two while others cover several pages. Some were repeated several times at different dates with only insignificant changes of wording; from time to time a private note became part of a letter. During various periods she kept diaries, but it is in the private notes that she reveals her inner self most clearly.[54]

In 1845 she made her first bid for freedom, quietly laying plans to go to Salisbury Infirmary for a few months to learn what she could of nursing, but her mother nipped those plans in the bud, and the failure of her plans left Florence in a state of dejection. She struggled with her religious beliefs; "To find out what we can do," she wrote as an annotation in Browning's *Paracelsus*, "one's individual place, as well as the General End, is man's task. To serve man for God's sake, not man's, will prevent failure from being disappointment."[55] She felt increasingly that only in a life of nursing could she find scope and reason for her life. In her diary (June 22, 1846) she wrote:

> The longer I live, the more I feel as if all my being was gradually drawing to one point, and if I could be permitted to return and accomplish that in another being, if I may not in this, I should need no other heaven. I could give up the hope of meeting and living with those I have loved (and nobody knows how I love) and be separated from here, if it would please God to give me, with a nearer consciousness of His Presence, the task of doing this in real life.[56]

She pursued her inquiries about nursing (Kaiserwerth on the Rhine, the Dublin Hospital, the Sisters of Charity's Maison de la Providence in Paris), but quietly, for to her family "it was as if I had wanted to be a kitchen-maid."[57] The condition of nurses at the time was hardly what a family would choose for a well-bred, refined daughter.[58] At the same time Florence was making progress in another way. She was studying information on hospitals obtained from Berlin and Paris and reports on public health in England, filling notebook after notebook with a mass of facts, compared, indexed, and tabulated, building a vast and detailed knowledge of sanitary conditions that was to make her the first expert in Europe.[59] But as her inner promptings and the requirements of life within the family continued at odds, she returned to the habit she called "dreaming,"[60] through which she also evaded the moment when she must decide another question—whether to marry Richard Monckton Milnes or, indeed, whether to marry at all.[61]

By the fall of 1847 her state of mind had affected her health. In hope that matters would improve with travel, she went to Italy for the winter, and in the fall of 1849 she went with friends to Greece and Egypt. She loved travel; it did not create the diversion her family had hoped, but it clarified something for her—her view of writing as a career. She was a constant letter writer and note taker, with a gift for self-expression and literary expression. Her mother used to praise her "beautiful letters," was proud of the "European reputation" she had gained among learned men, and wanted to know why she could not be happy in cultivating at home the gifts God had given her.[62] To Florence these things were not gifts to be cultivated, but temptations to be subdued. In a letter to Mary Clarke Mohl in 1844 she wrote:

> You ask me why I do not write something. I think what is not of the first class had better not exist at all; and besides I had so much rather live than write; writing is only a supplement for living. Would you have one go away and 'give utterance to one's feelings' in a poem to appear (price 2 guineas) in the *Belle Assemblée*? I think one's feelings waste themselves in words; they ought all to be distilled into actions, and into actions which bring results.[63]

On July 10, 1850, her diary records: "I had three paths among which to choose. I might have been a literary woman, or a married woman, or a Hospital Sister."[64] She had refused the first path; she also refused the second:

> I have an intellectual nature which requires satisfaction, and that would find it in him. I have a passional nature which requires satisfaction, and that would find it in him. I have a moral, an active nature which requires satisfaction, and that would not find it in his life. I can hardly find satisfaction for any of my natures. Sometimes I think that I will satisfy my passional nature at all events, because that will at least secure me from the evil of dreaming. But would it? I could be satisfied to spend a life with him combining our different powers in some great object. I could not satisfy this nature by spending a life with him in making society and arranging domestic things. . . . To be nailed to a continuation and exaggeration of my present life, without hope of another, would be intolerable to me. Voluntarily to put it out of my power ever to be able to seize the chance of forming for myself a true and rich life would seem to me like suicide.[65]

It was an act that required extraordinary courage. She was deeply stirred by Richard Monckton Milnes; she called him "the man I adored"; and she renounced him for the sake of a destiny that it seemed impossible she would ever fulfill. "I am 30," she wrote on her birthday, "the age at which Christ began his mission. Now no more childish things, no more vain things, no more love, nor more marriage. Now, Lord, let me only think of Thy will."[66]

It was now five years since she had attempted to enter Salisbury Infirmary. She was a woman of 30, and she had accomplished nothing toward her ideal—to train as a nurse. Only her determination persisted. "Resignation!" she had written in 1847, "I never understood the word!"[67] Now the final struggle for her emancipation began.

In a private note she said, "There are knots which are Gordian and can only be cut." She had done all that her family asked except give up her "call." They were not malicious in their opposition; they simply could not understand this headstrong, uncomfortable daughter and sister. Her father, apparently an amiable man of good impulses who was contented with his life of busy idleness as a wealthy, intellectual gentleman, was constitutionally unable to enter into her state of mind, but he supported and defended her as he could. Of her mother Florence once wrote in a character sketch, "She has the genius of order, the genius to organize a parish, to form society. She has obtained by her own exertions the best society in England."[68] They shared, these two, this genius for organization, but the use that each made of it exemplifies the gulf between them. The elder sister shared with the mother a focus of interest on Society. Parthenope was vivacious, inquiring, and highly gifted, both as an artist and as a writer and later as a hostess, and Florence felt the charm of all this. "No one less than I," she wrote, "wants her to do one single thing different from what she does. She wants no other religion, no other occupation, no other training than what she has. She has never had a difficulty except with me; she knows nothing of struggle in her unselfish nature."[69] But this was precisely the reason Parthenope could not empathize with Florence, because she could not comprehend her sister's difficulties. Florence, loving her sister and mother, struggled to meet their expectations for her, but the more she struggled, the more she failed.

> As the year [1851] advanced a more decided spirit of revolt begins to appear in her diaries. One of her perplexities hitherto had been a doubt whether the "mountains of difficulties" were to be taken as occasions for submissions to God's will, or whether they were piled up in order to try her patience and her resolve, and were to be surmounted by some initiative of her own. She now began to interpret God's will in the latter sense.[70]

As her guilt lessened, she wrote a private note on her family in a new vein (June 8, 1851): "I must expect no sympathy or help from them. I must *take* some things, as few as I can, to enable me to live. I must *take* them, they will not be given to me."[71] And she went to Kaiserwerth.

Kaiserwerth was followed by the Maison de la Providence, and now she was ready. Through a friend she learned of a suitable opening: The Institution for the Care of Sick Gentlewomen in Distressed Circumstances was in difficulty and was to be reorganized and moved to new premises. Would she be its superintendent? From Paris she accepted and kept up correspondence with the Committee of Ladies as to how things should be arranged:

> (Letter of Lady Canning, chairwoman of the committee, June 5, 1853): . . . The indispensable conditions of a suitable house are, *first*, that the nurse should never be obliged to quit her floor, except for her own dinner and supper, and her patients' dinner and supper (and even the latter might be avoided by the windlass we have talked about). Without a system of this kind, the nurse is converted into a pair of legs. *Secondly*, that the bells of the patients should all ring in the passage outside the nurse's own door *on that story*, and should have a valve which flies open when its bell rings, and *remains* open in order that the nurse may see who has rung.[72]

It is evident from the correspondence that the committee was far from easy to work with, and Florence was a demanding taskmistress and learning fast:

> (Letter to her father) 1 Upper Harley St., December 3 [1853]: Dear Papa— You ask me for my observations upon *my* line of statesmanship. I have been so very busy that I have scarcely made any resume in my own mind, but upon doing so now for your benefit, I perceive:—
> When I entered into service here, I determined that, happen what would, I *never* would intrigue among the Committee. Now I perceive that I do all my business by intrigue. I propose in private to A, B, or C the resolution I

think A, B, or C most capable of carrying in committee, and then leave it to them, and I always win.

In the next paragraph she details what she managed in this way. Then:

All these I proposed and carried in Committee, without telling them that they came from *me* and not from the Medical Men; and then, and not till then, I showed them to the Medical Men, without telling *them* that they were already passed *in committee*.

It was a bold stroke, but success is said to make an insurrection into a revolution. The Medical Men have had two meetings upon them, and approved them all, . . . and thought they were their own. And I came off with flying colours, no one suspecting my intrigue, which of course would ruin me were it known, as there is as much jealousy in the Committee of one another, and among the Medical Men of one another, as ever what's his name had of Marlborough. . . . so much for the earthquakes in this little mole-hill of ours.[73]

(To her father) I send you some more documentary evidence—the tail of my Quarterly Report. My committee are such children in administration that I am obliged to tell them such obvious truths as are contained in what *I make the Medical Men say*. This place is exactly like the administering of the Poor Law. We have cases of purely lazy fits and cases deserted by their families. And my committee have not the courage to discharge a single case. *They* say the Medical Men must do it . The Medical Men say *they* won't, although the cases, they say, *must* be discharged. And I always have to do it, as the stop-gap on all occasions.[74]

By such arts and such readiness to shoulder responsibility, she reduced chaos to order, and her management of the institution brought commendation in all quarters.

When she had been superintendent for five months, she wrote (January 10, 1854) to her Aunt Hannah Nicholson:

Our vocation is a difficult one as you, I am sure, know; and though there are many consolations, and very high ones, the disappointments are so numerous that we require all our faith and trust. But that is enough. I have never repented nor looked back, not for one moment. And I begin the New Year with more true feeling of a happy New Year than I have ever had in my life.[75]

She had found her vocation. The work on Harley Street did not fail, but:

. . . the scale of the undertaking was more restricted than Florence had desired, and she saw no means of widening it. She had wanted to receive patients of all classes, to enroll many volunteer nurses, to have opportunities for training them. Among a wide circle, both at home and abroad, her knowledge and her talents were well understood: . . . She was making the most of her present opportunity, but it was narrow. Some of her friends thought from the first that she was wasting her powers on unsuitable soil in Harley Street. . . . Her own primary object was to train nurses; and other friends . . .

advised her to leave Harley Street, since she found no scope for doing so. King's College Hospital had just been rebuilt, and another friend, Louisa Twining, opened negotiations in August 1854 for securing Miss Nightingale's appointment as Superintendent of Nurses there. . . . But the immediate future hid in it another fate for Florence Nightingale. . . . her good Aunt Mai had said it to her, "If you will be ready for *it*, something is getting ready for you, and will be sure to turn up in time." [76]

On September 20, 1854, the Battle of Alma was fought; the Crimean War had begun.

Florence was 34 now, a mature woman, trained in the calling she had sought so long, experienced as an administrator, with a growing reputation and a wide circle of influential friends. She "had at least as much of adroitness as of simplicity," [77] a keen intellect and a clear head, single-mindedness passionate dedication, [78] and a vision of how things should be. Now a task was at hand with scope to challenge her talents, and she was ready.

The Public Years: The Crimean War and Priorities

A letter of appeal [79] from an old and dear friend, the British Government's Secretary at War, Sidney Herbert, reached Miss Nightingale almost immediately after the London *Times* (October 9, 12, and 13, 1854) described the sufferings of the sick and wounded in the East: Would she accept the office of superintendent of the female nursing establishment in the English General Military Hospitals in Turkey? A letter from Florence [80] to the secretary through his wife reached him at the same time: She would like to be of service to the government by taking a group of women to nurse the troops in the East. In a matter of days she and 38 other nurses had embarked for Turkey.

The story of what happened in her 21 months of service during the Crimean War is history and legend. She was "the Lady with the Lamp," but she was also the sanitarian and administrator who reduced the mortality rate among the sick and wounded troops from 42 *percent* to 22 per *thousand*. [81] She drove herself until she fell ill of Crimean fever, [82] and her health was impaired for the rest of her life as a result. [83] In her struggle to overcome the ineffective medical administration of the British Army, her influential friends in London provided the authority to back her vision; the phrase for it in the Crimea was "Nightingale power." [84]

She knew she had the information and her friends had the power; by moving behind the scenes, she could accomplish the change she sought. In a long letter (August 25, 1856) to Colonel John Lefroy (a supporter in the War Office of her work since the Crimea and a constant correspondent with her on subjects connected with military hospitals and nurses) she explained her dilemma:

> Special difficulties, she wrote, confronted her. The first was that she was a woman—that was very bad; the second, that she was a popular heroine, which was worse. The two together formed a pill which officialdom would never swallow. Any scheme known to emanate from her would instantly be rejected because it came from her. Sir Benjamin Hawes [Permanent Under-Secretary for War, 1857-1862] had written inviting her to put forward sug-

gestions for improvements in the Army Medical Department. She had reason to believe the invitation was given with the object of creating an opportunity for registering an official rejection of her proposals, and she had refused. Dr. Pincoffs [a civilian physician who had been an eyewitness to her work in the Crimea] had asked her to be patroness and organizer of a scheme to provide treatment for discharged wounded men, and she told him that if he used her name the authorities would see to it that the scheme failed, "so great is the detestation with which I am regarded by the officials." Frankly, she continued, she did not know how to proceed. She might begin to work in the military hospitals at home as she had worked in Scutari and gradually reorganize the whole system. The Queen had written to her, and the Queen would certainly grant female nursing departments in all military hospitals. Again the difficulty was her position as a national heroine. It was nothing but an embarrassment. "The buzfuz about my name," she wrote contempuously, "has done infinite harm."

Suddenly she scribbled a postscript: "If I could only find a mouthpiece." She was convinced that she herself would shortly die—if only she could find someone to carry on the work! "If I could leave one man behind me," she wrote in a private note; and she returned to the idea again and again. "If I could leave one man behind me, if I fall out of the march, who would work the question of reform I should be satisfied, because he would do it better than I." She needed a man who would be acceptable to the official world, who would carry weight in official circles, but who would be ready to submit himself to her and be taught by her. Where could such a man be found? . . . [85]

The legend brought her one gift, but even that she had to put aside for a time: the Nightingale Fund, which "gave expression to the general feeling that the services of Miss Nightingale in the Hospitals of the East demanded a grateful recognition from the British people."[86] For the present her priorities must be revised; the welfare of the British Army took precedence over the organization and reform of nursing.

When she returned to England in July 1856 she went to her family in the country for a month to recuperate; but never again was she a permanent member of the household. Having won her independence at a great price, she meant to keep it. From that moment on her work came first, and the nature of it dictated that she live in or near London. Her father's generous money provision[87] permitted her to be financially independent and finally to have a comfortable house run by a competent staff. But no matter where she lived, she never materially altered the way of life that she established early in her career:

> She stayed in bed, with brief intervals, for more than fifty years. She believed she had heart disease; she believed, in 1857, that her life hung on a thread. She continued to believe that it hung on a thread, she made wills, distributed her possessions, not once but many times, but she did not die until 1910 at the age of ninety. . . .
>
> A great many people came to see her but her rules were strict. No one, not even a relation or a dearest friend, not the Prime Minister or the Commander-in-Chief, could see her without an appointment. . . . The amount of work that issued from her bedroom is staggering.

... How could Florence Nightingale possibly have accomplished all this unless she had been alone, and when and where could she be alone living a Victorian family life? That is something of which today we have mercifully no conception. ... One day after she had come back from the Crimea and was beginning her great work for the army and nursing, she broke out suddenly in the drawing room, 'I must be alone', and collapsed. It was the beginning of her invalidism. For where could she be alone, where could she find silence from chatter, freedom from interruptions, except in bed?[88]

As the summer of 1856 gave way to fall, she met and talked at length with the Queen and Prince Albert and began to assemble, man by man, her "Cabinet" of reformers, the men who could implement her vision.[89] There was Sidney Herbert, her "dear master," the "head and centre" of the enterprise[90] as chairman of the Royal Commission and Subcommissions on the Health of the Army; there was Sir John McNeill, a physician whom Miss Nightingale had admired since his work on the Commission of Inquiry into the Supplies of the British Army Government at Scutari and in the Crimea; and finally there was Dr. John Sutherland, a physician whom she met at Scutari and the main source of her wide knowledge of sanitary science. For the next five years she drove this trio like one possessed. Her own health was tenuous, but the weakness of body seemed only to strengthen the mind; for her "Cabinet", her special gift for inspiring her most intimate friends was trying indeed and for Sidney Herbert, the pace, together with a chronic kidney ailment, proved lethal.[91]

The thought of the work Miss Nightingale produced for the army leaves one with the feeling of profound fatigue. That any person should have driven herself to accomplish all she did seems too much. What must they have cost her, these letters and memoranda and reports without number, in physical, mental, and emotional stress? And yet the scope of her labors continued to expand; civilian hospitals and nursing followed these concerns in the military domain, and from the army she moved on to work for the nation and the world.

When her beloved friend and co-worker, now the Secretary for War and Prime Minister of her "Cabinet," Sidney Herbert, died in August, 1861, Miss Nightingale's most powerful link with the government was gone; her work with the government continued, but on a less intimate basis. In the years they had had together, she and her "Cabinet" had accomplished her goal: The medical administration of the army had been restructured, and her vision of improving the health of the British soldier was becoming a reality.

Now the other goal of her life—to raise nursing to the rank of a trained calling—could again become her first priority.[92] The money at the Nightingale Fund—£44,000—made it possible to open the Nightingale Training School for Nurses at St. Thomas's Hospital on June 24, 1860.[93] From that time on the status of nursing was the center of her world. New people entered her life, and, until the twentieth century opened, there were always new projects and concerns (the Indian sanitation plans,[94] statistics,[95] the National Association for the Promotion of Social Science), but at the heart of it all was nursing.

Nursing and the Nightingale Training School

The profession of nursing is at once very old and very new. The development of the nursing of the sick took place along three lines of influence—religion, war, and science—and Florence Nightingale came at an opportune moment to give it enormous impetus along each of these lines. Religion was being reassessed as to its relationship to humanity and, in the process, was becoming more closely allied to the service of humanity. Miss Nightingale was prepared, by cast of mind and by experience, to create new forms—an order of nurses devoted to their calling, but organized on a secular basis. The Crimean War gave further force to a movement for increasing the number and improving the qualification of nurses. Science was beginning to progress—sanitation was already making advances, and medicine and surgery were on the eve of great developments—and Miss Nightingale moved in the vanguard of this spirit. There was also a fourth line of influence which seems to have entered the equation with Miss Nightingale: her intense interest in seeing that a woman not be barred from entering a walk of life for which she is fitted simply because she is a woman, and nursing is certainly one such walk.

How, precisely, did she "found" modern nursing? "She made public opinion perceive, and act upon the perception, that nursing was an art, and must be raised to the status of a trained profession. That was the essence of the matter. Other things, such as the opening of nursing to higher social strata, the better payment of nurses, etc., though important and interesting, were only results."[96] The means she used were three: her example, her precept, and her practice. Her work in the Crimean War excited a passionate and affectionate admiration and set an example of commitment to a fuller and worthier life among her contemporaries that has hardly been equaled in the history of women. This was a woman of high ability and social standing who had forsaken all to be a nurse and who sought to raise nursing to the rank of a trained art. By her example she had moved closer to her goal.

Example had to be supplemented with precept. *Notes on Nursing*, her book of precepts on the art of nursing, was published in December 1859. Her feminist friend Harriet Martineau wrote of it, "This is a work of genius if I ever saw one; and it will operate accordingly. It is so real and so intense, that it will, I doubt not, create an Order of Nurses before it has finished its work."[97] Her prediction was correct: Miss Nightingale was the founder of the new order, and *Notes on Nursing* was the word. It was in this book that a doctrine, new to nursing and of great potency, first emerged: that "nursing the well" is even more important than nursing the sick, and that preventive hygiene is more important than curative medicine. The book is as cogent and thought-provoking a century later as it was at publication.

Following precept with practice, Miss Nightingale intended to use the Nightingale Fund to found or conduct "an Institution for the training, sustenance, and protection of Nurses"[98] and to become the superintendent of it herself. The scope of her labors for the army and the state of her health after her return from the Crimea soon made it obvious that she must work through other people and existing hospitals if anything was to come of the plan.

> Her choice fell, for the main application of the Fund, upon St. Thomas's Hospital. The Resident Medical Officer, Mr. R. G. Whitfield, was sympathetic. The Hospital was large, rich, and well managed. But, above all, the Matron was a woman after Miss Nightingale's own heart, strong, devoted to her work, devoid of all self-seeking, full of decision and administrative ability. . . . Mrs. Wardroper.[99]

When the venture was launched in June 1860, the scale was modest (15 probationers), but it was undertaken only after a vast amount of forethought, and it was destined to be the foundation of the modern art and practice of nursing.

The scheme had two basic concepts: "(1) that nurses should have their technical training in hospitals specially organized for the purpose; (2) that they should live in a home fit to form their moral life and discipline."[100] When their year of training was completed, the probationers were expected to enter service as hospital nurses or in some other public institution. This, too, was part of Miss Nightingale's scheme, for she expected that her school should, through its graduates, offer a means of training elsewhere. Although she was not among the students in person, she was deeply involved with them through the reports of Mrs. Wardroper and the diaries each student kept during her training.

In 1871 St. Thomas's Hospital was moved to new quarters, which she, with her usual meticulous attention to detail, had hoped to plan, and at the same time the training school had reached a crisis. Miss Nightingale's attention had been drawn from it by demands of the Poor Law reform and India, and early in 1872 she began an investigation of its organization and teaching. That summer, however, she had suddenly to deal with family crises as well: Her parents were ailing (her father was 78 and her mother 83), and the management of their affairs and property was in dishevelment. Moreover, Parthenope was suffering the first symptoms of arthritis, which would in a few years turn her into a helpless cripple. For eight months, Florence was imprisoned again. By this time she was 52, but she had lost none of her capacity to suffer. In a private note of the late summer 1872 she wrote:

> Oh to be turned back to this petty stagnant stifling life at Embley. I should hate myself (I *do* hate myself) but I should LOATHE myself, oh my God, if I could *like* it, find 'rest' in it. Fortunately there is no rest in it, but ever increasing anxieties. *Il faut que la victime soit mise en pièces.* Oh my God![101]

Back in London she flew into the reconstruction of the Nightingale School. From 1872 on she set forth to become personally acquainted with every probationer. All influences were secondary to the influence of Miss Nightingale; she dominated the school. It was work with human beings, the work she longed for. Family problems continued to plague her until 1880, and there was the loss of dearly loved friends, but her life, after the tedious years of administration, was suddenly rich again.

With each year the area of influence of the Nighingale Training School grew as its graduates went off to various posts in Great Britain and the colonies, Europe, the United States, and other parts of the world, and with these women went the influence and encouragement of Miss Nightingale.

> The Lady in South Street was not only the queen of the Nightingale Nurses, she was also their mother. The principal lieutenants who went out on important service,[102] and many members of the rank and file, maintained constant correspondence with her—sending to her direct reports, consulting her in difficulties, looking to her, and never in vain, for counsel and encourage-

ment. Miss Nightingale took especial pains to help and to influence the Lady Superintendents who went from St. Thomas's in command of nursing parties. Among her earlier papers containing thoughts about her future work, there is more than one reference to "Richelieu's 'Self-multiplication.'" She strove to extend her work by creating lieutenants in her own image.[103]

She advised them, helped them, planned for them, with extraordinary thoroughness. Was a Sister returning to work in the North after a holiday in London? She would remember how careless girls sometimes are of regular meals, and her Commissionaire [manservant] would be dispatched to see the Sister off and put a luncheon-basket in the [railway] carriage. Miss Nightingale was an old hand at purveying, and amongst her papers are careful lists of what such baskets were to contain. She heard of a member of a certain nursing staff being run down. "What Miss X. wants is to be fed like a baby," she wrote, sending a detailed dietary and adding, "Get the things out of my money." She was constant in seeing that her "daughters" took proper holidays; sometimes helping to defray the expense, more often having them stay with her in South Street or in the country. She was constant, too, in sending them presents of books—both of a professional kind likely to be of help to them in their work, and such as would encourage a taste for general literature. To those who were in London hospitals or infirmaries, her notes were often accompanied by "fresh country eggs," game, or flowers. She always remembered them when Christmas came round and sent evergreens for the wards. At one or two of the London Infirmaries there is a Matron's Garden, planted with rhododendrons. The plants were sent by Miss Nightingale from Embley [her father's country home near Romsey, in Hampshire]. . . . Her pupils, wherever they might be, referred to their "dear Mistress" or "dearest friend" [or "beloved chief"] in all their trials, difficulties, perplexities, and she never failed them—sending them words of encouragement, advice, and good cheer. "Should there be anything in which I can be of the least use, here I am": this was a frequent formula in her messages. In these letters a religious note is seldom absent. . . . letters in which a high ideal was . . . continually and persistently presented. But letters . . . not less conspicuous for shrewd practical sense and wordly wisdom.[104]

The Later Years

In 1887 Queen Victoria celebrated her Jubilee, and for Miss Nightingale, too, it was a Jubilee, for it was 50 years earlier, in February 1837, that her "voices" had called her to service. On August 5, 1887, she wrote to her Aunt Mai:

Thinking of you always, grieved by your sufferings [widowed and completely crippled by arthritis], hoping you have still to enjoy. In this month 34 years ago you lodged with me in Harley Street (Aug. 12) and in this month 31 years ago you returned me to England from Scutari (Aug. 7th). And in this month 30 years ago the first Royal Commission was finished (Aug. 7). And since then 30 years of work often cut to pieces but never destroyed, God bless you! In this month 26 years ago Sidney Herbert died, after five years of work for us (Aug. 2). And in this month 24 years ago the work of the second Royal Commission (India) was finished. And in this month, this year, my powers seem all to have failed and old age set in.[105]

She accepted old age and seemed to find peace in its coming. The storms of her earlier years were over, her mind was at rest, her health better than it had been since the Crimea, and her work bearing fruit in abundance as she entered into the last period of active work. Indian schemes still required her attention and she became involved with district nursing, but she was to fight one last battle. A proposal in 1886 by the Hospitals' Association taken up in 1888 by the British Nurses' Association was aimed at determining a standard of technical excellence in nursing. Miss Nightingale opposed the proposal for two reasons: She thought it premature for the infant profession, and the method proposed—qualifying a nurse by examination—took no account of the character training which she held to be as important as the acquisition of technical skills. The decision, which was reached at last in May 1893, was a victory for neither side. It was a quiet end to her last battle.

In these later years, life gave compensations for earlier anguish. She was treated by the world at large with a deference that bordered on veneration, and she who had never married enjoyed the position of respected matriarch in the lives of a wide circle of young people. She had been reconciled with her mother earlier; now came a reconciliation with her sister and pleasure in the sister's stepchildren. Again and again old friends left her world, but new ones entered. It seemed as if she might go on forever. Her spirit had not dimmed. In 1889 she wrote to Sir Robert Rawlinson (an old friend from the Crimea Sanitary Commission): "No, no a thousand times no. I am not growing apathetic!" But by 1901 the occasional difficulty with her sight had developed into total blindness, and in 1906 the India Office was informed that it was no longer useful to send papers to Miss Nightingale. Her memory had failed and she could no longer comprehend the material. She lingered on as honors were showered on her—the Order of Merit bestowed on her by King Edward VII in 1907, the first woman so honored, the Freedom of the City of London, the Jubilee of the founding of the Nightingale Training School in 1910—but she knew nothing. On the 13th of August, 1910, she was gone.

CONCLUSION

Florence Nightingale was a woman of resilience and enormous tensile strength, of vision and deep conviction, and she moved the immovable as few people, men or women, do—but at the price of stress which seemed never to end.

Hers was a world of wealth, affection, secure social position, and education, but it was a world laced with incongruities and ambiguities. She was educated in a manner that broadened and sharpened the mind—but it was to be used in the paths of social grace. She chose to work in a profession whose members were women, while experiencing most women with whom she dealt as a sore trial to her endurance.

From the perspective of her own time, she was physically feminine and mentally masculine, a patently unacceptable combination. She refused to submerge the masculine side of herself, thereby creating a dichotomy between society's expectations of women (as exemplified by her mother and sister) and her inner promptings. It was from this basic dichotomy that the stresses she experienced arose.

How did she deal with these stresses? She dealt in three areas: the mental, the emotional, and the physical. Over the years she had voluminous correspondence with several men and women with whom she could match intellects, John Stuart Mill, Benjamin Jowett (tutor at Balliol College and Regius Professor of Greek, Oxford), and Harriet Martineau among them. From time to time there were letters moving between Miss Nightingale and such friends daily. She sent copies of her works for their critique and discussed ideas proposed on both sides, seeming to find it invigorating and a catharsis to put thoughts on paper in this way. She turned to this as a means of renewal often, particularly when she was involved in considering her thoughts on religion. Her friendships with such men as Sidney Herbert and Benjamin Jowett she characterized as being the relationships of "man to man," of comradeship; they were interactions on the mental plane, where she was at her best. She had a passion for statistics and facts in the areas of her interests, and she turned to amassing this material with an almost religious fervor when answers were needed or when, as in the winter of 1850 when she could not move into the work she longed to do, she wished to immerse herself mentally in what she could not experience physically. Her finely honed mind also expressed itself in wit. Her private comments on others were caustic on occasion, but her public wit was in the best sense trenchant. Furthermore, she enjoyed and practiced with skill the art of maneuvering behind the scenes. She realized the power of her legend after the Crimea, but, rather than use it as a sledgehammer to subdue the opposition, she employed the more subtle tool of persuasion. Her references in letters and personal notes to the considered choice and use of this method say much about her mental processes and understanding of others' motivations and sensitivities. Her mind was extraordinary in its uncompromising clarity and realism, and when she moved in this aspect of her being she was enormously powerful.

The emotional area of her life, however, was another world—violent, exaggerated, and unreasoning. Here the atmosphere in which she was brought up prevented her from achieving balance. A life that appeared to be serene and peaceful seethed beneath the surface with overblown reactions to the least situation. Her ragged emotionalism spent itself repeatedly in written words—private notes and letters to friends who understood and could deal with the violence of her feelings. With Mary Clarke Mohl and her Aunt Mai Smith in particular Miss Nightingale over the years was able to work through her feelings and gain a measure of peace and composure.

Her response in the physical area to the stress of her life is perhaps most characteristic of the age in which she lived. There seems to be no question that she was weary and physically at low ebb when she returned from the Crimea, but her resolution was unfaltering; she had work to do for the army, and time was short. So rather than allow herself time for physical recuperation she pushed herself until August 1857 when, the report of the Sanitary Commission completed,

> . . . she collapsed and could do no more. She went to Malvern, where she could be alone and take the 'water-cure.' The doctor found that her heart was palpitating and beating rapidly. He told her that she must lie down and not get up till her heart had become normal. From that time on to the end of her life—fifty-three years—she lived on a couch or in a wheelchair.

> When she returned to London the expectation of a visit from her sister was sufficient to bring on an attack of palpitation, rapid breathing, headache, and pain in the heart region. Her sister put off her visit. For some time

the prospect of any unpleasant occurrence, or unwanted visit, or even opposition to her wishes or non-agreement with her opinions, was sufficient to bring on an attack. She was thus prevented from doing anything she did not want to do, or from meeting anyone whom she disliked. Thus was formed the habit of life which became confirmed and continued long after the immediate crisis was past. She concentrated on her work, had no desire for anything else other than the big schemes which occupied all her waking hours.[106]

No one has ever stated that Miss Nightingale suffered from any organic disease, and she was not paralyzed. She did, however, begin to speak of her weakness and severe pain with a kind of morbid pleasure, but they in no way curbed her intellectual activity. Although she virtually boasted of her weakness, she obviously had great staying power, and she herself realized this. She was overworked and tired as well, for writing is a tiring occupation and she wrote voluminously, but she was not physically invalid.

Retiring to her bedroom was an acceptable way of coping with the stress of the mission she had set for herself:

> She hated publicity, though she undoubtedly loved power. She disliked company, except such as would help her in her work. She found her invalid state enabled her the more easily to induce those whom she wished to interview— statesmen, generals, viceroys, distinguished doctors, nurses—to come to see her at her own time under the most convenient conditions. Much of her work was secret, and secrets are best kept in seclusion. Moreover, those who were opposed to her did not feel justified in openly opposing an invalid.[107]

Wherever the truth may lie as to the need for her sojourn in bed, she was not alone in finding this a functional answer to the pressures of the Victorian life, for among those who "stayed in bed" were Elizabeth Barrett Browning, Harriett Martineau, and Charles Darwin.

Given the competing aspects of the woman, the era, and the vision, one marvels at Miss Nightingale's innovation in coping with the stresses that were her companions through eight decades of change.

NOTES

1.   Walter E. Houghton, *The Victorian Frame of Mind: 1830-1870* (New Haven: Yale University Press, 1957), p. 1.

2.   Ibid., pp. 1-2.

3.   William Makepeace Thackeray, *Works of Thackeray* (New York: Charles Scribner's Sons, 1911), Vol. 22, "De Juventute," *Roundabout Papers*, p. 82.

4.   John Stuart Mill, *The Spirit of the Age*, ed. F. A. von Hayek (Chicago: University of Chicago Press, 1942), pp. 2, 6.

5.   Cf. Edward Dowden, "Victorian Literature" (1887), *Transcripts and Studies* (London: Kegan Paul, Trench and Co., 1888), p. 159.

6.   John Stuart Mill, "The Subjection of Women," *On Liberty, Representative Government, The Subjection of Women*, The World's Classics, Vol. 170 (London: Oxford University Press, 1912), p. 445.

7. John Stuart Mill, "Democracy in America," *Dissertations and Discussions*, 4 vols. (New York: Henry Holt & Co., 1874), 2: 62-71.

8. Houghton, *Victorian Frame of Mind*, p. 5.

9. Cf. Thomas Henry Huxley, "The Progress of Science, 1837-1887," *Method and Results: Essays by Thomas H. Huxley* (New York: D. Appleton & Co., 1899), p. 42.

10. Houghton, *Victorian Frame of Mind*, p. 6.

11. William Rathbone Greg, "Life at High Pressure" (1875), *Literary and Social Judgments*, 2 vols. (London: N. Trübner & Co., 1877), 2: 272.

12. Houghton, *Victorian Frame of Mind*, p. 6 and chap. 8, pp. 183-195.   '

13. Joseph A. Banks, *Prosperity and Parenthood: A Study of Family Planning Among the Victorian Middle Class* (London: Routledge and Paul, 1954), chap. 6.

14. Cf. Mark Pattison, "The Age of Reason," *Fortnightly Review* 27 (1877): 357.

15. Houghton, *Victorian Frame of Mind*, p. 7.

16. Greg, "Life at High Pressure," p. 263.

17. Frederic Harrison, *Autobiographic Memoirs*, 2 vols. (London: Macmillan & Co., 1911), 1: 12, 18-19.

18. Greg, "Life at High Pressure," p. 268.

19. George Eliot, *Works*, Cabinet ed. (Edinburgh: William Blackwood & Sons, [1878]), vol. 5, *Adam Bede*, 2: 341.

20. Frances Power Cobbe, "The Nineteenth Century," *Fraser's Magazine* 69 (1864): 482.

21. Arthur Penrhyn Stanley, *The Life and Correspondence of Thomas Arnold, D.D., Late Headmaster of Rugby School* (New York: D. Appleton & Co., 1846), p. 324 (letter of October 5, 1838).

21a. Houghton, *Victorian Frame of Mind*, pp. 9-10.

22. Hugh Stowell, "The Age We Live In," *Exeter Hall Lectures*, vol. 6, London, 1850-51 pp. 45-46, cited in Houghton, *Victorian Frame of Mind*, p. 9.

23. Matthew Arnold, "Bishop Butler and the Zeit-Geist," *Last Essays on Church and Religion* (New York, 1894), p. 287, cited in Houghton, *Victorian Frame of Mind*, pp. 9-10.

24. James Anthony Froude, Preface to *Short Studies on Great Subjects*, 4 vols. (London: Longmans, Green & Co., 1888), pp. v-vi, cited in Houghton, *Victorian Frame of Mind*, p. 10.

25. John, Viscount Morley, *Recollections*, 2 vols. (London: Macmillan & Co., 1917), 1: 100.

26. John Stuart Mill, *The Letters of John Stuart Mill*, ed. H.S.R. Elliot, 2 vols. (London: Longmans, Green & Co., 1910), 2: 220.

27. Cf. W.H. Auden and N.H. Pearson, eds., *Poets of the English Language*, 5 vols. (New York: The Viking Press, 1950), 5:xxii-xxiii, in which Auden discusses aspects of the impact of these disciplines.

28. Houghton, *Victorian Frame of Mind*, p. 14.

29. Ibid., p. 20.

30. Mill, *Spirit of the Age*, pp. 12, 13.

31. Houghton, *Victorian Frame of Mind*, p. 342.

32. Mill, "Subjection of Women," p. 540.

33. Stanley, *Correspondence of Arnold*, p. 151.

34. Houghton, *Victorian Frame of Mind*, p. 343.

35. John Ruskin, *Complete Works* (New York: Thomas Y. Crowell & Co., n.d.), vol. 12, sec. 68, "Sesame and Lilies," Lecture II of *Queens' Gardens*, pp. 59-60.

36. Cf. Barbara Frankel, "The Genteel Family: High Victorian Conceptions of Domesticity and Good Behavior" (PhD diss., University of Wisconsin, 1969), for a consideration of the Victorian middle-class home as a bulwark against social chaos.

37. Leonore Davidoff, *The Best Circles: Women and Society in Victorian England* (Totowa, N.J.: Rowman & Littlefield, 1973), p. 15.

38. Ibid., pp. 16, 17.

39. Cf. M. Jeanne Peterson, "The Victorian Governess: Status Incongruence in Family and Society," in *Suffer and Be Still: Women in the Victorian Age*, Martha Vicinus ed. (Bloomington: Indiana University Press, 1972), pp. 3-19, for an examination of the peculiarly tenuous position of the employed "lady."

40. Davidoff, *Best Circles*, p. 95. For the middle-class spinster who was both financially independent and unencumbered by relatives there was the possibility of charitable work. Cf. Harriet Warm Schupf, "Single Women and Social Reform in Mid-Nineteenth Century England: The Case of Mary Carpenter," *Victorian Studies* 17, no. 3 (March 1974): 301-317.

41. Cf. Diana Hopkins, *Family Inheritance: The Life of Eva Hubback* (London: Staples Press, 1954).

42.   Davidoff, *Best Circles*, pp. 98, 99.
43.   Sir Edward Cook, *The Life of Florence Nightingale*, 2 vols. (London: Macmillan & Co., 1914), 1: 307.
44.   Cecil Woodham-Smith, *Lonely Crusader: The Life of Florence Nightingale* (New York: McGraw-Hill Book Co., 1951), p. 183.
45.   Cook, *Life of Florence Nightingale*, 1: 12.
46.   Ida B. O'Malley, *Florence Nightingale, 1820-1856* (London: Thornton Butterworth, 1931), p. 17.
47.   Ibid., pp. 24-25.
48.   Cook, *Life of Florence Nightingale*, 1: 10-11.
49.   Ibid., p. 31.
50.   George Pickering, *Creative Malady* (London: George Allen Unwin, 1974), p. 100; Woodham-Smith, *Lonely Crusader: The Life of Florence Nightingale*, p. 13.
51.   Cook, *Life of Florence Nightingale*, 1: 42.
52.   Ibid., pp. 63-64.
53.   Ibid., pp. 41-42, from Florence Nightingale, *Suggestions for Thought to Searchers after Truth*, 3 vols. (London: Eyre and Spottiswoode, 1860), 2: 385.
54.   See Cook, *Life of Florence Nightingale*, 1: vi, for further comments on her papers.
55.   Cook, *Life of Florence Nightingale*, 1: 54.
56.   Ibid., p. 60.
57.   Ibid.
58.   For a description of the life in nursing at that time, see M. Adelaide Nutting and Lavinia L. Dock, *A History of Nursing*, 2 vols. (New York: G. P. Putnam's Sons, 1907), vol. 1, chap. 14, and vol. 2, chaps. 1, 2; see also Woodham-Smith, *Lonely Crusader: The Life of Florence Nightingale* pp. 40-41.
59.   O'Malley, *Florence Nightingale, 1820-1856*, p. 90; Woodham-Smith, *Florence Nightingale 1820-1910*, p. 43.
60.   Cook, *Life of Florence Nightingale*, 1: 92. Woodham-Smith, *Florence Nightingale, 1820-1910*, pp. 43, 32, 52.
61.   Cook, *Life of Florence Nightingale*, vol. 1, chap. 7; Woodham-Smith, *Florence Nightingale, 1820-1910*, pp. 29-31, 46, 50-51.
62.   Cook, *Life of Florence Nightingale*, 1: 94.
63.   Ibid., pp. 93-94.
64.   Ibid., p. 96; Woodham-Smith, *Lonely Crusader: The Life of Florence Nightingale*, p. 55.
65.   Cook, *Life of Florence Nightingale*, 1: 100.
66.   Ibid., p. 101.
67.   O'Malley, *Florence Nightingale, 1820-1856*, p. 130.
68.   Cook, *Life of Florence Nightingale*, 1: 105.
69.   Ibid.
70.   Ibid., p. 107.
71.   O'Malley, *Florence Nightingale, 1820-1856*, p. 182; Woodham-Smith, *Florence Nightingale, 1820-1910*, p. 60.
72.   Cook, *Life of Florence Nightingale*, 1: 131.
73.   Ibid., pp. 135-136.
74.   Ibid., p. 136.
75.   Ibid., pp. 137-138.
76.   Ibid., pp. 140-141.
77.   Ibid., p. xxxi.
78.   O'Malley, *Florence Nightingale. 1820-1856*, p. 149, note 1.
79.   Cook, *Life of Florence Nightingale*, 1: 151-154.
80.   Ibid., pp. 150-151.
81.   Ibid., p. 254.
82.   Ibid., p. 258; Woodham-Smith, *Florence Nightingale, 1820-1910*, pp. 151-152.
83.   Cook, *Life of Florence Nightingale*, 1: 371-373.
84.   Ibid., p. 206.
85.   Woodham-Smith, *Lonely Crusader: The Life of Florence Nightingale*, pp. 182-183.
86.   Cook, *Life of Florence Nightingale*, 1: 269; Woodham-Smith, *Florence Nightingale, 1820-1910*, pp. 163-164.
87.   Cook, *Life of Florence Nightingale*, 1: 130, 504.
88.   Cecil Woodham-Smith, "They Stayed in Bed," *Listener*, 55, no. 1407 (February 6, 1956); 245-246.

89.   Cook, *Life of Florence Nightingale*, 1: 312-412.

90.   Ibid., pp. 312, 407.

91.   Ibid., p. 312 and chap. 5, pp. 401-412.

92.   Cook, *Life of Florence Nightingale*, 1: 307.

93.   Ibid., pp. 456-467.

94.   Ibid., 2: 145-184.

95.   Ibid., 1: 428-438.

96.   Ibid., pp. 445-446.

97.   Ibid., p. 448.

98.   Ibid., p. 456.

99.   Ibid., p. 458.

100.   Ibid., p. 460; *British Medical Journal*, December 31, 1892, p. 1448.

101.   Woodham-Smith, *Florence-Nightingale, 1820-1910*, p. 327.

102.   The life and work of six of the most influential of these "lieutenants" is considered in Zachary Cope's *Six Disciples of Florence Nightingale* (London: Pitman Medical Publishing Co., 1961).

103.   Cook, *Life of Florence Nightingale*, 2: 191.

104.   Ibid., pp. 257-259. A selection of these letters is present in Cook, *Life of Florence Nightingale*, 2: 259-262, and throughout Cope's *Six Disciples.*

105.   George Pickering, *Creative Malady*, (London: George Allen & Unwin, Ltd., 1974) p. 161; Woodham-Smith, *Florence Nightingale, 1820-1910*, p. 348.

106.   Zachary Cope, *Florence Nightingale and the Doctors* (London: Museum Press, 1958), p. 157.

107.   Ibid., p. 161.

2

The Progress of Women and Nursing

Parallel or Divergent?

LAURIE K. GLASS
KAREN PAULSEN BRAND

Throughout history, women have sought means of expressing themselves, developing their opportunities, and expanding their experiences. Much evidence supports the contention that the development of nursing and the status of women were interdependent and often parallel; the advances of one affected the advances of the other. Evidence also suggests that the advancement of women and nursing may no longer be parallel but perhaps divergent. Nurses have struggled not only to create a profession but to be a profession of women. Accepting the assumption that the present exists as it does because of the past, the authors will explore the historical development of the relationship between women and nursing. Current concerns affecting this relationship will then be addressed.

HISTORICAL OVERVIEW*

The first opportunity for women to leave the home and work for a cause came during the Middle Ages with the establishment of religious orders in Europe. Work within religious orders was considered socially acceptable for virgins, widows, and women without means of support. The tasks of these women included providing care, food, spiritual guidance, and support to all who needed it. Nursing care as it existed at that time emphasized primarily care of the soul. Care of physical ailments was characterized by compassion and a lack of scientific knowledge and skill.

Work in religious orders continued until the Reformation in the early sixteenth century, when there was a reduction in the number of predominantly Catholic religious orders and hospitals.[1] The sick continued to require care, but charity and a spiritual obligation no longer inspired the nature of nursing care. With few church-supported hospitals, nursing lacked organization and control.

Until the nineteenth century, nursing care was disorganized, degenerate, and sporadically provided by women who lived by gambling, prostitution, thievery, and bribery. The sick were virtually left to fend for themselves, preferring to die at

---

*Portions of this chapter were previously published in *Nursing Forum* 14, no. 2 (1975): 160-174, under the title "Perils and Parallels of Women and Nursing." Reprinted with permission from Nursing Publications, Inc., Park Ridge, N.J.

home rather than subject themselves to the filth of hospitals or the abuse of its caregivers. Women and nursing were relegated to a low, ineffectual position in society.

During the nineteenth century a change began in society that emphasized the value of human life. With the rise of humanism, major concerns such as slavery and reforms for prisons and the insane became popular movements. The status of women and the status of nursing were also affected by the social climate. The novels of Charles Dickens, reflecting the existing social conditions, were widely read and greatly influenced the awareness of the public. The deteriorated state of nursing was expressed through such Dickens' characters as Sairy Gamp and Betsy Prig in *The Life and Adventures of Martin Chuzzlewit.* With nursing thus portrayed, action was needed.

One attempt to improve nursing care was the establishment of a hospital and training school at Kaiserwerth, Germany, in 1836. However, nurses' training continued to adhere closely to the philosophies of the old religious orders, founded on monastic ideals of self-abnegation, strict obedience to authority, and dedication to duty.[2] Any type of creative or independent action by women was repressed. Although nursing took a step forward, the status of women was not directly improved.

Not until two American women were denied seating and the privilege of publicly speaking at an antislavery convention in England, in 1843, did organized movements for the rights of women gain momentum. Realizing that women were now placed one step below slaves and that even illiterate men were allowed the vote, a number of women gathered at Seneca Falls, New York, in 1848, to consider their situation. In this first public gathering, led by Elizabeth Cady Stanton, women asked for the vote and the "right to be people."[3] Women were acutely aware of the need for women and child labor laws, sanitation laws, quality health care, and other social reforms. They formulated corrective plans but found effective action impossible without the support of men.

The Crimean War, in 1854, gave impetus to women's attempts to gain a foothold in the operation of society. Florence Nightingale, seeking to make nursing an art and a science, had a positive effect on raising the status of women. As a woman from the upper class in England, she capitalized on the humanism of the day and developed an occupation deemed appropriate for women. To improve the status of nursing (which would also affect the status of women) it was necessary to establish high standards for education and practice as well as strict rules and regulations governing the character and morals of the nurses Florence Nightingale proposed to teach. She insisted that "to be a good nurse, one had to be a good woman first" and "to be a good woman at all, one must be an improving woman."[4] She firmly believed that women should have the same rights as men and that equal rights meant equal responsibilities. "If women could have educational and vocational opportunities, then suffrage would resolve itself."[5] Nightingale maintained that women should have a profession in which they could be fulfilled, independent, and contributing members of society. Furthermore, she was instrumental in ensuring that nursing care would no longer be gratuitous because a profession not well compensated would not attract the kind of intelligent, independent women it required. Her influence and the prevailing social climate contributed to the development of nursing not only as a profession but as a proper activity for women.

Nightingale's first training school for nurses opened in 1860 at St. Thomas' Hospital in London and provided professional opportunities for women of all classes. The lower-class woman found in nursing an alternative to working in the mines or factories for her livelihood. For the upper-class woman, whose degree of idleness reflected the position and status of her husband, nursing provided an opportunity to direct her pent-up energies into an avenue of reform popular at that time. Florence Nightingale's philosophy and methods served as a model for the establishment of schools throughout Europe.

The Nightingale method of training gained popularity in the United States as schools of nursing opened at Bellevue, Massachusetts General, and New Haven hospitals in 1873. The early graduates of these training schools became directors of nursing service and were expected to start schools of nursing in the hospitals. The history of nursing was inextricably linked with the growth and development of hospitals. Schools, created to serve the needs of hospitals, could not afford independence. When the hospitals required the pupil nurse to provide nursing care in exchange for her training, the student was forced to comply. Such exploitation was further evidenced by long working hours (as many as 105 hours per week) and little or no pay (about three dollars per day or twenty cents per hour).[6] Regimented life styles, crowded living conditions, and authoritarian male supervision yielded no freedom and little power for the working nurse.

Nevertheless, control of the profession was a major concern to nursing leaders in the late nineteenth century. The American Society of Superintendents of Training Schools for Nurses (forerunner of National League for Nursing) organized in 1893 to propose standards for admission to the schools. Later, it also dealt with standards for curriculum and practice. Registration policies were sought to protect the public and to ensure quality care. In addition to the efforts of the society, the initiation of college courses for nurses at New York's Teacher's College, Columbia University, in 1899, facilitated the development of nursing. The school philosophy and administration supported female leadership and recognition for women, which contributed to the success of the program. The first nurse professor, M. Adelaide Nutting, provided strong leadership, organized the faculty women's club, and obtained the funds necessary for the continued survival of the nursing courses at Teacher's College. Early financial support was provided by nurses who demonstrated their confidence in the school by drawing from their own resources: an example of women helping women for a common effort.

Nutting constantly struggled with the general public attitude that nurses were being overtrained and that, knowing too much, they would be unfit for essential nursing tasks. She and other nursing leaders sought to inform the public that education was necessary for quality nursing care. The quality of education was frequently studied and attempts were made to initiate necessary changes.

When the Flexner Report (1910) revealed the existence of substandard schools of medicine and resulted in the closing of the inferior schools, nursing leaders proposed a similar study to disclose substandard nursing schools. Since hospital nursing schools required nursing students to provide patient care and closing schools meant closing hospitals, the resultant Goldmark Report (1926-1934) never achieved such an impact. Because men (physicians) controlled the training setting, women (nurses) did not even control the only profession they had.

Women actively protested their situation by speaking out not only for the vote but for greater and more equal opportunities. Susan B. Anthony, one of the early suffragettes, assembled and submitted what was to be the Fourteenth Amendment to the Constitution (suffrage), although it was not acted on until 1920 (as the Nineteenth Amendment). One way in which women could wield power became apparent in 1891, when the Johns Hopkins Medical School desperately needed funds in order to open. Certain daughters of the trustees and other prominent citizens formed the Women's Fund Committee, raised the needed amount, and made it available with stipulations. The stipulations were that women receive equal consideration for admission, that everyone admitted meet certain standards, and that the medical classroom building be renamed the Women's Memorial Building. The funds were accepted and the stipulations met.[7] Dr. Elizabeth Blackwell established another means of wielding power. Having fought to obtain a medical degree only to be faced with the opposition of the men in medicine and the hesitation of women to join her profession, she became a women's rights supporter focusing on nursing. Her friendship with Florence Nightingale influenced her decision to establish a hospital for women and children managed and staffed by women. Tactics such as these were not new; the fact that women were using them was.

Organization and support were necessary for women and nurses to meet their ideals. Lavinia Dock recognized the importance of organized effort to create or influence public opinion. In 1896, she was instrumental in forming the Nurses Associated Alumnae of the United States (the forerunner of American Nurses' Association), an organization in which nurses could share their professional concerns. The nurses involved in the women's movement looked toward this organization as an ally. Dock, nursing's most ardent suffragette, was disappointed in the alumnae's refusal to support a suffrage resolution at a 1908 convention. In a letter to the editor of the *American Journal of Nursing* she wrote:

> It was a shock, because, though I know many nurses have never given the subject a thought, yet I believed that they might always be depended upon, in their associations, to take instinctually the intelligent and above all the sympathetic position on large human questions. I am far from thinking that nurses have time or strength for work outside of their own field, and do not expect to see them actively engaged in the equality movement, but to give moral support and endorsement takes no time; to feel intelligent sympathy costs no money.[8]

For a few years all Lavinia Dock's financial and physical resources supported the suffrage movement. She achieved great satisfaction in going to jail (three times) for suffrage. Nurses' concern with the status of women became evident in letters to the editor in the *American Journal of Nursing* (1907-1908). That concern was heightened when attempts were made to legislate control of nursing practice. Met by ignorant, rude, and unconcerned male legislators, the nursing leaders concluded that a woman's profession would not exert influence nor gain support until women had a bargaining agent and the power behind it (i.e., the vote). In 1910, nurses and their leaders, Lavinia Dock, Isabel Stewart, and M. Adelaide Nutting, joined the ranks of women who marched down 5th Avenue in New York City in support of suffrage. The forces of women and nursing had met.

With World War I came an endurance test for the schools of nursing. Governmental pressure to lower or waiver admission standards and to intensify and shorten the training course met the resistance of nursing leaders. Three major projects were developed and implemented: the Army School of Nursing, the Student Nurse Reserve, and the Vassar Training Camp. Through the perseverant questioning, planning, and acting undertaken by nursing leaders, thousands of women fulfilled a demand for supporting the troops with assurance of quality. During the war, women became the sustaining force in the country's economy, assuming responsibility and work normally reserved for men. At last, in 1920, women were given the vote and, in 1923, the Equal Rights Amendment was formulated. Women had shown the ability to meet the demands placed upon them, and the status of women and of nursing rose significantly.

The depression years threatened the hard-won gains of women and nurses. Women, forced to give up their independence and work opportunities, returned to the home, thus allowing men to fill the limited number of jobs. Most nurses were without patients, since nursing was still predominantly private duty, and few people could afford such care. Opportunities for women were scarce and, although nursing schools continued to open and operate, the graduates of these schools received no guarantee of finding employment.

Although the training remained apprenticeship in nature, concerned nurses continued to establish and improve standards for curriculum and practice. Led by the University of Minnesota, in 1909, the educational preparation of nurses increasingly took place within the university setting. A basic tenet of Florence Nightingale, that professional nursing required a liberal education, was finally being implemented. Education in a university became increasingly available to women in a variety of fields; the placement of nursing within universities helped nursing keep pace with the advances of women.

After the experience of World War I, nursing was much better prepared to meet the demands of World War II, as evidenced when 40 percent of the nation's nurses volunteered for military service. With the large number of doctors involved in the war effort and the evolving medical advances, nurses assumed more responsibilities for patient care and for the implementation of new technical skills. A significant event, the delegation of non-nursing tasks to ancillary personnel, made more time available for activities commensurate with the nurse's level of preparation and at the same time opened more job opportunities for women with less education.

The establishment of the U.S. Cadet Nurse Corps, in 1943, increased the public's awareness of the need for federally supported education and brought thousands of women into accelerated nursing programs. Attention was directed to broadening the base of nursing service for the American people. The recruitment of blacks into nursing and the increasing equality of educational and employment opportunities for all nurses indicated progress. Women in general enjoyed greater equality and independence, although an organized women's movement was not active as in World War I. It was due to the efforts of women that industry and the economy continued to function and the health needs of the nation were met.

Although men resumed a greater responsibility for maintenance of the economy immediately after World War II, many opportunities continued to be available for women educationally and in the labor force. Even with an emphasis on the family unit, a woman's decision to combine a career and a home slowly achieved social acceptance.

Activity on the national level indicated nursing's intention to keep pace with social changes. The American Nurses' Association became the first professional organization to racially integrate, in 1946. The International Council of Nurses met in 1947, in Atlantic City, amid protests that it was too soon after the war for such an international gathering. The meeting provided a model for all nations and an asset to the United States when it proved to be a productive and amiable event. Through the nursing profession women received national recognition for the progressive efforts of their organizations.

A number of studies by nurses and non-nurses, many at the request of the national organizations, explored nursing functions, accreditation, registration, and curriculum standards and attempted to arrive at a comprehensive definition of nursing. Esther Lucille Brown, in 1948, published a report, *Nursing for the Future,*[9] urging that the designation "professional" be reserved for college-prepared nurses and that a differentiation among levels of preparation be defined in education and practice. She pointed to the persistent difficulty of obtaining public funding because of the old apprenticeship idea attached to hospital schools. A criticism leveled against nursing was that "no other profession has been developed on the assumption that an education can be secured in exchange for service."[10] Financially, nurses were still insecure because of the tradition that hospitals offered charity services and the ingrained reluctance of people to pay for their care even if they were able to do so. Following the Brown report, accreditation of schools and standard testing were implemented under the direction of the National League for Nursing. Research by nurses and higher education received greater emphasis to meet the increasingly demanding standards that society required of a profession.

As evidenced repeatedly throughout history, nursing's struggle to be a profession was an integral part of the women's rights movement, and the post war years were no exception. Having been active in the civil rights movements, fighting for rights and against oppression in the late 1950s, women once again activated their own rights movement in the 1960s. Women frequently made the news. President Kennedy chose a woman for his personal physician and appointed a committee to study the status of women. Women authored books calling for social reform and social equality. College education became increasingly available, and highly educated and skilled women demanded entry into a variety of work areas previously closed to them. Parallels in the progress of nursing were evidenced as nurses pursued masters and doctoral levels of education. They demanded an equal voice in health care planning, and insisted on a collegial relationship with physicians and others on the health care team. Equality in all aspects of the lives and professions of women emerged as the issue. In 1972, almost 50 years after it was first proposed, the Equal Rights Amendment passed in the U.S. Senate and continued on its way to possible ratification by the states. No longer was nursing the only profession open to women.

Throughout history the development of nursing and the status of women have been parallel and affected by similar influences. Today, the continuing parallel development of nursing and the women's movement is uncertain.

WOMEN AND NURSING:
WITHIN THE SOCIAL FRAMEWORK

Women's efforts to change society's attitudes have resulted in changing women's expectations of themselves. Rather than aligning themselves with nurses, women in the women's movement seem embarrassed by the meekness and subservience of their sisters in the nursing profession. Nurses seem to be held in low esteem by progressive, assertive women. Although historically the nursing profession represented women's means for self-expression, creativity, independence, and education, it no longer occupies that status in the eyes of women today. Commenting on the *History of Nursing*, written in the early 1900s by Lavinia Dock and M. Adelaide Nutting, Nutting said that it was "one of the liveliest and finest histories of the women's movement yet published."[11] Yet, today, the relationship appears weakened. Are the nurses themselves different? Are the emerging valued characteristics of women different? Why is it that, after the progressive, aggressive activities of the early nursing leaders, nursing once again assumed a meeker, more subservient role which only recently has begun to change?

Consideration of the current relationship between women and nursing and the factors affecting the nature of that relationship may clarify the direction the relationship is taking.

There is evidence that the women-nursing relationship is diverging. Nursing is a profession basically responding to society's needs and shaped by societal changes; it does not shape society's attitudes or values. Women, however, are taking an increasingly active role in shaping the attitudes, norms, and values of society. They correctly identified society's foundation as male dominated and directed their efforts to changing the previously unquestioned acceptance of this foundation. Now women are insisting on equal rights and opportunities through judicial, educational, occupational, and political means. They are characterized by a strong, outspoken leadership; they are articulate, forceful, and organized under a common goal.

Nursing is not in this "shaping" position; by nature it responds to the trends taking place in society and is thus shaped by it. Few nursing leaders questioned the male dominance in the health field. Lavinia Dock was an exception who recognized the threat of male dominance as a major problem confronting the profession and women.[12] Even before 1910, nursing leaders did wonder why the training school was always the handmaiden of the hospital, why nursing education always had to pay its own way or be the object of philanthropy, or why it could not be tax supported as was education for the professions of medicine, law, and engineering.[13] But the profession did not acknowledge the underlying cause to be male domination, nor did it consider male influence to be a concern of high priority. Dock complained that nursing "has not made itself a moral force; is not a public conscience; takes no position in large public questions; is not feared by those of low standards; allows all manner of new conditions and developments in nursing affairs to arise, flourish, succeed, or fail."[14] Even today, efforts to change attitudes constitute a great struggle. Women, especially nurses, may accept the need to change intellectually, but the need is not internalized emotionally nor demonstrated by action.

Rarely does it occur to one to question the foundation of one's social framework. The women who enter nursing are a product of society's values and attitudes. From a very young age, a girl is profoundly influenced by the behavioral patterns society deems proper and necessary to maintain the status quo—patterns enforced by a male-dominated culture. Societal attitudes are ingrained in the young girl's formulation of her goals, values, education, activities, and thought processes, although she may be fully unaware of the power that fashions and pervades every aspect of her life. Male dominance itself is not doubted—only the problems the girl confronts as she tries to arrange her life in a manner consistent with the foundation on which her existence is based. If the girl is "successful," she will adhere to the attitudes and values instilled in her by the male-dominated society. Women who dare to question the rationale for the social foundation are labeled "unsuccessful." A reactionary society views these women as radicals, deviates, and mavericks, and it moves swiftly to curtail the unacceptable behaviors. The power wielded by society is intimidating and fearful; few women have the stamina or fortitude to withstand the determination of a society bent on maintaining the status quo. The consequences of staunchly refuting the male domination are severe: How many women can tolerate the ostracism, protest, and ridicule leveled against them by the very society that exerted such a profound influence during their impressionable years? The values and attitudes of gentility, dependence, passiveness, and the need for social approval are difficult to repudiate, especially when the rewards for compliance are so great.

The nurse's image that Florence Nightingale conveyed as she developed modern nursing did not deviate far from what society considered proper behaviors in women. Modern nursing promoted the feminine traits still cultivated today. Nightingale also insisted vigorously that women *did* have a brain and could intelligently utilize a systematic thought process to make decisions. She firmly believed that women should have formal training that emphasized scientific principles. But intelligence had to be couched in the feminine characteristics deemed appropriate for women—a situation she did not consider inconsistent. Although Nightingale was widely recognized for her progressive ideas related to hygiene and improved health care, the prevailing image of her through history was that of a woman who built a profession on the natural feminine characteristics of nurturance, compassion, and submissiveness.

A major reason that the trainee nurses' preparation emphasized desirable feminine characteristics was that Nightingale attempted to develop a profession for the gentlewoman of the day. Very fresh in her mind was the image of the degenerate, decadent, detestable nurse of the seventeenth to the early nineteenth centuries. In order to improve the dismal reputation of nursing, Nightingale had to require saint-like qualities in her nurses. The public's image of a Nightingale nurse was of a selfless, endlessly toiling woman who valued gentility and respect for the physician. Nightingale further reinforced this view when she wrote that "nurses are there solely to carry out the orders of the medical and surgical staff, including the whole practice of cleanliness, fresh air, diet, etc."[15] She held that the emphasis of nurses' training was to understand how best to carry out orders. When she stated that "nurses cannot be registered and examined any more than mothers,"[16] Nightingale demonstrated how closely related she saw the role of mothering to that of nursing. Thus, the public did not see women systematically testing out theories or basing their practice on scientific principles, although Nightingale placed considerable emphasis on this also. The image of an intelligent woman was not promoted, and nursing quickly grew into an acceptable occupation for women compatible with society's male-dominance framework.

It is interesting that the early healers were women. It was women who learned by trial and error and who were empirical and rational in their approach to healing. Whereas they treated the sick on the basis of experience, men utilized superstition and faith. Men tended to take heroic measures like massive bleeding and potent laxatives, while women employed dietary changes and herbs. Although history suggests that women were more successful in their healing art than men, they were judged to be witches relying on witchcraft and the devil to effect their cures. Religious fervor, fanned by threatened males, encouraged the belief that one should be healed through faith, not through direct experience, and that death was preferable to cure by the devil. The empirical health-promoting activities of women were discredited. Women had the right ideas, talents, and tools, but the timing was wrong, and society rejected their efforts. Of course, when men "discovered" the practical use of scientific principles and empirical data in health, social attitudes changed accordingly. Women who quietly accepted their secondary place and deferred to men and who did not participate in the healing based on validated data were praised by society as occupying the proper place of women.

What happened? Why did women, who had utilized systematic inquiry valued by men, fail to gain a foothold in the shaping of positive societal attitudes toward women in the health field?

Perhaps part of the explanation is that men actively and unashamedly manipulated. They spoke loudly, and they engaged in spirited arguments and debates that established opinions as fact. As men reinforced aggressiveness in discussion and in practice, social pressures continued to effectively reinforce the quiet, meek, and nurturing characteristics in women. Women may have intelligently based their practice on scientific principles, but they failed to speak loudly; they did not publish nor engage in lively debates; they did not insist; and they did not value as feminine the aggressive spirit necessary to convince people of the worth of their ideas or to have them implemented. Instead, women tended to be quiet doers.

In recent years, the difference between the roles of men and women in health care has been further institutionalized. The cure role (male) of diagnosis and prescription is active, manipulative, and intellectual. The care role (female) of nurturance and compassion is passive. Women are praised for assisting nature but not interfering with it.

Women, and nursing, worked within this framework of society. Women sought men's cooperation to achieve goals for nursing. In order to raise educational standards, procure financial aid, and participate in the health care delivery system, women worked with men. Instead of liberation from men, women sought their approval and permission for the privileges and freedoms they desired. Although women's efforts were apparent and distinct from men's, women still deferred to men, to the physician's orders, to male dominance for much of their decision making.

Women themselves foster this dominance when they accept as desirable and internalize the traditional feminine characteristics. Their socialization is perpetuated from within when women reward each other for demonstrating these traits. Certain expectations and stereotypes are powerful influences on the progress or the lack of it in a profession. Stereotypes linked with long traditions are difficult to change and outlast the realities on which they were based. Since nursing tends to reflect slow-to-change prevailing social attitudes, even idealistic young women who enter the profession find themselves unable to shake off the influence of its traditional nature. Either they meet the expectations of fellow nurses, or they become disillusioned and bitter and eventually leave. The women who conform place much emphasis on the behaviors of collaboration, team work, and mutual agreement rather than on dominance, their enormous potential power, or change. These behaviors are instilled in nursing education, which tends to be a sex-segregated system, and then are solidified when there is a lack of interaction with men in the work environment. As a result, women consider working with and being with men as two separate forms of activity. The predominance of women in nursing and the hierarchy within nursing do not promote autonomy. Nursing may be weak in part because it includes very few men; thus, nurses are not able to see the applicability of male behaviors to the progress of the profession. Nurses can scarcely congratulate themselves for upward mobility when they move within a narrow system comprised almost exclusively of women. Power and prestige reside with the men, and an all-woman profession either lacks the power or fails to utilize its power to convincingly wield enough influence to change the prevailing social norms.

At the turn of the century, women believed that the inequality existing between men and women could be resolved if women obtained the right to vote. Once the vote was obtained, many women assumed that the problem ceased to exist. Only a few women correctly concluded that the basic problem (i.e., male domination in society) had not been identified. As the years passed, other aspects of freedom and independence took high priority as women reached a readiness to deal with them. With increasing confidence, women are now refusing to view male permission as necessary for those things they consider to be their rights. With the refutation of male dominance, social norms, values, and attitudes are undergoing a pronounced change. Women's efforts are gaining influence in shaping society's attitudes, directions, and expectations.

The present momentum of the women's movement may widen the gap between itself and nursing unless nursing also demonstrates a readiness for change, acknowledges the impact of male dominance on the profession, and aggressively confronts the issues concerning women.

WOMEN AND NURSING:
PARALLEL OR DIVERGENT PROGRESS?

It has been shown historically how nursing provided women with a vehicle for self-expression and independence in a manner compatible with the norms of the times. When woman's place was in the home, nursing was an acceptable occupation in which to seek training and employment. Job availability, variety of work hours, part-time employment, and the nurturing nature of the work were depicted as ideal aspects of employment for women. Bearing and raising children influenced the enter and exit pattern of nurses as they dropped their employment for years at a time. The socialization of women at this time led to the belief that these aspects of nursing made it an ideal way of making women useful outside the home. Also, the income, small as it was, provided some extra purchasing power for growing families. While this mode of employment relieved personal and financial stress within the family, it created considerable stress within the profession. Nursing, attempting to maintain its responsibilities as a profession, found progress difficult to achieve with a large portion of the membership working part-time and sporadically. How many other professions equate marriage and family responsibilities with professional responsibilities?

Besides attempting to manage a profession with part-time commitments, nursing is also plagued by myths and stereotypes accepted by the public and perpetuated by those within the profession. A long tradition of involvement with religious orders and war has resulted in an impression that contrasts with reality. Some common myths include the following:

1. Nursing is for single women who are either recovering from a love affair or looking for a husband (i.e., a doctor).

2. Nursing provides a domestic service (i.e., scrubbing, laundering, and feeding).

3. Nursing is a good rehearsal for mothering; one will always be able to use it in raising a family.

4. Nurses meet their sexual needs through prostitutional practices (with patients and physicians).

5. Nurses can exit from nursing for years at a time and always reenter.

6. Nursing is a natural function; since it can be done by intuition, one must avoid overeducation.

Besides persistent traditions and myths, the media's interpretation and representation of nurses have been of no assistance to the profession. Dixie McCall, of the television series "Emergency," is seen working all hours and in all areas of the hospital, accomplishing feats impossible even for the most energetic and intelligent nurse. This wonder woman represents an unreal picture of a profession so technically and intellectually advanced that specialization is almost a must. On the other hand, there is Consuela in the "Marcus Welby, M.D." television series. Several viewings of the program are necessary to determine that Consuela is, in fact, a nurse. Her functions of phone answering, appointment scheduling, and physician seeking could be handled by one with much less education. Would these programs portray these images if nursing as a profession took a stand and demanded a more up-to-date image? Consider a weekly 30-minute show on the life of an inner-city public health nurse!

Society, represented by the health care consumer and public awareness, places controls on nursing's development and on the nature of its practice, thus restricting its progress to a conservative and slow pace. Mythic stereotypes and media misrepresentation instill in society ideas that are difficult to change. For too long, nurses have quietly accepted this situation, not wanting to create a disturbance or "rock the boat." Traditionally, nurses within the profession have lacked the autonomy, ingenuity, initiative, and adaptability to strive for a change in society's attitudes and values. With the gaining momentum of the women's movement, one would hope that nurses, too, will benefit, if not as shapers of society, then by being advantageously shaped by society. Being too busy with long hours, poor pay, lack of recognition, lack of support, and often divided commitments, nurses have had little time to be actively involved with improving the status of women.

Nursing's response to society's image of it has been generally conservative and certainly not dynamic or progressive. "Make do with what one has" seems to be a prevailing thought. An example of this is nurses thinking that they should be able to give good patient care no matter what the nurse-patient ratio is or the number of hours they have in which to work. Rather than recognize an intolerable situation and take action to rectify it, nurses persistently work overtime (without pay) and carry out important technical skills while relegating tasks of professional care and patient teaching to such a low priority that they are virtually never carried out. It is no surprise that hospitalized members of society perceive nurses as hurried, overworked pill passers, bedpan pushers, bath givers, and bed makers. Powerful change-making strategies are available to nurses if they can get beyond the stereotype and the socialized thought pattern of women as subservient, submissive, nurturing, and kindly in all acts.

Recent strikes by nurses over issues of quality patient care are an example of one of the change-making strategies available. The power is there if the profession is willing to take it and use it. Simply by virtue of their comprising the largest group of health care providers, nurses should be able to wield influence and changes. When Inglenook wine produced and displayed a television advertisement depicting nurses as subordinate to physicians, an outcry by nurses resulted in a new, acceptable version.

Now women are insisting on changes at a rate more rapid than can occur in nursing, which is bound by the rate of change in society as a whole. If the women's movement succeeds in bringing about change in society, nursing will benefit. However, nurses are not in the forefront insisting on these changes. A schematic representation of social change appears like this,

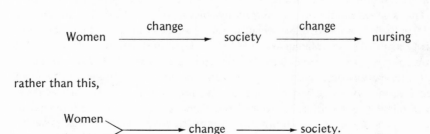

rather than this,

Women are forging ahead utilizing the tools of politics and the law to obtain what they believe is their right. Nurses in the past few years have also organized to use these tools. Nevertheless, nursing continues to follow a few years behind, and the idea of separateness persists.

Not only are women and nursing progressing at different rates, but women are entering other professions where they are presently in the minority. Engineering, trucking, mining, law, and medicine, among others, currently offer expanded choices to women interested in employment. A certain mystique and uniqueness characterize minorities of all sorts, and women are no exception. Hardly a day passes when one does not read or hear of a woman in an "unusual" occupation—"unusual" because for years that occupation was considered unsuitable for women. Conferences and counseling programs aimed at high school and early college women emphasize opportunities in all fields. Industry and big business eagerly recruit women to fulfill minority quotas and pacify women's organizations.

Women in nursing do not constitute a minority and cannot, therefore, claim the uniqueness of women in other professions. Nursing has weathered a history of domination and control by men (physicians and hospital administrators). A constant striving for independence from this subordinate role has resulted in women rising within their own system and assuming control of a hierarchy of women. Within the profession of nursing and the health care delivery system, women have developed a caste system which interferes with the advancement of the profession and the delivery of health care. Within nursing, constant verbal battles are also fought between the educators and the service nurses, between the administrative nursing leaders and the staff nurses, and among the graduates of the three different preparatory programs (i.e., baccalaureate, associate degree, and diploma). Conflicts and jealousy among the nursing levels (RN, LPN, and aide) often jeopardize effective team functioning. As an oppressed group of women, nurses have experienced stresses through frustration, internal bickering, and dissension within nursing.

The women's movement points to nursing as a prime example of sex discrimination. If a woman is intelligent and capable, she could be a physician; however, sexual constraints are strong, and she resigns herself to entering nursing. To combat this, women's organizations encourage women to be physicians, dentists, and scientists. Nursing is hampered when intelligent, creative, and independent women go into other professions—nursing is no longer the first choice of women who want to work, who want an education, and who want responsibility. Nursing education must maintain high admission standards, and the nursing profession must update society's image of nursing if the profession is to survive.

Strong leadership within nursing is not as visible today as it was at the turn of the century. As the number of nurses increased, the ability to control decreased and lines of communication faltered. Many of the current leaders entered nursing during an era when nursing was viewed as a part-time occupation rather than as a career requiring ongoing commitment and when the women's movement was inactive. Consequently, little activity is demonstrated today by these leaders in regard to women's concerns. But, in the last ten years, the women's movement has gained momentum and more nurses have committed themselves to a professional career. A newer, younger group of women with interests in the future of nursing and women are striving to break into the leadership circle. If they succeed, the status of women and nursing may once again be parallel.

With nursing's historical background and internal problems, it is not surprising that the women's movement lacks any motivation to include nurses as allies. Action is further hindered through a general lack of information about nursing by members of women's groups. If more nurses became active within women's organizations, this problem would be alleviated. Historically, nursing has provided numerous firsts for women and, for a full perspective, this fact must be acknowledged. A brief review of a nursing history textbook adds to one's ability to educate women on the merits (past and potential) of the nursing profession. Alignment with the women's movement could ease the struggles of the profession. Strength comes with numbers and, if nursing could receive the support of the existing 51 percent of society, it would undoubtedly enjoy greater prestige and attract intelligent, capable women necessary to guarantee progress, quality, and full accountability in the health care delivery system.

WOMEN AND NURSING: THE FUTURE

Reflecting on the associations between women and nursing and the advancements of both, one is bound to ask certain questions. Are the women presently in nursing already shaped by an earlier society in which women played a different role? Are the changes in nursing dependent on the types of women who enter the profession, on the women who are changing attitudes of society at so many different levels? Does this suggest that women entering nursing today are the shapers of society who will determine the focus and nature of the nursing of tomorrow? Can nursing continue to advance without an alliance with the women's movement? Even though nursing is a socially defined necessity, will society (women included) permit a change in the definition so that better health care will benefit all people?

Nursing is still primarily a profession of women and has available to it all the power, resources, and energy characterizing the women's movement today—providing that the women in nursing recognize these as strengths and realize the potential impact that can be exerted on the profession. The women in nursing can shape the social climate, which could, in turn, significantly influence the focus and nature of nursing. Will there be continued parallel development or divergence? Nursing must not separate itself from the efforts of the women's movement.

NOTES

1. G.J. Griffin and J.K. Griffin, *Jensen's History of Professional Nursing* (St. Louis: Mosby Co., 1969), pp. 24-30.

2. M. Rawnsley, "The Goldmark Report: Midpoint in Nursing History," *Nursing Outlook* 21 (June 1973): 381.

3. B. Clemons, "Women's Liberation and Nursing: Historic Interplay," *American Operating Room Nurse Journal* 13 (June 1971): 74.

4. Florence Nightingale, *Florence Nightingale to Her Nurses.* (London: Macmillan & Co., 1914), p. 5.

5. E.R. Barritt, "Florence Nightingale's Values and Modern Nursing Education," *Nursing Forum* 12, no. 1, (1973): 12.

6. National League for Nursing, "Three Score Years and Ten," Paper, presented at 1963 NLN Convention, Atlantic City, May 13-17, 1963), pp. 8-9.

7. H.E. Marshall, *Mary Adelaide Nutting, Pioneer of Modern Nursing* (Baltimore: Johns Hopkins University Press, 1972), p. 55.

8. L. Dock, "The Suffrage Question," in letter to the editor, *American Journal of Nursing* 8 (August 1908): 925-926.

9. E.L. Brown, *Nursing for the Future* (New York: Russell Sage Foundation, 1948) pp. 62-137.

10. M.M. Roberts, *American Nursing, History and Interpretation* (New York: Macmillan Co., 1954), pp. 61, 134.

11. Marshall, *Mary Adelaide Nutting*, p. 155.

12. J. Ashley, "Nurses in American History: Nursing and Early Feminism," *American Journal of Nursing* 78 (September 1975): 1466.

13. Marshall, *Mary Adelaide Nutting*, p. 164.

14. L. Dock, "The Duty of This Society in Public Work." In *Proceedings of the Tenth Annual Convention of the American Society of Superintendents of Training Schools, Pittsburgh, October 7-9, 1903* (Baltimore: J.H. Furst Co., 1904), pp. 77-78.

15. L. Dock, "History of the Reform in Nursing in Bellvue Hospital," *American Journal of Nursing* 1 (November 1901): 2.

16. B. Ehrenreich and D. English, *Witches, Midwives and Nurses* (New York: Feminist Press, Glass Mountain Pamphlets no. 1, 1973), p. 35.

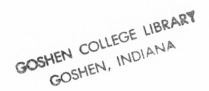

3
The Nurse's Self-image

MARY ANN BUSH
DIANE K. KJERVIK

Women and nurses have not systematically learned to value themselves. In this male-dominated society, females learn to care for others rather than themselves and, as a result, have not nurtured their own self-images. Adult women are faced with the incongruity of being expected to perform professionally and autonomously but at the same time to play the traditionally feminine, passive role. This incongruity leads to stress upon the self-concepts of women and nurses.

The authors will examine this subject by defining self-image, discussing the development of one's self-concept (including nurses' self-image), and considering assertiveness as a way to build one's self-concept.

It is useful to share thoughts and convictions about nurses with other nurses. This is based on a belief that nurses have much to offer the health care system in the forms of creative thinking, different types of organizational structures, promotion of health care, and the provision of excellent nursing care.

Numbering almost 1.5 million persons, nurses embody tremendous energy, knowledge, resources, and power among themselves. Nursing constitutes more than half of all personnel providing health care.[1] Working collectively, nurses can play a major role in making health care available to all persons and can also begin to concentrate on promotion and maintenance of health, which is sorely lacking in our present system. It is much more easy, practical, and logical to expend energy maintaining health than it is to cure illness.

But to have an impact on the changing health care system, which is being so carefully studied and scrutinized throughout the country, nurses need to be convinced of their personal value and their professional value. Nurses need to be visible and assertive. They need to be identified as members of an autonomous profession with a unique knowledge and expertise to offer the persons they serve.

To be accepted as collaborators and professionals in their own right, nurses need to present themselves in an assertive manner as professionals who are convinced of their self-worth. Their behavior will then belie their beliefs, and the health care system will find in its midst nurses who do indeed place patient care as their primary goal. Nurses will then cease to see themselves carefully suggesting rather than stating what they think, cease to see persons discharged before they are able to care for themselves, cease to see persons reach death with no chance to deal with one of the most important experiences of their life because the physician says it will upset the patient. The present status of nursing's professional self-image rests in its history and in the socialization process of our culture. Nursing's image is based on anonymity and a position of secondary status, and this has not served nursing, society, or nursing's clients to advantage. Nurses are in the midst of an inequitable health delivery system in which care is dictated by physicians, hospital administrators, university administrators, and insurance companies. Yet nurses comprise the largest group in the health care industry. It is appropriate and essential that nurses improve their self-image and take control of their own profession. They need to do this both for themselves as individuals who have chosen to be nurses and for the people whose health is their commitment and concern.

SELF-IMAGE

Self-image is one's conception of the sort of person one is. It is built up from one's beliefs about oneself and an awareness of oneself, and this knowledge has been consciously, unconsciously, or even subliminally formed by each person's experiences—the successes, failures, humiliations, and journeys into oneself as well as other persons' feedback responses. From these experiences each person constructs a picture of herself which she feels to be true, and then she behaves accordingly. It is well known that if a child is labeled "bad" and treated as "bad," she will behave badly, and thus a vicious circle will have been wrought. Put another way, one's self-concept is very simply "how one perceives oneself," and each person is constantly telling herself and others what her self-image is. Each person communicates her self-concept by the way she stands, sits, talks, gestures, looks, feels, responds, asserts herself, or remains silent. As each person sends out these messages, they are, for the most part, received and returned in an affirming or negating manner. On the basis of these responses and one's self-knowledge, a person esteems herself to be worthy or unworthy and then expresses this personal judgment in the attitudes she holds toward herself. Thus, a circular pattern is established. A person behaves in accordance with her beliefs.

There are two aspects involved in establishing a sense of selfness or personhood: (1) personal experiences and personal feedback in relation to other persons and (2) each person's journey into herself or an intrapsychic sense of self.

These experiences incorporate what people tell us, what people tell others, how people respond to us generally, and how people respond to specific behaviors. For example, a nurse hears feedback that she is a capable, knowledgeable nurse, and then when she gets home and turns on the television set she watches a program telling her that a nurse is a passive, unintelligent, anonymous person whose role is to look pretty and to please. (In a script of the television program "Colombo," a nurse takes an assertive role and challenges the quality of care a physician is rendering. Her body is found later!) Or, if a person in the first five minutes of meeting a nurse begins to tell her his ills, she knows she is being told because she is a nurse, not because of the person she is. To stop at a car accident and administer first aid elicits a more specific feedback response. The message will probably be affirmative. The responses a nurse receives from all these incidents have an effect on her self-image, and, whether or not she validates the responses within herself, they are imprinted in her consciousness and/or her memory. If each response imprints itself then each response lends self-respect or diminution of self-respect.

What, then, of a nurse's role? What does this role in the health care system tell people about how nurses feel about themselves? Because most nurses are women and have grown up in American society, they have been socialized to believe that the white male is superior, not so much by verbal statements as by attitudes that are clearly although indirectly communicated. They have been raised to believe that the male ego is fragile and that they must protect it by not winning, by not being "too" smart, not being "too" successful, by not stealing the limelight. This is an insult to both men and women because it negates the personhood, uniqueness, strengths, and self-worth of both sexes. But because it is familiar, it is secure. In the hospitals and other health care institutions, this male-female role has taken on the caricature of the doctor-nurse game. This caricature has been perpetuated by Cherry Ames, Sue Barton, most of our news media, as well as nurses themselves. This game was well defined by Leonard Stein in 1967.[2] In this game of subtleties, nurses are communicating to others and habituating themselves to secondary status and value. The object of the game is to make the doctor feel in control at all times. The nurse is to be actively helpful yet appear passive. An illustration of this game is presented by Tricia Kushner in an article entitled "The Nursing Profession: Condition Critical." She uses an example typical of many incidents occurring in nursing: A nurse specializing in coronary care may well know emergency responses better than a physician not involved in acute coronary crises; but, as the physician arrives on the scene, the nurse will not, in all likelihood, tell him what to do. She may instead offer a suggestion about what has worked before in a similar situation, and the doctor may then authoritatively order what she has suggested. The scene will probably end with the nurse saying, "Thank you, Doctor."[3] People might respond favorably to an example like this, but what is good about it? It is a good illustration of what has kept nursing an unrecognized profession and has subtly reinforced the physician's image as sole decision maker in the health care field. The patient is helped, and all would deem this "good." The patient, however, could still be helped without the nurse playing down her knowledge and expertise by carefully couching what she knows in terms of a suggestion. It seems that the nurse is taking care of the doctor almost as though he were sick. Smoyak points out that nurses, because of their caring, sympathetic, and humanitarian natures, often see other people as ill. Nurses take care of physicians who are "forgetful," "rushed," or "overburdened." Smoyak suggests that nurses learn to distinguish between workers and patients and begin to believe that well people are in a sense "fair game" for confrontation.[4] Although the doctor-nurse game is almost second nature to nurses (and played under the weighted factor of "good patient care"), it does continue to perpetuate the second-rate status of nurses in health care. A second-rate role is bound to lead to frustration, high attrition rates, and nurses leaving the field, and often the reason is never ascertained. As both Maslow and Sidney Jourard attest, a person who is living a role not based on inner striving and desires will become dispirited, and because one's inner nature cannot be annihilated or forever negated, it will press forward.[5,6] It is important to note that one's inner nature is not bad; it is neutral at the least and considered good by most. It pushes for identity, self-esteem, and autonomy for all persons. To resist is to deny this inner nature, and these resistances take their toll—now, next year, or many years from now.

Abraham Maslow in *Toward a Psychology of Being* has addressed this issue. It seems quite clear to Maslow that personality problems are sometimes "loud protests against the crushing on one's psychological bones," or one's inner nature. He feels that what is sick is to not protest. Unfortunately, many people don't protest and end up paying years later in neurotic or psychosomatic symptoms of various kinds. Or, what might be worse, some people never realize that they have missed true happiness, true fulfillment of promise, and a serene old age. These people miss the joy and wonder of a creative, aesthetic, and fulfilling life.[7] Self-actualization, high-level wellness, and transparent self were not written for one-half of the human race. They were written for all persons, and put forth very clearly that maturity, self-actualization, and high-level wellness are dependent on a high degree of self-esteem in which the person knows who she is, what she wants, and what is realistic for her, and she has the choice to strive for what will make her whole. The following questions, which are based on Hamachek's assessment criteria for low self-concept, may help in assessing one's sense of self-worth:[8]

1. Do you feel inferior to many of your colleagues in the work setting?

2. Are you crushed by negative criticism from others?

3. Is your whole day "made" if someone compliments you about something, no matter how small?

4. Do you blame others for your own problems?

5. Do you shy away from competitive situations?

6. Do you avoid other people rather than relating to them honestly?

If a person answers affirmatively to most or all of these questions, her self-image may be negative and she probably needs some uplifting experiences.

In order to develop a positive self-image, one must be able to be still with oneself and, in that silence, search for answers and identify what one really feels and who one really is. It means that one may need to say, "I really don't feel this way or want this for myself." It means *choosing* to stay home and care for the family after coming to grips with one's being and inner nature, but not acting in a given way because it is expected and pleases others. If a nurse finds herself in a crisis situation in dealing with a particularly difficult doctor in regard to patient care and knows that, if she doesn't word a request in the right manner, the patient will suffer, then she will in all likelihood *choose* to suggest a change in care. But she has made this choice for a particular reason, in a particular situation, and she has not negated herself in doing so. Valid choices have as their basis and prerequisite the freedom to make the choice.

So much of learning has been based on rewards for total self-giving in the form of caring for others and negation of self, and such behavior has been promoted under the guise of humility, dedication, virtue, and good patient care. The Catholic Church has for years admired and paid homage to persons who attained sainthood because of heroic lives of self-abnegation. In recent years, the Church has acknowledged that many of these persons never existed, and the Christian Church, which has for centuries lauded selflessness and self-negation in the name of virtue, has as its leader one of the greatest teachers and self-actualized persons of all time. Christ is recognized by Christians and non-Christians alike as a fully mature, self-actualized person, a transparent self who attained high-level wellness. If one were to study theology and scripture, one would not find incidents in which Christ negated Himself, sold Himself short, or did not challenge a social system that was dishonest. Perhaps those who always put others' desires, thoughts, feelings, and needs ahead of their own are not being virtuous or selfless. Perhaps instead they are guilty of another sin, that of accidie—the failure to become all that one is capable of becoming.

What relevance, then, does a positive self-image have to what we as nurses do in our professional lives? There is evidence that people who are self-accepting are more accepting of others.[9] If nurses could accept themselves, perhaps they could be more open and tolerant of the behavior of their patients. A study published in 1975 showed that nurses with positive self-concepts were rated as giving better patient care then nurses with negative self-images.[10] The study indicates the importance of considering a nurse's self-concept as a significant variable affecting patient care. Only by becoming a full human person can a nurse influence the health care system in a way that will make health available to all persons in the best possible sense. Only by being as full a human person as possible can a nurse provide good nursing care for the total good of the individual by promoting his/her health, by helping him/her cope with his/her illness or suffering, by helping him/her find meaning in suffering, and/or by helping him/her prepare for death. Much of nursing care demands that nurses act as change agents. Nurses cannot help patients and their families change if they refuse change in their own lives, and it is very difficult, if not impossible, to change if one does not feel good about oneself. Nursing has a great deal to offer the health care system. Nurses have an important role in promoting health. A nurse is able to teach patient care, to assess a person's total being, to act as a change agent to help make the world a healthier place in which to live. Nurses have been selling themselves short and grossly underrating their abilities and importance. Professional licensure and status demand accountability and responsibility, and nurses have a responsibility to acknowledge the major role they play in health care. This will surely be in the patient's or client's best interests, but it means that nurses must develop more positive self-images. It means that nurses must start perceiving themselves as capable providers with knowledge and expertise. It means that nurses must start viewing themselves as autonomous professionals collaborating with other professionals. These beliefs about abilities, expertise, and knowledge will be communicated to all who work with and relate to nurses. These convictions will give nurses the courage to act as change agents for themselves, to endure the resistances they will encounter, and to eventually achieve the status they deserve from the knowledge and abilities they possess.

This present-day role in nursing is firmly rooted in history, and the feelings associated with this role are deeply embedded in social and cultural values. As the past grew out of the social and political climate of the times, so will the present. To better understand the avenues presently open to nurses, it is necessary to look at nursing history in an attempt to understand from whence nursing has come.

HISTORICAL FACTORS

The beginning of nursing as we know it today flowed from Florence Nightingale's entrance into the Crimean War in the mid-1800s. Nightingale ordered the women who accompanied her not to assist physicians who did not ask for their help, which was significant in two respects. First, Nightingale defined nursing as women's work, whereas in previous centuries both men and women had performed nursing duties. Second, she set up a subservient relationship to the physicians on the battlefield whereby the nurses would care only for those patients whom the doctors ordered them to see.

Nightingale acted, however, in the context of the political climate of the time. She was aware of the powerlessness of women in society and supported the movement for women's suffrage. Her view of power and women is apparent in the following statement, which she made in support of equal suffrage rights: "I am convinced that political power is the greatest that it is possible to wield for human happiness, and I neither can approve of women who decline the responsibility of it nor of men who would shut them out from it. Until women do wield it, in an open, direct manner, I am convinced that the evils can never be satisfactorily dealt with."[11]

Nightingale supported power for women and for nurses during a time when neither group had any significant influence. Women, who had acted as health care providers for centuries, had been systematically and thoroughly removed from these roles by males who wanted control over health care as well as economic, social, religious, and political systems in society.[12] By the time Nightingale came along, males were frowning at the idea of women aiding sick or wounded people; so she found that the one way she could gain ingress to helping the wounded soldiers was by seeking the physician's approval. The flattery to their egos must have been enough to please the physicians and get the nurses into the helping arena again. The primary goal of helping the patient was achieved, but the self-determination of the nurses' practice was damaged.

These historical roots are still apparent in nursing practice today. Over 98 percent of nurses are female, which means, today as it did then, that the characteristics attributed to women are considered typical of nurses as well. How often are nurses and women described (in the media, for instance) as weak, passive sex symbols whose primary need is to help others at their own expense? How often do nurses believe this about themselves without hearing it from anyone else?

The abnegation of self is manifest in numerous ways in nursing and in society's view of the nurse. Take, for example, the 1976 thirteen-cent U.S. postage stamp which pictures a woman who was a nurse—Clara Maass. The contribution she made was not small; written on the stamp is the epitaph "She gave her life." Clara Maass died during tests proving that the mosquito was the yellow fever vector. Consider that there have been very few women who have appeared on postage stamps and no nurses that can be readily recalled. How was Clara Maass selected? Of all the nurses and women in the world who have created works of art, developed new systems of technology, or created a new profession such as Florence Nightingale did, how was Clara Maass selected? For what activity are women and nurses rewarded? Clara Maass was commended for her death; she was honored for self-sacrifice.

How often does this same self-denial happen when, in a small way, nurses defend the questionable actions of a physician to an inquisitive patient. Not only do nurses give up their own important perceptions of what happens to the patient (self-denial), but they also abnegate their advocacy role for the patient, so that the patient suffers.

The control of nursing practice by nurses that was lost during the inception of the nursing profession is being steadily regained. Lobbyists are working for direct reimbursement for services rendered and changes in legal definitions of nursing. Collective bargaining agents are negotiating for higher wages and a greater voice for nurses in decisions affecting patient care. But what about the nurse by herself? Is she ready and willing to assume more responsibility after years of taking orders and being steadily lulled into a passive feminine role?

An analogy can be drawn to what is happening in this society to women as a whole. Laws to end sex discrimination are on the books, and gradually hiring practices, credit practices, social security benefits, and child custody decisions are changing. But many individual women are not ready for or do not want these changes.

Because of their low self-confidence, they don't think that new hiring practices will help them. Changes will only add to their feelings of inadequacy, because they'll think that they should have gone into engineering or medicine or law to improve the lot of women. And now it's too late—too late to learn all that math and chemistry or too late to get into law school. Thus, they feel that they'll be "a disappointment to everyone." In other words, legal changes add to some women's feelings of guilt. This is probably why they resist these changes so vigorously: "Why should I have more choices? I'll just have more failures to deal with."

Women suffer from an inordinate amount of guilt. Anne Schaef from the Women's Institute of Alternative Psychotherapy in Colorado is developing a new theory of the psychology of women based on her psychotherapeutic practice over a 15-year period. She believes that women are afflicted with, as she calls it, "the original sin of being born female." Because she has to live with this original sin, a woman tries to overcome it by pleasing the white males in society by seeking their approval. It is not enough to give approval to herself because she herself is a female. Schaef finds that her female patients have an overwhelming sense of rage, which is localized and experienced in the stomach area and, when unexpressed, turns inward as guilt.[13] Dr. Fritz Perls, a Gestalt therapist, directed his patients to ask themselves what they resented when they were expressing guilty feelings verbally.[14]

But guilt is a passive response, and rage is more active. Is this why women and perhaps nurses experience guilt and not rage? Guilt, of course, feeds a low self-concept, and one might think, "Well, that's easy. We've identified the problem—guilt. Now let's terminate it!" It's not easy to do away with, because a low self-concept has become part of the woman's or the nurse's self-image. When it is given up, a part of the woman dies, and, with the death of a part of oneself, there is grief. Does this sound strange—to grieve for the loss of a negative opinion of oneself?

Think of it this way: The woman's image of herself as a woman is related to her passivity. She values her femininity. Her relationships with males flourish because of this image, and she may lose more than a low self-concept when she changes. She fears the loss of approval from other females, but especially males. Therefore, the decision to give up guilt must be weighed carefully by each individual woman or nurse. Laws or policies cannot dictate giving up guilt. Each women must choose.

ASSERTIVENESS

Giving up guilt must, if it is going to succeed, include a choice for a more active pattern of response. Recognizing and knowing one's thoughts, feelings, and behaviors would be a first step toward more active patterns of behavior. Owning these thoughts, feelings, and behaviors in the sense of claiming responsibility for them would be the next step. Such owning would result in being able to give direct expression to oneself, regardless of the situation. Such direct expression of thoughts and feelings is termed "assertive behavior." Assertiveness is giving expression to one's rights, thoughts, and feelings *without* degrading, insulting, or interfering with the reasonable rights of others. Assertiveness attacks the problems and attempts to deal with the issues at hand in a way that resolves problems and will establish precedents for dealing with future problems.

Assertiveness is a prerequisite for achieving self-esteem. It is necessary for autonomy and growth toward self-actualization. It is the quality and the behavior that expresses the belief that each person is important. Each person is important enough to be recognized and acknowledged and have her needs responded to. As such, assertiveness is a very important personality trait. It is also a very elusive personality trait. Some persons are fortunate. They grow up in an environment that fosters rational verbalization of both thoughts and feelings. Most people, i.e., white women, black men, and other minorities, have unfortunately been taught that only white men have a right and an obligation to be assertive.

Although most people profess to believe in the statement that all men are created equal, if not in ability, at least before the law and as human persons, they do not, in fact, believe that all human persons are created equal nor do they treat all human persons as equals. The following examples reflect this stereotypic dichotomy of values:[15]

1. Parents are better than children. Parents can be arbitrary, inconsiderate, and demanding of their children. They can order a child to "come here this very minute," and the child must stop midsentence and run immediately to his parent's side. Any child who responded by treating his parents in similar fashion would in all likelihood be punished.

2. Administrative personnel are better than employees. Bosses are allowed to be grumpy, have bad days, organize their work poorly, and demand inhuman work loads from their secretaries as a result. Bosses deserve smiles, hellos, and good mornings. Employees may or may not get them.

3. Whites are better than blacks. History speaks for itself here.

4. Married women are better than single women and certainly better than divorcees. Divorcees have failed in one of the most important pursuits of womanhood; they have lost their identity with a man.

The following examples are closer to home:

5. Physicians are better than nurses.

6. Nurses are better than nurse's aides and on down the line of nursing degrees.

This type of illustration could go on ad infinitum. The point is simple. Certain people are assumed, on the basis of education, age, sex, marital status, etc., to have more rights than others. When one thinks of it in this way, the hierarchy that persons live by really doesn't make much sense. A physician is better prepared than a nurse in the area of disease pathology, but both have equal rights to respect, dignity, feeling, thoughts, and ideas. It is in this context that women have been slighted and put down, and, as a result, they have generally learned that their role is to accept the way they are treated and be nonassertive in their quest for their goals. The point of talking about these stereotypes is to enhance one's awareness of them and then to begin to try to act differently. By becoming more assertive, nurses improve their self-image and, consequently, their image as nurses.

Because the concept *assertiveness* has been used a number of times, it should be defined along with its two opposites, *aggressiveness* and *nonassertiveness*.[16] Assertiveness is thinking and acting in ways in which one stands up for one's legitimate personal rights. It is the act of giving expression to one's positive and negative thoughts in a way that defines one's perspective without subtracting from the legitimate rights of others. A person who is nonassertive allows other people to treat her, her thoughts, and her feelings in whatever way they want to. It means that a person does what others want regardless of her own desires.

Aggressiveness is standing up for what one wants regardless of the rights of others. It can be difficult to see the differences between aggression and assertion. Aggression can be physical or verbal. Except in relation to children and behavior related to drug dependency, most people are not physically aggressive. Verbal aggression, however, is all too common. This can be illustrated by an example many workers might have experienced. In an excused absence from a meeting, a person's colleagues agree that it is that person's turn to do some extra after-hour duties once a month. The feeling response is that of being taken advantage of, and the person very likely feels angry. This situation can be handled in one of the three ways.

The person could assertively and in a firm tone of voice state that she would prefer that the group not make decisions about her personal time. She might then agree to check her calendar to determine if she is able to perform the duties and accordingly decide whether she will do the task and then let the committee know of her decision.

To handle the situation nonassertively, she could say nothing and simply do the job. While doing the job, however, she might well be tied in knots.

Handling the situation aggressively would neither help her win friends nor influence people, but she would probably not be expected to perform the duties. The scene might include some shouting about people who interfere with a person's personal life, perhaps pounding a fist on a table, and maybe a quick, determined exit signaled by a slamming door.

In the previously cited example in which the nurse noticed changes on a patient's electrocardiogram and called for any available physician, there were also alternative approaches. Encountering the young physician who did not know the best course of action, she could have chosen the nonassertive stand of silence and waited, to the patient's detriment. She could have threatened the doctor with a malpractice suit if he didn't do something quickly. Or she could have made an assertive statement such as, "Doctor, I think the patient needs 50 mg of Xylocaine."

In summary, an assertive person attempts to deal with the issues at hand in a way that resolves the problem and establishes a precedent for dealing with future problems. Assertiveness gives expression to a person's rights and feelings without degrading, insulting, or interfering with the reasonable rights of others. Assertiveness attacks the problem. It is a mode of dealing with both positive and negative feelings.

Nonassertiveness also establishes a pattern for future interactions. It is a pattern of avoiding problems and denying one's rights and feelings. People who are nonassertive are often taken advantage of and consequently become dispirited.

An aggressive person attempts to solve problems by trampling on the rights and feelings of others. In terms of future relations, aggressiveness will probably instill fear and even hatred in others, and these people will then avoid contact with the aggressive person. In an aggressive exchange the aggressor often draws on irrelevant information to down the opponent. Behaviors also reflect attitude; an aggressive person need not shout or harrass to convey aggression.

Each of these approaches has positive and negative aspects. People who are nonassertive get what they want from relationships by sheer luck, because successful, intimate relationships are dependent on people being open and honestly communicating. A person who is unable to be assertive about her likes and dislikes will probably not be able to develop or maintain a genuinely intimate relationship. In addition to interfering with intimacy, nonassertiveness often leads to feelings of resentment. Nonassertiveness is a passive resistance to the strivings of one's inner nature, and this resistance will take its toll, now or in the future. The only positive aspect of this approach seems to be that, unless they are passive-aggressive, most nonassertive people are viewed in positive ways by persons they relate to casually. They do not rock the boat or alter the status quo.

Aggression, or dealing with problems by attacking the other person, has rather obvious drawbacks. Often aggressive people get what they want from life; however, the cost is high. Although their rights are seldom violated, they have as much difficulty building rewarding, intimate relationships as nonasserters. Most acquaintances have little respect and little liking for aggressive people.

Assertive people run the risk of being resented by some people, especially nonasserters who are passive-aggressive. They also, however, are able to attempt to get what they want from relationships and from life. They have the capacity to solve problems and to therefore build meaningful relationships. Asserters are respected by most acquaintances. They are seldom taken advantage of and probably feel good about themselves most of the time. They do, however, disturb some people by upsetting the status quo. They may be called aggressive, and they do not always get what they want.

Before talking about increasing assertiveness, it is important to note that there are two kinds of nonasserters. Situational nonasserters usually are able to stand up for themselves and appropriately express their thoughts and feelings, but they have a few weak spots. These weaknesses include inability to give positive or negative feedback to spouses, friends, neighbors, employers, sales persons, repair persons, etc. Most people have weak spots. General nonasserters seldom stand up for themselves. They are the people who can never say no, who are shabbily treated and taken advantage of. These people often have complicating emotional problems and need professional help in order to be more assertive and realistically self-oriented.

A person who identifies herself as a situational nonasserter and wants to make a change can do so. One way of doing this is by becoming more aware of nonassertive behavior and the frequency with which it occurs. The next step is choosing an area of nonassertive behavior and setting up a hierarchy of behaviors leading to the assertive behavior desired. The goal would be owning the assertive behavior and putting it into practice. To do this, a person starts with a behavior that is very easy and gradually increases the difficulty of the behavior to be practiced. The important fact is that a person takes small steps at a time in order to ensure success. Experiencing success is the best motivator for subsequent attempts.[17] For example, if a person is annoyed because a close friend never pays for coffee when they are on a break, that person might start the hierarchy with a base behavior of disagreeing with the friend in a general conversation. That would be a number 1 behavior. A number 4 behavior might involve disagreement on a sensitive issue, and a number 8 might include telling the friend something unpleasant about her daughter's behavior. A number 10 behavior would be the desired goal, telling the friend about feeling irritated when she does not pay for her coffee, and then going on to offer some means of rectifying the situation.

Once a hierarchy is set up, it helps to practice the difficult area with a friend, a mirror, a tape recorder, or preferably by role play. Many people who feel they are being assertive are in fact by tone of voice, gesture, or posture being either nonassertive or aggressive. It helps to elicit feedback.

It is important to remember that increasing assertiveness will be upsetting to some people, because they may not like the change and may call it aggressiveness. Some relationships may be shaken up, especially marital relationships. It often helps to talk with another person who may be affected by the change and let him/her know what is being done and thus to some extent decrease the threat. The positive aspects of increasing assertiveness are an increase in self-confidence, a decrease in anxiety, and an increased feeling of self-worth. Assertiveness training seminars can be quite helpful for persons who want to increase their assertiveness, and they are often available through local organizations such as the YWCA.

Changes do cost, and such changes can involve pain, giving up feelings of guilt, and taking many risks. For nursing to develop as a profession on its own right, it seems essential that nurses take the risk and elevate their self-images to recognize themselves as persons with a knowledge and expertise that is valuable and beneficial in giving direction to our evolving health care system.

The following prayer written by Shirley Smoyak summarizes best the intent and message of what is written here:[18]

A NURSE'S PSALM

Colleagueship is my guide; I shall not want.

This maketh me to demand equal pay for equal work.

To visualize a new day of equal exchanges; it comforth
my soul.

This guides me to see that the rights of one mean
obligations of another; I am ready.

Yea, though I walk through the valley of the shadow of
medical male domination, I will bear no long-lasting
grudges—

Retribution for past grievances is not my aim—

Only acknowledgment as a colleague in health care delivery.

Human capacity to do good gives me courage.

Many physicians are ready for the new day — in spite of
their training and prejudices.

They speak for sharing, for cooperation, for collaboration.

Hope springs eternal.

Only positive, respectful interaction and joint practice
will lay before me the rest of my life.

And I shall work, refreshed and renewed, for the common
good of all, till the end of my days.

Amen

NOTES

1. Shirley Smoyak, "The Changing Role of Nursing Today," *Occupational Health Nursing*, October 1974, p. 12.

2. Leonard Stein, "The Doctor-Nurse Game," *Archives of General Psychiatry* 16 (June 1967): 699-703.

3. Tricia Kushner, "The Nursing Profession: Condition Critical," *Ms.* 2, no. 2 (August 1973): 75.

4. Smoyak, "Changing Role," p. 13.

5. Sidney M. Jourard, *The Transparent Self* (Princeton, N.J.: D. Van Nostrand Co., 1964) pp. 99-108.

6. Abraham Maslow, *Toward a Psychology of Being* (New York: D. Van Nostrand Co., 1968), pp. 3-8.

7. Ibid., p. 8.

8. Don Hamachek, *Encounters with the Self* (New York: Holt, Rinehart and Winston, 1971), p. 236.

9. Ibid., p. 232.

10. E. Dyer, M. Monson, and J. Van Drimmelen, "What are the Relationships of Quality Patient Care to Nurses' Performance, Biographical and Personality Variables?" *Psychological Reports* 36, no. 1 (February 1975): 255-266.

11. Minnie Goodnow, *Nursing History* (Philadelphia: W. B. Saunders Co., 1942), p. 101.

12. Barbara Ehrenreich and Deirdre English, *Witches, Midwives and Nurses: A History of Women Healers* (Old Westbury, NY: Feminist Press at SUNY, 1973), pp. 25-32.

13. Anne W. Schaef, Lecture given at Unity Church, St. Paul, Minn., May 3, 1976.

14. Frederick Perls, *Gestalt Therapy: Verbatim* (Lafayette, Calif.: Real People Press, 1969), p. 48.

15. Center for Rational Living, 2130 Fairways Lane, St. Paul, Minn., 1974.

16. Ibid.

17. Ibid.

18. Smoyak, "Changing Role," p. 13.

4
Nursing's Future Role

MARY WEISENSEE

Human beings do have a genuine freedom to make choices.
Our destiny is not predetermined for us; we determine it
for ourselves.

Arnold Toynbee

What will the health care system consist of in 2025? Will we recognize any of the participants as we know them today, or will there be computers, robots, automats, and telecare? It has been forecast* that nurses will be phased out, physicians' roles will change dramatically and the majority will meet their demise, and pharmacists and physicians' assistants will become obsolete.[1] Forecasts such as these should stimulate one to consider some of the preferable alternatives for the future.

In this chapter some of the past values and practices of nursing and their influence in the present health care system are discussed. Alternatives for the role of nursing in the future are explored, and the following question is addressed: If nursing is to exist, will it be a profession or a technological handmaiden to medicine; will it be subsumed by other health care workers and by a better educated public? Also included is a discussion of how changed values and views of work and leisure in postindustrial society interact with education, technology, and health and how changed needs and associated stress factors influence the demands and roles of health care providers and recipients in the next 25 to 50 years.

THE PRESENT DILEMMA

Since members of the medical profession have exerted major control over nursing in education and practice, a discussion of nursing must include its relationship to medicine in the health-sickness care enterprise. The public has had to resort to expensive malpractice suits to give physicians the message that they are not infallible. Some physicians adhere to humane and altruistic principles, and some are control, power, money, and status hungry and regard patients as another number in the file and dollar signs in their accounts. Many physicians have been inculcated with the idea that they, having received a medical degree, are expert and responsible for everything and that they are the captain of every team with which they are associated. On the other hand, nurses are "instilled with fear of

---

*The terms "forecast" and "prediction" will be defined as used in futures literature. "Prediction" refers to something that *will* happen, whereas a "forecast" is a "probabilistic," reasonably definite statement about the future, based upon an evaluation of alternative possibilities.[2]

independent action"[3] in order to protect the fragile ego of the physician. Even though physicians have virtually no skills for running a team, they attempt to operate the health care train looking backward out of the caboose.

In the past, the status, integrity, and superior position of the physician have been held beyond question by the layperson. This has been changing with the increased numbers of malpractice cases and investigations into Medicare and Medicaid frauds. Nursing homes and hospitals have been vehicles for medical and pharmaceutical scandals, which have tarnished the image of other members of the health professions. Nursing has remained clear of these undesirable practices and scandals, possibly because nurses have not enjoyed the fee-for-service payment system and opportunities for becoming involved in these dishonest practices have therefore not been as available to this profession. The vices of nurses are apparent in other avenues, such as the alarmingly high numbers of license revocations that occur because of chemical abuse and the omissions and apathy manifested by lack of political sophistication and involvement.

BARRIERS TO THE ADVANCEMENT OF NURSING EDUCATION

The advancement of the status of nursing education, even though still chaotic and multifocused, has historically survived some monumental obstacles. Not only does nursing have the distinct disadvantage of being primarily a profession composed of females; physicians (predominantly male) have vigorously protested the education of nurses in the university setting.[4]

The influential Dr. Charles Mayo of the famous clinic was of the opinion that nurses spent too much time being educated and not enough alleviating the pain and suffering of humankind.[5] In 1906, the New York Academy of Medicine attacked the overeducation of nurses and even influenced some three-year schools to decrease their "training" to two years for a period of time.[6] The physicians were threatened because nurses were receiving almost as much education as the physicians of that era. One physician is recorded as being a proponent of the liberal education of nurses in the university setting. He was Dr. William Menninger in 1949.[7] This is an interesting contrast, as his specialty area was mental health. One wonders why physicians were not busy keeping their own house in order rather than interfering with another profession.

The collegiate school of nursing in a community often receives little support from the professional community and usually resistance from the physicians. The majority of staff nurses in the clinical practice agencies (hospitals) with the exception of community health are three-year diploma graduates from hospital programs who view graduates of baccalaureate programs as a threat. Therefore, many retaliate with sarcastic comments when the already anxious student makes a mistake or asks a naive question.

Physicians do not always look favorably upon baccalaureate students because they are taught to question and challenge anything that seems unclear or violates principles. Physicians are accustomed to the three-year diploma nurses who are

in awe of the status and prestige of the physician and are ready and willing to follow his* orders without question in accordance with the male-female (dominance-
submission) role playing that has been traditional until recently.

These situations can be detrimental to the students, faculty, and administrator
of the nursing school, especially when an irate physician uses his clout to influence
health and political decisions that favor the medical point of view rather than considering what is best for the patient's or client's total health care.

ANTI-INTELLECTUALISM AND
SUSPICION OF THEORY IN
COMMUNITY-PROFESSIONAL RELATIONS

Nursing administrators and educators have to work doubly hard at being accepted
in the professional community of practicing nurses. Practicing nurses often feel that
the faculty are far off and isolated in the ivory tower away from the "real" world,
dreaming up farfetched and unworkable theories instead of caring for patients and
clients, which is what really is important. They forget that students are people and
that they were once students.

The conflicting relationship between nursing education and nursing service exists
in almost every setting. Some of this conflict is an inherent, antitheoretical, anti-
conceptual trait which also exists in other areas of education and against the so-
called innovators. Even though university faculty members consider themselves
avant-garde in curriculum and many of their practices, there are those areas of
"vested interest" that are supremely resistant to change even though there is no
theoretical rationale for adhering to the traditional practice.

This anti-intellectualism is not unique to nursing, but this does not make the
problem any easier to deal with. In fact, it compounds it according to Theodore
Sizer, former dean of education at Harvard. Sizer discusses some of his dissatisfac-
tions with education and expounds on his disappointment with those who "prefer
to fiddle with things we understand and can manipulate."[8] This is frequently seen
as a method of procrastination, due to inability or fear of proceeding into the abstract and making a mistake or statement that others may question and/or criticize.
It is easier to deal with concrete data than to plan for an abstract and uncertain
future of nursing education. For example, Barritt stated that the dean's major task
was "crisis intervention."[9] Perhaps, if she and her faculty could plan ahead in a
more organized fashion, there would not be so many crises that required intervention. Many nurses somehow feel that dramatic, crisis intervention makes them more
worthy of their salary than quietly delineating a methodical scheme for proceeding
on a long-range scale and meeting crises day to day.

Sizer's comment that "we worship experience" certainly finds a corollary in
nursing and nursing education. Hospitals and schools of nursing advertise for those
who are "experienced." They must assume that quality is analogous with the num-

---

*In this chapter to save space "he/she" will not be used. He will be used to refer to
physicians and "she" to refer to nurses with the realization that these stereotypes are
changing.

ber of years of work. The status of experience is almost as absurd as the opposite: requiring only a certain degree to qualify for a position. This relates to Sizer's second frustration, that "education is more than schooling."[10] The individual differences, such as ability to conceptualize, set priorities, and solve problems, are some of those qualities that an administrator must make judgments about when interviewing a potential faculty member for her staff. It may not mean that, simply because an individual has had ten years of experience, she has learned and grown with this experience each year. It is possible that the individual has had one year of experience ten times.

Sizer's third frustration, "the relative inability of the education profession to connect the ideas of those working on curriculum matters with those involved with policy,"[11] was perfectly exemplified in a comment by a nursing director in her administrative frustrations of working with the faculty in current curriculum revision. She asked the faculty whether the revised curriculum would require any additional faculty positions. The faculty replied that they did not yet know. The administrator, however, had to know immediately in order to prepare the budget request for the next year. This is a recurrent dilemma and an example of the administrative-faculty schism due to the mutual lack of understanding of the pressures and expectations of each.

FACTORS CONTRIBUTING TO THE PRESENT CHAOS

Nursing, as a profession or occupational category, has had the distinct disadvantage of being a low-status female group. It has been plagued with the traditional, religious, and subservient dedication. Change has been almost as difficult as it would be to install a woman in the Pope's position.

The duties of nurses have to a great extent, especially in hospitals, come under the category of medically delegated tasks (carrying out physicians' orders). A good nurse was one who knew when to call the doctor. If she called him too early or too late she was a poor nurse, and she would be reprimanded. In this light, nursing became known as a "noncognitive occupation,"[12] leaving decision making to the physician. Since the American Medical Association has more power and influence than the American Nurses' Association, why would anything change this system?

The longevity of a staff nurse in a hospital position is rather short. This presents a great and expensive dilemma to the administration, and the cause is quite obvious. What intelligent, young female in this liberated age is going to find job satisfaction in being ordered (by a physician) to perform every action. Even shampooing a patient's hair, in many hospitals, must still be preceded by a physician's order. The traditional assumption is that the patients are the physician's, and nurses must abide by the orders. Other factors, such as shift rotation, low salaries, bureaucratic inertia, and a reward system that does not reinforce the values learned in school, also contribute to the short duration in a staff nurse position.

CONCEPTION OF THE ASSOCIATE
DEGREE NURSING PROGRAM

After World War II, there was an acute shortage of nurses. In her doctoral dissertation, Mildred Montag, in 1951, conceived the idea that, since there were two-year colleges, a nursing curriculum could also be planned to educate a nurse in a shorter period of time. This would quickly produce more nurses since the other programs took three years for a hospital diploma and four years for a baccalaureate. This plan was utilized on an experimental basis in several states and met with enormous success (according to Montag). The ADN programs mushroomed, just as did junior and community colleges. The original concept of the ADN program was a technical nurse preparation to fill the gap in hospital bedside nursing. The program was designed as a terminal type of education. The premises of Montag's ADN program[13] were the following:

1. Nursing functions can and should be differentiated into technical and professional categories. The technical program should be "unlimited in depth, but limited in scope."[14]

2. The educational preparation of technical and professional workers must be different. Technical nursing shares characteristics of other technical programs, and professional education belongs in the university.[15] The main difference is that nursing is dealing with people and the engineer deals with objects, and this basic assumption creates problems in splitting the patient to care for him/her.

3. If the functions are different, the two groups must be taught to work together. To accommodate this Montag suggested team nursing.[16] Ideally, the team would be comprised of persons of various skills and led by a professional nurse.

Problems

The ADNs soon grew weary of no advancement and were dissatisfied with being on a dead-end street. They began inquiring as to how they would enter the baccalaureate program for a degree that would allow them greater opportunities and advancement. Mildred Montag maintains that the ADN program was the only nursing curriculum that was deliberately planned,[17] although the plan did not provide for transfer or articulation from the two-year to the four-year college or university, nor did it indicate how they would influence the long-range future of nursing.

Uses and Abuses of the ADN

The ADN team has not functioned well, and according to Montag it is because of inadequate leadership.[18] In the author's experience, this may be partially true, but a leader cannot lead if the members will not follow or are not competent and reliable. This leads to another problem area: The ADN, who was not taught to lead the team, is often expected in the employment situation to function as the team leader. When assigned according to their educational preparation, ADNs are usually valuable and contributing members of the nursing staff. These graduates frequently have the misfortune of being placed by their employers in positions of leadership for which they were not prepared.

Much of this misuse of the ADN was attributed to the acute shortage of nurses, and the BSNs were not in adequate supply to always fill the positions that were intended for them. There was also mismanagement of the professional nurse in assigning her to pass medications only or to transcribe orders. This was especially prevalent prior to the use of the ward clerk to perform paper work and answer the telephone. There were other aspects of the situation: The BSN wanted to use her creativity and talent in more independent positions than in the bureaucracy of the hospital structure. She preferred to be employed in community health positions, which offered more independence and challenge. There, the BSN would be encouraged to think and utilize the knowledge she had learned in school rather than merely obey orders. In the hospital, the team leader was the "checker-upper" and coordinator. She checked on the ADN, LPN, and aide to be certain that all of the nursing care and diagnostic tests were adequately performed. She was responsible to so many bosses that to relate to and keep them informed and content was in itself a mammoth task. After conferring with the physician, the head nurse, supervisor, and all of the workers on the team, she barely had time to even meet the patients.

Another factor contributing to the inadequate number of BSNs in the hospital was the fact that the motivated were needed and encouraged to attend graduate school to become faculty and directors of nursing. They were also needed to further develop theory and engage in research.

In summary, there were several reasons for the "shortage" of nurses: inappropriate assignments (misuse), incompetent team members and leaders, changing motivation and goals, and need for advanced education.

Controversy and Lack of Acceptance of the ADN

Although nurses identified as technical nurses have existed for 25 years, the concept of technical nursing has never really been accepted. "Because so much emphasis has been placed on professionalism in nursing and because the term profession has been applied to nursing almost ever since the beginning of modern nursing, anything which seemed less than professional seemed to be a lowering of standards and status."[19] The ADNs have in many respects been viewed as second-class citizens in the nursing ranks or ignored altogether. This has caused them to either become bitter and calloused or seek a route to becoming a BSN. Their efforts to advance educationally have met with much resistance. Since the ADN program was originally intended to be a terminal program with no provision for transfer into upper-division courses at the university level, university faculties have responded as if they were being invaded by the enemy.

It may seem workable on paper to plan a terminal program, but it does not function so easily with the human element in the actual situation. Even when students are in the ADN programs, there is a certain stigma about being in a program that is categorized as terminal. This is an especially distasteful term in nursing, as the word "terminal" usually refers to a patient who is near death.

The lack of recognition of the ADN by the public is evidenced by the fact that many state laws do not even mention the technical nurse. The statutes refer to the registered nurse and then discuss the qualifications and duties of the professional nurse. Thus, a registered nurse is a nurse prepared at the associate degree, diploma, or baccalaureate level.

There is another problematic area, that of state board examinations. This plan of educating persons in two-, three-, and four-year programs and testing all of the graduates with the same examination is a ludicrous and incongruous practice. That they all be certified with the same credential seems demeaning to some and an unfair source of stress to lesser prepared persons. Why should a person who has two years of education and is to function at technical levels be expected to pass the same examination as a person who has four years of education and is to function as a professional? The high failure rate of the ADN on state board examinations is depressing psychologically and unsound both educationally and economically.

Confusion Regarding Roles

The ADN concept as it currently exists has outlived its usefulness. The program was created at a time when there was an acute shortage of RNs, and it met the need then and filled the gap. Now it is time to look at quality rather than quantity. The situation is analogous to the ice box and the Model T. They were good products and served a function at the time, but how marketable and useful are they today (except as additions to antique collections)?

Furthermore, team nursing has met with failure, and now hospitals are implementing primary nursing. This system again does not utilize the ADN as she was prepared, to function under the supervision of a professional nurse. The primary-nursing system is designed so that the professional nurse can practice holistic patient care and function independently. This means that she is responsible for the nursing care of her patients and is accountable for it. The ADN has not been educated for this role, and it is not fair to her or the patients to expect this professional level of performance.

Also, the bed-occupancy rate in hospitals is decreasing, and the large number of bedside nurses will not be needed in the future. Maxmen forecasts that, as soon as 1990, professional nurses will be even more widely used to deliver primary health care.[20] Finally, the cost of hospitalization is becoming almost prohibitive. The public is becoming more sophisticated, and they do not enter the hospital for the simple (noncomplex) types of care that the ADN was conceptualized and educated to perform.

CONTROL OF NURSES AND NURSING CARE

I share many of Kinlein's frustations of hospital nursing as I recall my experiences as a hospital staff nurse. The setting of my first position was a midwestern, 200-bed hospital in which the attitude of the nursing hierarchy was that giving direct patient care, except for "sterile" treatments, was nurse aides' work, and when an extra RN happened to be on duty or the census was low, the RNs could get caught up on "their work," such as taking inventory and counting bedpans and linen. This hardly seems possible, but in this modern age, it was an actual situation in the 1960s. Nurses passed medications, did the charting, carried the charts, and followed the physician when he made his rounds.

One example of a frustrating incident in which I was attempting to implement patient-centered care is as follows. I was caring for an 18-year-old girl who had knee surgery in the morning and whose leg was in a cast. I was on the 3:00 p.m. to 11:00 p.m. shift, and throughout the evening I had attempted to make her comfortable by implementing all of the nursing measures I had learned in nursing school, such as positioning, application of ice, massaging, exercise, and analgesics. Still, at about 10 p.m., she complained of pain in her leg and foot. I had decided that, since none of my measures had relieved the pain, the cast must be too tight and the physician must be notified to come to the hospital, as there were no residents or interns to bivalve the cast. Because of the bureaucratic red tape of the hospital, the staff RN on the 3:00 p.m. to 11:00 p.m. shift had to have the supervisor's permission to telephone a physician. I called the supervisor. She came, and I explained my assessment. She glanced at the girl's leg in a cursory fashion and stated that there was no need to call the physician. My better judgment would not let me sign off that evening without calling the physician, which I did. He immediately came and bivalved the cast. The patient's pain was relieved and so was mine. I received no verbal reprimand for the action, but I became aware of subtle repercussions several years later when I discovered that in my reference letter the director stated that my "technical skills were competent but [my] attitude was poor." How could an RN who had the patient's interest as top priority have an agreeable attitude toward an administration with such restrictive policies and practices that a nurse had to break the rules to provide safe patient care?

It is for such reasons that I left the hospital for further education, hoping that somehow I could influence changes in this archaic, patient-demeaning environment where there was no hope for change against the ingrained system of technical servitude of first keeping physicians contented and then the patients.

In the hospital, the nurse has very little control over nursing. She must submit to the unpredictable demands and schedules of physicians' rounds, physical and occupational therapy, and x-ray schedules, at any time, and then on weekends be ready, willing, and able to perform physical and occupational therapy and pharmacy duties that physicians and other health care workers hold on to so religiously during the convenient hours of 9:00 a.m. to 5:00 p.m. on Monday through Friday. Hospitals should either close or fully function on weekends and holidays and not expect the nurses to perform all of the health care functions of workers who want the day off. The charges to the patient do not decrease on Saturday, Sunday, and holidays; neither, therefore, should the quality of services.

Hans Mauksch contrasts the functioning of a hospital when a person enters for care and cure with a car entering a mechanic's garage.[21] He elaborates on the complexities of the situation thusly: "According to the principles of institutional processes—according to the laws of human organization—the hospital ought not to be able to function. In seeking an answer to the question as to why the hospital does function despite all the built in dilemmas, the effectiveness of the informal organization of the hospital in maintaining its processes becomes obvious."[22]

The plight of the patient in this structure is described and vivid situations of stress for patients and nurses are brought to mind as one reads the irksome experiences of Norman Cousins when he recalls his patient status in a hospital in which there was no coordination of activities with his specific needs in central focus so that he could obtain some much needed rest. After noting that the activities were performed at the convenience of the hospital staff he states, "I had the fast-growing conviction that a hospital is no place for a person who is seriously ill."[23] He further laments the poor nutrition, sanitation, and personal recognition. Therefore, in order to recuperate he transferred to a hotel, which at one-third the cost allowed him the rest he needed to recover.[24]

Other evidence of the deplorable and stressful conditions in hospitals and nursing homes was verified in a recent publication which received national press coverage. The probe by *Nursing 76* received an opinion of more than 38 percent of the nurse respondents stating that they would not want to be a patient in the institution where they were employed.[25] What does this sort of testimony convey about the changes that are so desperately needed in our sick, sickness care system? Kalisch and Kalisch comment: "Health care in the United States is currently in a drastic state of flux. Nurses are under attack from both above and below."[26] To their comment, I would add that the attacks are also from within, as illustrated by the above *Nursing 76* finding. As has been discussed, nurses are not isolated when the health care system is attacked, but nursing certainly has perpetuated many of the problems.

COPING WITH THE STRESS

For the nurse who cannot afford either economically or psychologically to take risks, the ultimate reality of the hospital employment is as follows, according to Friedson: "They must either learn to find satisfaction in such subordination or find some independent source of legitimacy. In the former case they remain part of the medically dominated hierarchy; . . . in the latter, . . . they assume a position outside though parallel to the medical hierarchy."[27] This happens to nurses at all levels of preparation as is discussed by a nurse prepared at the master's level who laments the varied range of non-nursing tasks that she performed when she was employed in an emergency-room situation. Her tasks kept her from giving psychological support to anxious patients and their families in this highly stressful setting. Her conclusion is a caveat to all of us: "If we're not careful we'll expand ourselves right out of a job."[28] It is apparent that nurses are forced to perform the tasks that are left over as well as the delegated medical tasks, and little or no time is left for the functions that are the essence of nursing and utilizing the education that they have obtained. It is not difficult to lose sight of the forest when pressures to perform are intense. Nurses are required to be pleasant and cooperative co-workers for day-to-day psychological survival as well as the realities of economic survival which can itself be threatened if an unfavorable reference would be written by a supervisor.

This submission happens not only to nurses in staff positions but also to directors of nursing service who seem to occupy a second place and succumb to the dictates of the medical director and chief of staff of the hospital or institution, especially when there is a situation in which a physician desires a change in some aspect of nursing intervention or policy.

The following phrase often comes to mind in relation to nurses: "We have met the enemy and they is us." It is disheartening to experience or read about the numerous situations and nasty games that nurses play on other nurses, especially when one is attempting to do something that is unique and innovative. In addition to the tales of woe and hurdles that Kinlein speaks of so vividly in her book, *Independent Nursing Practice with Clients*, nurses with information and medical records personnel attempt to exert control by withholding information.[29] There is another nurse who has been attempting to provide some nursing services in an "interdependent" manner, as Wong calls it. The restrictive policies issued to her by so-called nursing colleagues were seemingly quite discriminatory when she attempted to visit a patient in the hospital and discuss some of the problems with the family, even when the physician in charge of the patient asked Ms. Wong to come. She was even advised that she must receive permission from the hospital administration. It seems that a nursing service that cannot or will not stand up and support other nurses is not worthy of its position or status of being a profession. As Wong reiterates, "What further proof of nursing's second class, subservient status in the hospital hierarchy, dominated by medicine, is needed?"[30] Wong's experiences as related in her article seem typical of the barbaric types of behavior that one is confronted with when entering a hospital unit as a researcher or as one who supposedly has goals in common with other health care workers, that of assisting the patient and his/her family. The stresses that Wong has faced have been caused not only by physicians, public health agencies, and hospital administrators, but by the crass attitudes of nurses. She avows, "The root of the problem is not within other disciplines but within our own."[31]

The discrepancies between what is practiced and what is preached seem ironic, especially when one notes in an issue of *Nursing Outlook*[32] an advertisement for a hospital stating, "A good nurse is love made visible," after one has just read the insensitive reception and anything but love that Ms. Wong has received from nursing colleagues. What, then, will become of nursing, its intensity of stress, and its future role?

The only consolation for the plight of the innovator is that society has never been very kind to those who have benefited society with their inventions, changes, and creative thoughts. Pasteur, Simmelweis, Galileo, da Vinci, and numerous others had ideas that were ahead of society's values. They were therefore persecuted or killed, or their ideas were ignored until someone rediscovered them many years later when society "needed" them. In many respects, we have not advanced in our regard for our fellow human beings whether we consider ourselves workers in a profession, occupation, or vocation. Only when a discovery or invention assists in an immediate crisis do we accept and honor the innovative individual, as was the case with Salk, who provided us with polio vaccine and made polio a disease of the past.

CHANGES IN HEALTH CARE PRACTICES IN THE FUTURE—PHYSICIAN CONTROL VERSUS NURSE CONTROL

If a physician is overworked, he will probably welcome some assistance from a nurse practitioner or a physician's assistant, providing that he still believes he is in control. Lovett and Bashshue of the University of Michigan School of Public Health convey this attitude: "With increasing numbers of nonphysician manpower types involved in the delivery of care, the responsibility of the supervising physician for communication and control of the care has been heightened."[33] Whenever another health care worker is delivering services, the physician seems to be of the opinion that it is within the medical realm and that these people need to be under his supervision. Once physicians realize that there is such a thing as *health* care and that all care is not sickness or pathology oriented as is the focus in medical care, then the medical and nursing professions can communicate and function on a colleague basis—and the client can make a decision as to whether health care or sickness care is needed at a particular time.

Kinlein describes this disease approach as compared to her practice of nursing: "The use of the word 'positive' conveys health to the client; in medicine the use of the word 'positive' conveys illness. From the client's perspective, something that is positive is good for him, so a subtle change in viewpoint occurs, removing the impression that 'positive' findings have 'negative' implications for his health."[34] Attitudes are also exemplified in relation to this negative outlook in the physican-initiated *Problem Oriented Medical Records* approach in contrast to the nursing goals of promoting some positive outcome. Another attitudinal example of control of the physician is apparent in the term applied to the consumer of the physician's services.

The approach of medicine is disease focused, as the names allopathic and osteopathic imply, and the person served is the patient. The word "patient" denotes one who is sick, suffering, or "one that is acted upon."[35] Therefore, when health care is sought and given, the term "patient" is clearly inappropriate to describe the individual seeking services. That is analogous to calling a suspect of a crime a prisoner before trial and conviction of guilt. Semantics may seem a small thing, but semantics can certainly influence people's attitudes or goals they are striving for in their interactions. It seems that the word "patient" is appropriate only when a person is being acted upon, for example, when he/she is under general anesthesia during surgery, is unconscious, or has identified himself as sick and has sought the services of the physician but is not an active participant in his/her care.

Most of the time in which an individual is in a hospital, he/she is there to receive nursing care, not medical care. The physician may perform an hour of surgery and make a five-minute daily visit, but the majority of the intervention and reasons for hospitalization rather than being discharged is for nursing care. Ideally according to rehabilitation principles, nurses attempt to involve the individual in his/her care to promote independence after discharge rather than dependence.

The physician may willingly give up some control by delegating the routine and less desirable tasks to either of his new co-workers, the physician's assistant or the nurse practitioner. For a time they may be excited about the new role that challenges them, until they master the techniques and, in analyzing the situation, discover what has happened to them. In interpersonal relationships they will always be secondary or, when there is an opportunity for overlapping and competition, the physician will assume that he has first choice, opportunity, and control, and if the census is low the nurse practitioner and physician's assistant will be dismissed like any other salaried employee. Maxmen recognizes that this bizarre situation of unclear, overlapping duties will have to be overcome, "if rationality, cohesiveness, and coherence are to be brought to bear upon future health and delivery systems."[36]

Thomstad, Cunningham, and Kaplan discuss many of the conflicts and difficult decisions of a physician and nurse collaborating in a working relationship. The two members of this successful team are described by the sociologist as "atypical,"[37] and the situation is an excellent example of the stresses involved in compromising and working closely together for the best interests of the patients and clients rather than for self-interest. How many atypical persons of this caliber can we find to make needed changes? How can more be produced?

Changes in a society may be introduced by professionals, but unless there is a crisis or a definite need felt by the population for which the change is intended, the change will not "catch on" and will diffuse throughout the group and become the established norm. A change may be bitterly fought until it is forced upon a population group, and then they will take advantage of it in every way possible. For example, some physicians fought Medicare until they found that it could be lucrative for their business in that they could give minimal service and send enormous bills, which were paid by the government. Some incomes became so immense that they were investigated and the physicians were found to have billed for services never rendered.

Although Maxmen disagrees, it seems that an idea whose time has come is independent nursing practice such as that recently established by Kinlein. With a better educated public and with the technology available to store knowledge and assist in decision making, the nurse can function quite competently as a primary health care provider, adviser, and counselor, part of the role that Maxmen gives the future medic.[38] When there was illness, she/he would know whom to consult or which computer program to call upon for the required expertise. Maxmen's traditional medical education is apparent as are the inconsistencies in the responsibilities he proposes for medics and nurses: "Nevertheless, the fact is that some individual ultimately must be in charge of the patient's care. Although admittedly some nurses are more knowledgeable and resourceful than some physicians, for the most part the latter are better equipped to coordinate and to make critical decisions affecting a patient's treatment. Thus, for the nurse to practice independently of the physician is usually neither possible nor desirable."[39]

NURSING EDUCATION IN THE FUTURE— THE PARADOX OF TRADITION VERSUS INNOVATION

There is extreme pressure on all types of education from students and the public to prepare the individual for the appropriate roles for the future, but if education is too idealistic, innovative, or futuristic or deviates from the norms of the past it is ridiculed and accused of not being practical. Since educational institutions must convince public officials of their worth and their purposes for being funded, it is often difficult to be innovative and yet traditional enough to maintain the confidence of the legislators, administrators, and those who have a voice in the appropriation of finances to the universities.

There have been long and heated debates on the issue of diversity, uniqueness, and academic freedom versus the cost effectiveness and standardization of the product, the graduate of the program, be it nurse, physician, hospital administrator, or engineer. The author does not foresee any satisfactory universal resolution to this controversy. It will depend upon which side can obtain the most votes on election day.

Many changes may be desirable and technologically, sociologically, psychologically, and economically sound and reasonable, but if they are not politically advantageous to the policy makers, whose decisions are largely dictated by lobbyist pressures and reelection popularity potentials, the changes in legislation to facilitate changes will not occur, whether they be in health, energy, or transportation.

EXAMPLES OF RECOMMENDED REVISIONS FOR NURSING EDUCATION IN THE FUTURE

1. Of foremost importance is to include information and experiences so that nurses are politically informed and involved. The lack of political participation has been alluded to previously, but if nursing is to attain and maintain a voice in health or sickness care and not be superceded by Maxmen's "medic," physician's assistant, or some other health care worker, nurses must get into the political arena, where the decisions of survival of educational programs are made. Since politicians control the purse strings, and funding determines the survival or demise of a program, this would seem to be the key to survival of nursing in any professional form. It does not seem reasonable that the threatened medical profession will suddenly turn altruistic and vote for nursing to practice in any form except under its control. Nursing then would exist as a handmaiden and nurse the physician rather than their patients and clients. One could argue that independent practice would still be an option, but the author could foresee the AMA sponsoring legislation to prohibit nurses from practicing independently. If nurses are not acutely aware and involved, they will be forced into the control of the physician in all aspects of their functioning and of course would not qualify to be called professionals.

In addition to including courses and experiences in political involvement at the undergraduate level, the author suggests that nurses be encouraged to develop expertise in political science, economics, and law at the doctoral level as they have been in other areas such as anthropology, psychology, and physiology.

2. If nursing does not have a political voice, it will not survive. Assuming that nursing *will* survive and that there is a future to mold, the author believes that there should be courses which stimulate students to think futuristically, giving consideration to possible, probable, and desirable alternatives for both their personal and professional lives. There has been an overwhelmingly positive response to this type of course when offered by the author as an elective to undergraduates. For more advanced students, courses and experiences related to research and long-range planning techniques should be available. There are arguments by some in opposition that the techniques of futures research are not always right, so why bother? It would seem that they are certainly better than nothing, as is evidenced by the botched up system or "nonsystem" of health care that we are involved in now. Arnstein, of the National Center for Health Services Research, describes some of the

benefits of the holistic type of policy research called technology assessment: "A comprehensive assessment can narrow the usual vast range of uncertainty by distinguishing what is known from what is not known; what is true from what is verifiable; what is feared from what is welcomed, and what competing and sometimes conflicting perspectives need to be taken into account."[40]

We should think futuristically rather than allow ourselves to be preoccupied with reassessing the past and becoming paralyzed with the complexities of the present. We should "think the unthinkable" and set ourselves to creating a desirable future in education and service for the benefit of students and clients rather than for our own convenience. Faculties must revise their thinking to be prepared for students who are taking "future"-oriented courses in their secondary school.

3. Nursing students should be selected on the basis of the qualities that are desirable for the graduate of the program to possess. If they are empathy and creativity, then the student should be given an empathy and creativity test prior to admission to the program. This would be preferable to basing admission on criteria not directly relevant to the goal for the outcome of the profession. Perhaps identification of talents for processing information and adapting to uncertainties of the future are the desired skills for the nurse of the future rather than the past grade-point evaluation and desire usually summed up in the phrase which stated that "I've always wanted to help people."

When one reads Kinlein's and Wong's poignant examples of the inhumane and destructive behavior exhibited by nurses toward other nurses, one questions whether such nurses are victims of the "burnout" syndrome or whether they ever had any empathy. If nurses don't have empathy and show concern for their fellow nurses, how then can they be a recognized, powerful, unified, and politically influential profession?

Arguments against the use of the grade-point average for admission to school are supported by studies on records of college graduates with high academic achievement which have suggested that these graduates are less effective and less competent than students who had lower averages. According to Douglas Heath, psychology professor at Haverford College: "Thus a student's high-school average and aptitude scores may predict his freshman grades in college, but not much beyond that. Similarly, college grades and tests such as Graduate Record Examinations, which are used to forecast success in graduate school, generally are not considered reliable predictors of future professional accomplishment."[41]

4. Computer simulations of clinical experience will be an especially useful tool to decrease expenses of teaching and travel time in this energy-conservation era, and they will also spare patients and clients the trauma of the trial and error experiences of beginning students. Computer simulations will allow the experience of potential situations and will help students to determine whether they are in the type of specialty that is appropriate for their interests, goals, temperament, and abilities.

Computers have a potential use in almost every area of nursing education and in the practice of providing accurate and efficient care to the client. They are powerful tools in instruction, as described by Silva,[42] and in evaluation and research as well as numerous other areas, according to Meadows.[43] In practice computers have the potential of being as useful as antibiotics, the stethoscope, and x-ray techniques.[44] There are those who argue that technology promotes impersonal instruction or care. On this point the author agrees with Maxmen, who believes that computers can improve and personalize care to patients and clients[45] and that in certain tasks the computer is more accurate, efficient, and complete than the human being. After a person performs the same task repeatedly he becomes machine-like, bored, and inefficient, whereas the computer does not forget or become bored or tired.

5. Students need to learn decision making and priority setting in their personal lives that can be compatible with the needs and expectations of a career, recognizing that repeated learning and unlearning will be the trend to avoid obsolescence. They need to learn to base decisions on minimal crucial data since by the time all of the possible data can be collected and evaluated the decision will be useless and archaic. Drucker advises that we obtain results by utilizing opportunities rather than by merely solving problems.[46]

Liberal education of the professional is of vital importance for the future. Donald Michael, a social psychologist and futurist, suggests that, with the increasing number of variables that one must consider other than cause and effect possibilites, a broader outlook is imperative for long-range planning. He further recommends the following: "With regard to the education of the feelings, the self, the emotional: we must educate for empathy, compassion, trust, nonexploitiveness, nonmanipulativeness, for self-growth and self-esteem, for tolerance of ambiguity, for acknowledgement of error, for patience, for suffering."[47]

6. Credit should be given for selected life experiences that will contribute to the competencies that should characterize a nurse. It has been demonstrated in several circumstances that informal life experiences are often more important than formal classroom experiences for which college credit is traditionally given. Provisions must be made for experimentation with nontraditional forms of education, such as one 3-hour class session rather than three 1-hour sessions and use of technology, as mentioned previously.

7. Education must decrease the stress of transition from student role to practitioner role with a more future-focused curriculum and experiences. Students should not be filled with ideas and ideals that are outmoded for the career of a student who will be practicing in the next 25 years rather than the last 25.

8. The concept of baccalaureate education should be reevaluated. As 1985 rapidly approaches and confusion is rampant in the field of nursing education, it is time to make some sense out of the nonsense whose existence has been so prolonged. Many excuses can be made for not moving to the baccalaureate degree as the initial entrance requirement to professional practice. But we must examine the true needs—separate the emotional from the intellectual and make some decisions about the future of nursing education. The cost-of-change factor always comes to the surface. Some educators as well as workers in nursing service think only in terms of dollars and cents. Others can see beyond this to the consequences of *not* changing the present chaotic system of short-range planning or no planning at all. The economic issue arose at the June 1976 American Nurses' Convention during a discussion of the high cost of paying for a staff with increased education. Luther Christman, dean of Nursing and Allied Health Services at Rush University, Chicago, stated that the most economical classification of RN with which to staff the

hospital is the nurse prepared at the master's level.[48] In relation to this indecision and costs, Nyquist commented: "It will be my thesis that this is a decade of decision for the nursing profession; that nursing and nursing education stand on a threshold of danger and that the present danger is, in part, the result of professional conservatism, indecision and disunity; widespread misunderstanding of the development of nursing as a profession and general abysmal ignorance of the economics of health care."[49]

The cost of change may be great, but what is the cost of not changing? The educators blame the people in nursing service and vice versa, but it would seem that the basic purpose of education is to prepare people to function in the future. Then developing a rational system and communicating it to the public (future students especially), so that they can make informed decisions, is vital.

In many situations the educators appear to be the most prominent barriers to change, yet paradoxically they teach it and talk about it frequently. According to Swanson:

> Since vested interests are very large in education, and since any significant educational development is a threat to some type of investment, the favorite type of attack is on conceptual or moral grounds.
>
> Each new educational development or emphasis finds a few educators scurrying to their cognitive, affective, or psychomotor roots of thought and planning.[50]

Fagin examines the chaos of nursing education from recommendations of studies 30 years ago to the present predicament: "It is clear that nursing's so-called solution to the problem has heightened, rather than lessened, the profession's disunification." The confusion within the profession has been conveyed to the public, which tends to group nurses as "uninformed, unintelligent, undereducated, inarticulate, and other-directed workers."[51]

As a result of nursing's attempt to be all things to all people, professionals muddle through and don't do anything very well. McGriff states that society cannot afford to educate, nor is it necessary to have, all BSNs.[52] The author could not disagree more. In this country, what is valued *will* become reality. Going to the moon was expensive, too, but it was accomplished. The ideals that are valued can and will be accomplished when the profession unifies to operationalize a goal. If the profession begins to think positively rather than about what is wrong and cannot be done, great changes can be made in upgrading nursing education. For too long nursing has operated with the anonymous author's "Seven steps to Stagnation" as quoted from Braden and Herban:[53]

1. We're not ready for that
2. We've never done it that way
3. We're doing all right without it
4. We tried it once before
5. It costs too much
6. That's not our responsibility
7. It just won't work.

In the author's opinion, the nursing profession should apply some of its teachings about change to the present professional dilemma. It seems clear that, if nursing is going to remain a viable and useful profession, it must move to the baccalaureate degree as a minimum level of education for entrance into the profession. The rationale for this is as follows: (1) expanding body of knowledge, (2) necessity of liberal education for a professional, (3) opportunity to function on a collegial basis with other professionals, (4) necessity of maintaining nursing's self-esteem as a profession, and (5) opportunity to be of greater service to society.

The preceding is not intended to be an exhaustive discussion, but only to give some suggestions for changes in preparation for the future.

PROFESSIONAL AND SOCIAL INFLUENCES ON NURSING

The author certainly sees nursing's future role as stressful to all of the members of the profession (if it is a profession; this will be discussed later). From the viewpoint of both the innovators who want to make things happen and the status quo keepers who cannot cope with the rapid pace of change and adhere to the nostalgia of the "good old days" (that never really were), there are and will be additional issues to be resolved. There are and will be changes regarding education and roles, and there will be grappling with who we are as nurses and what we should do in 25 years as compared with what we are doing at the present: either fitting into or changing the system. Does nursing have a future role in health care delivery? If so what will it be? Will the society of the twenty-first century live in a disease-free world and need only health teaching in order to prevent maladies. This health teaching could be provided in the public schools at kindergarten through twelfth-grade levels.

Today many of the common diseases are preventable, such as those associated with human compulsions and their complicating sequelae, for example, overeating (obesity), heavy smoking (emphysema and lung cancer), and various forms of legal and illegal consumption of alcohol and drugs (chemical dependency). These diseases do not have to exist in most instances because the knowledge and technology are available to prevent them if individuals would take responsibility for their own health. But that is not the way many human beings function. They ignore warnings and deny the facts in the hope that they will not be affected. Even if individuals possess the correct knowledge, it does not follow that they will apply it, be they professionals or laymen. As one notes the extensive numbers of physicians, nurses, and other health care workers who smoke, are obese, and use chemicals indiscriminately, one wonders how much credibility health professionals have with the public since they do not always practice what they preach and provide good role models in health care practices.

The reactions of some professionals to high stress levels are described by psychologist Christina Maslach as the "burnout" syndrome, which contributes to an individual's emotional and physical ailments and professional inadequacy:

> There is little doubt that burnout plays a major role in the poor delivery
> of health and welfare services to people in need of them. They wait longer

to receive less attention and less care. It is also a key factor in low worker morale, absenteeism and high job turnover (for a common response to burnout is to quit and get out).

Further we found that burnout correlates with other damaging indices of human stress, such as alcoholism, mental illness, marital conflict and suicide.[54]

This raises serious questions as to how health professions can keep their own bodies and minds healthy in order to assist the public in coping with their stresses and distresses. Sometimes they act as if the rapid pace of stress and change is a phenomenon of this decade, but past literature indicates that this is not so. It is interesting to note the comments to a 1913 class of graduating nurses in which Hotvedt emphasizes: "One of the main characteristics of our present and, let me say, American life, is its overwhelming intensity. This peculiar high pressure is evident on every side. It has a great practical bearing which merits careful study."[55]

Is nursing a profession or is it a group of occupations? Freidson suggests that nursing is a paramedical occupation which takes orders from physicians and that nurses, therefore, cannot expect to be equals of physicians.[56] The issue of the criterion of autonomy does cause much stress and heated discussion in the health care arena, especially nursing. Nursing meets some of the qualifications of a profession in that it has some concocted abstractions that it calls theory and has the educational status of a baccalaureate degree in a university setting.

Nursing can and does maintain some control in its own regulation, more so of licensure and presently of the mandatory continuing education of graduates than of the numerous levels of basic educational preparation. For example, after over a quarter century of discussion about phasing out three-year hospital schools of nursing, some are still holding onto every last thread of existence and pretending that the 1965 position paper was never written. What does this convey about the ability of the profession to exert its own control? Or is nursing not really a profession, and should it stop pretending that it is a profession to make the situation more palatable?

Who determines the image, functions and status of a profession or an occupational group? In the literature that discusses professions, nursing is not mentioned as one of the professions; it may be referred to as a semiprofession or quasi-profession, but that is as near to profession as the author has noted in literature.[57] Goode excludes nursing because he feels its training is no more than a "lower level medical education."[58]

Schumacher's view of inflation is another example of an author's image of nursing: "Garbage collectors, airline pilots, coal miners, oil exporting countries, power station maintenance men, even nurses, railwaymen, postmen, teachers, in various places at various times have discovered that they can successfully insist on much higher incomes than society or the so-called market mechanism had hitherto granted them"[59] The word "even" implies that one would not expect nurses to demand a reasonable salary along with other salaried workers in our society. This would seem to relate to the political naivete of nurses, which has been identified and discussed in excellent articles by such authors as Kalisch and Kalisch,[60] Mullane,[61] and most recently by Hott.[62] Even though the problems and concerns have been identified, political participation by nurses must increase beyond the present handful who are informed and active. This aspect must be emphasized more in future curricula and is elaborated on in another section of this chapter.

If nursing is to survive as a viable helping profession, it must first help itself through a peaceful settlement as to the role and purposes it desires to achieve rather than through an attempt to be all things to all people and doing a haphazard job at all of them. If the energy that was spent on in-fighting over trivial matters could be eliminated, there would be time and energy for accomplishing the bigger and better things that are waiting to be done. The situation is so chaotic that students, the public, counselors, and even other health professions do not know how to help a potential student to assess the merits of each program and the goals and potential benefits of it. Meanwhile the credibility of the professional or occupational groups ascribing to the title of nurse is declining. There must be unification of the goals of the group of nurses if it is to attain and maintain professional status with some concrete goals and directions, or the divide and conquer tactics that have predominated thus far will witness the demise of nursing to the medic or physician's assistant.

CAN TRULY PROFESSIONAL NURSING BE PRACTICED IN THE HOSPITAL OF TODAY?

Because of the hierarchy of the hospital, in which the physician issues orders for the nurse to carry out for his patient, it is doubtful whether professional nursing can be practiced in the hospital setting as it exists in the majority of situations today. Nurses can practice with some new titles and focus on professional aspects to make the situation more palatable, but at present nurses are secondary, subservient, and dependent on the physician's orders for most actions. It is the desire of the hospital bureaucracy to entice physicians to admit patients to their particular hospital because that is the hospital's means of livelihood and existence. Every empty bed is a loss of money to the organization, and therefore hospital administrations will not assist in initiating any changes in policies or procedures that will give nurses more autonomy or decision-making power—nurses are only one group of the many salaried employees of the organization and do not constitute a source of revenues as do the physicians, who admit patients. We can change the name "nurse" to "primary nurse," but how much autonomy will they *really* have?

EXAMPLES OF SOME CHANGES NEEDED IN FUTURE NURSING PRACTICE

1. The licensure examinations must be appropriate to the program and the goals of the program. They are preferable to educating with an integrated program and testing with the medical model approach based on diploma program curricula.

We may say that we are a profession, but when it comes to credential and licensure time with the state board examination, the test is still based upon the traditional diploma program orientation. Is it not rather incongruous to educate with an integrated curriculum and license according to tests based upon the medical model of obstetrics, pediatrics, psychiatry, medicine, and surgery?

It seems that examination and licensure should be more closely related to the type of position one occupies. If a nurse is employed in a public health agency in an inner-city area, certainly the needs of the clients and competencies of the nurse would be much different than if she were employed in a coronary care unit in a large teaching-research hospital. Having passed an examination "once upon a time" is not in step with the competencies needed today.

2. Education and the recency of experiences must be taken into consideration. With the rapid pace of change and information explosion, continual reeducation and reexamination must be instituted and related to the type of employment. If a nurse is employed in community health it does not seem to be the best use of her time if she attends classes on techniques and procedures not relevant to the client in the home and community. Mandatory continuing education, which has been legislated in several states, is a step in the right direction, but merely being physically present in a class or seminar does not insure assimilation of the content.

3. The nursing department in each agency should take education and experience into consideration for each position and administer an examination (both written and practical), whether it be for initial employment or for promotion or transfer within the agency or institution. This is *not* to be confused with institutional licensure, because this would be controlled by nurses for nurses and give better assurance of competence to the public. This might assist in the elimination of those nurses who would not want to become patients in their own institutions as was referred to previously.[63] It is hoped that this would decrease the prevalent and deplorable evidence of the "Peter Principle" that we observe commonly operating. One example frequently observed is the most competent staff nurse being promoted to head nurse, a position for which she may not be best suited. If the opportunity were given to express interest in and take competency examinations for the position, the individual could take courses or undergo experiences that would enable her to prepare adequately for the position.

Rather than each hospital setting up these assessment-type centers, perhaps several hospitals or agencies in a region could collaborate to use the services of one center or university with their individual competencies tested and taught. Thus the expense of duplication of many of the services could be eliminated for each agency. It is important to be aware of cost, especially since the costs of health-illness care are soaring and the quality of care does not seem to be increasing in proportion. If one pays for a Cadillac and receives a Volkswagen, she/he has a perfect right to complain. Would it not be more humane to be tested at an assessment center and learn the correct skills rather than muddle through at the expense and discomfort of a person who is under a great deal of stress in illness and hospitalization?

4. Reference letters may become passé with the rapid changes, and the assessment of an employer from a few years previous may be as useless as a birth certificate to prove that one is still alive.

5. The importance of nurses in giving the emotional support that physicians have been lax in providing will be given a greater emphasis and rewarded rather than the task and "doing" orientation, which has been a higher priority in many institutions.

6. The agency ombudsman role has been heralded as a valuable innovation in

many institutions. The author's opinion of the need and establishment of this role is based on the fact that nursing has not been performing its duties adequately and providing holistic care for the patients, clients, and families who are the recipients of services of the institution. The addition of this "checker-upper" person to the hierarchy is evidence of the gap in services of the nursing department. The author would eliminate this position and make it possible and rewarding for nurses to give holistic care.

SPECULATIONS ON CHANGES IN HEALTH CARE PERSONNEL AND TECHNOLOGY

What are some possible, probable, and desirable alternatives for the future role of nursing in health care? Speculation about an abstract, uncertain future is beyond the comprehension of many of those who dwell upon the concrete, crisis-oriented world. Many people are suspicious and reject any unusual forecasts which may change their comfortable role. Maxmen declares, "Our identities are threatened by living in a nation where the only constant is change and the only tradition is transience."[64] Many well-educated people will never advance beyond the creativity of their doctoral dissertation or beyond the achievement of their initial education. More and more they will find themselves obsolete in a very few years or that the position for which they were educated has been eliminated. A lifetime career from the initial preparation to retirement could become a phenomenon of the past.

Upon reflection, one can realize that the once "far out" science fiction of yester-year is the reality of today. This may help to bring credibility and consideration to many long-range forecasts. Initially, Maxman's *Post-Physician Era* may seem like science fiction, and the skeptics will say, "radical," "impossible," "it can't happen," "never," "not in my lifetime," etc. But who thought a century ago that there would be airplanes and spacecraft to the moon, that horse and buggy makers would become passé, that ice boxes and wash boards would become museum pieces, and that common pest houses would be outmoded along with tuberculosis sanitoriums, polio wards, and common deaths from diphtheria and pneumonia?

As one recalls the pattern over the century of physicians delegating many of their less desirable, less lucrative, and repetitious tasks to nurses and other health care workers, it seems that it could be a rather natural cycle of events if physicians, except possibly those who performed limited complex surgery, became extinct.

But what about the issue of control that physicians now have and have had over nurses and other health care workers? This sort of provocative and sensational forecast certainly opens numerous questions regarding responsibilities of other personnel, legal and economic perspectives, and the empire that physicians have been controlling.

The next natural question is, Who and what technology would perform the duties of the physician? What impact would this have, legally and economically, on hospitals, nurses, other health providers, and the state of health and illness of the clients and patients of the nation? How much money could be saved? For example, the cost of educating one medical student is $100,000.[65] "The myth of MD necessity"[66] might as well change as many other "unthinkables" have been shaken and changed. As Maxmen states, "We may be unable NOT to afford an automated medical care system."[67]

Another question is whether physicians will allow their demise to occur. Maxmen proposes that "they will not only permit but facilitate their own obsolescense."[68] This seems somewhat difficult for many to believe in view of physicians' past attitudes of control and omnipotence.

It is of interest to contrast the forecasts of the neurologist Stanley Lesse, who believes that medicine will become more health oriented and attuned to stress prevention.[69] Maxmen, on the other hand, comments that "doctors, with their extensive scientific training, would not seem to be eager to devote their major clinical efforts providing emotional comfort to patients"[70] and would be willing for the medic to assume this responsibility for the psychosocial aspects of patients and clients. Possibly Maxmen does not realize that nurses are already educated to quite capably assume this role.

Maxmen forecasts that computers will be able to store and retrieve the scientific information necessary to diagnose the illnesses that may still exist in 2025.[71]

The author projects that there will be many fewer illnesses and that such diseases as cancer will be cured and eliminated, just as smallpox, polio, and diphtheria have become rare. Spare-parts replacement surgery will be the most common, and former long hospitalizations will consist of only an overnight observation before the individual is released to his/her home for the remainder of the convalescent period, where she and his/her family can be taught to perform any care with the use of a computer and phonovision and the guidance of a nurse.

Each individual's health and illness records will be available on an international computer file. Each person will select a nurse for assistance in reviewing his/her health status each year. The computer-obtained history will be client initiated, and a health status report will be compiled by the computer with the data from other blood and specimen profiles.

Regarding the accuracy and completeness of computerized histories, Maxmen cites studies that have shown them to be more complete and accurate than those performed by a physician. Many patients and clients prefer them and state that they tell the truth more frequently to the computer than to the physician.[72] In many instances the computer can correlate information such as the heart rate and latency to questions and the tone of voice to detect illness that would be missed by the usual patient-physician interview.[73]

One immediate question most nurses will ask in reaction to the concept of the postphysician era is, Who will assume responsibility for the legality of ordering medications? How will nursing practice acts be revised to insure the legal means for another professional to order medications? Perhaps nursing and pharmacy will enter a new collaborative relationship. It seems only natural that the previously overeducated, underutilized pharmacists will, in the postphysician era, finally be in a situation to utilize the education of pharmacology and chemistry that they have acquired. It has always seemed so wasteful for a pharmacist with four or five years of education to count pills and copy labels from big boxes onto little boxes. The postphysician era would seem to be the arrival of a golden age of opportunity for both the nurse and the pharmacist. The author forecasts that most of the other responsibilities previously performed by the physician could be assumed, except surgery, possibly, by nurse practitioners, computers, and technicians, such as the physician's assistants, to perform technical tasks such as suturing minor lacerations and cast applications.

How appealing will these changes be to the AMA, ANA, pharmacists, hospitals, policy makers, and the general public? On a gradual, progressive basis, acceptance would be feasible and realistic. If the system were all changed tomorrow there would be some violent opposition. The AMA officials would suffer from apoplexy and the disbelief that anyone could contemplate the world surviving without them. And, of course, what would the medical school faculty find for a new role? Maxmen transforms them into researchers.[74] If nurses are politically astute enough to take advantage of forthcoming opportunities and not spend their time trying to define nursing and continually in-fighting, they will be able to assume control over their practice and arrive at a full professional status in the future.

AN OUTLOOK ON CHANGES IN
VALUES FOR WORK AND LEISURE

Staggering ranges of choices now confront us in the areas of both work and leisure, and the changes that will take place before the end of the century will alter our values phenomenally. Much of the science fiction of yesterday has already arrived, and we must learn to cope or "cop out."

In primitive societies the environment and technology changed very little between the birth and death of an individual, but now the changes are of such significance that there is increasing danger that one's education for an occupation will become obsolete by the time she/he is fully prepared to perform it.

Cooperative planning for education is a key to survival for the next 25 years and beyond. Burt Nanus, director of futures research at the University of Southern California, believes "one cannot successfully design a program of education without projecting the environment within which those being educated will have to function."[75] This suggests that educators at all levels must plan not only with educators, but with many key persons in society in order to prevent many "misfits" from graduating from any educational program. Values will have to be explored for the young to fit into the world as it changes, and older people will have to continually return to school in order to function effectively in this age of rapid change. What is fact today will be supplanted with new evidence and information tomorrow: therefore, persons of all ages will need to retool. This may lead to the disappearance of academic degrees because no one will ever complete an education. Many of our accepted traditions will be stored in mothballs or museums. The elderly will no longer be the source of wisdom and experience, because they will be obsolete if they do not continually unlearn and relearn. That is not to degrade the elderly for there will be ample opportunity for them to keep up, but age will no longer be synonymous with wisdom and experience, the qualities often required for promotion. It has been noted in some corporations that the age of business executives has been decreasing in the past decade, which corresponds to the trend of new ideas being valued rather than older age being more important for promotion.

Value changes are further discussed by Berger: "Though the Protestant Ethic is by no means in its grave, there is a clearly growing consensus (more apparent, of course, on the lower levels of the occupational ladder than on the higher) that the major satisfactions in life are to be sought through leisure, not work."[76]

The level of occupational importance (central life interest) for industrial workers was found to be 24 percent by Dubin,[77] and the central life interest of registered nurses as reported by Orzack was 79 percent,[78] which is an interesting contrast in that their work was the major life interest of these registered nurses. Since these data were collected in the 1950s it would be enlightening to know whether these trends are consistent or whether values of work and nonwork (leisure) are changing markedly.

Persons in professional groups receive more personal rewards and satisfaction from their interaction with clients than do industrial workers. The relationship with some peers and colleagues is different from that of the assembly-line workers, as explained by Edward Gross: "The major function of colleague groups is to prevent one from cracking up in face of significant failure."[79] This is certainly apparent to a member of the health professions when observing and experiencing the highly contrasting emotions that must be dealt with in day-to-day life and death situations. The value of each life and the consequences of action or inaction cannot be as easily measured as the number of pieces produced on the assembly line.

Strom suggests that the child's answer to "What do you want to be when you grow up?" is "I already am—and you should recognize me as a person whether I'm employed or not, whether I'm through with school or not."[80] Education is important from several perspectives: "In the sphere of education, Riesman argues that the schools will have to concern themselves increasingly with preparing the young for their future leisure life rather than for occupational roles, if education is to continue to be a meaningful experience."[81] Brightbill highlights the focus of education: "Leadership of the future begins today with those who educate tomorrow's leaders. Among the momentous tasks of higher education is that of designing an educational experience which will contribute effectively to the intelligent use of leisure."[82]

So frequently in the past we have heard and used the phrase "terminal education." This type of thinking must be discarded, because no one's education is ever terminated as long as he/she is living. Brightbill comments in regard to learning and knowledge: "Learning and education will continue to inform in order to develop thinking and knowledge. But more than ever, they will have to *inspire*. We will not benefit from tomorrow's opportunities by applying today's formulae for success."[83]

Many nontechnological or social value changes in our society have to be instituted when there is an opportunity created by a crisis; for example, changes in education were made following the student riots and sit-ins of the late 1960s. The attention now given to equality and antidiscrimination was fostered by racial unrest and the women's liberation movement. The legislation and attention given to mental health and improvement of conditions for the retarded were greatly influenced when politicians were in power whose families (such as the Kennedys and Humphreys) had been influenced by such tragedies. And recently we have experienced a phase of the energy crisis that has forced us to reexamine some of the values and traditional practices that we had accepted as fact for many years.

In regard to the role of education in preparing society for the future, Brightbill states: "When everything is carefully considered, when we trace civilization's patterns, we see that it has been education which has given us . . . leisure . . . The first purpose of education is to discover truth. Its second purpose is to leave a larger personality in its wake. Another purpose should be to enhance the well-being of all mankind."[84]

In the future of our postindustrial, service-oriented, knowledge-age, work society, leisure, education, and health care will assume new roles and values. Just as the once essential horse has been transferred to the arena of leisure and entertainment so will other accepted practices, beliefs, and products change. McLuhan believes that the arrival of more automation will make a liberal education mandatory[85] in order for humankind to use its intellect and imagination for the benefit of society rather than allowing these resources to be destructively channeled into violence and crime, which would erode and eradicate our society.

CONCLUSION

In conclusion, I refer to the epigraph. There are choices for nursing that are yet to be determined by the values of the profession and the values of society. It may be that this postindustrial age, or as some call it the knowledge age, will be followed by a health age, in which people will spend much of their nonwork time in pursuit of activities that are beneficial to their health, rather than an age of "overindulgence" such as we are experiencing now. With shorter working hours, society will quite naturally have to find some activity to occupy the hours. Possibly people will focus upon themselves in a somewhat narcissistic manner, spending more time and effort in health-promotion activities in which nurses will have an active teaching and counseling role. Although something seems farfetched now, one cannot say that it will never occur. We have seen numerous accomplishments in the past few decades which people of previous centuries would never have believed were remotely possible.

NOTES

1. Jerrold S. Maxman, *The Post-Physician Era* (New York: Wiley, 1976) pp. 274-282.

2. Roy Amara and Gerald R. Salineck, "Forecasting: From Conjectural Art toward Science," *Futurist* 6, no. 3 (June 1972): 112.

3. Leonard Stein, "The Doctor-Nurse Game," *American Journal of Nursing* 68, no. 1 (January 1968): 104.

4. Vern Bullough and Bonnie Bullough, *The Emergence of Modern Nursing*, 2nd ed. (New York: Macmillan Co., 1969), p. 170.

5. Ibid., p. 181.

6. Roy Bixler and G. Bixler, *Administration for Nursing Education* (New York: G. P. Putnams Sons, 1954), p. 143.

7. Charles H. Russell, *Liberal Education and Nursing* (New York: Columbia University, Teachers College Press, 1959), p. 36.

8. Theodore Sizer, "Three Major Frustrations," *Phi Delta Kappan* 53, No. 10 (June 1972): 634.

9. Evelyn Barritt, "The Art and Science of Being Dean," *Nursing Outlook* 22, no. 12 (December 1974): 750.

10. Sizer, "Major Frustrations," p. 634.

11. Ibid.

12. Bonnie Bullough, "You Can't Get There from Here: Articulation in Nursing Education," *Journal of Nursing Education* 11, no. 4 (November 1972): 7.

13. Mildred Montag, "The Associate Degree Nursing Program: Idea and Concept," in *Technical Nursing: Dimensions and Dynamics*, ed. Sandra Rasmussen (Philadelphia: F. A. Davis Co., 1972), p. 6.

14. Ibid.

15. Ibid., p. 7.

16. Ibid.

17. Ibid., p. 5.

18. Ibid., p. 7.

19. Ibid., p. 8.

20. Maxmen, *Post-Physician Era*, p. 277.

21. Hans O. Mauksch, "It Defies All Logic—But A Hospital Does Function," in *Social Interaction and Patient Care*, ed. James K. Skipper and Robert C. Leonard (Philadelphia: J. B. Lippincott, 1965), p. 250.

22. Ibid., p. 250.

23. Norman Cousins, "Anatomy of an Illness," *Saturday Review*, May 28, 1977, p. 4.

24. Ibid., p. 48.

25. G. Ray Funkhouser and *Nursing 76* Part I, "Probe—Quality of Care," *Nursing 76* 6, no. 12 (December 1976): 26.

26. Beatrice J. Kalish and Philip A. Kalisch, "A Discourse on the Politics of Nursing," *Journal of Nursing Administration* 6, no. 3 (March-April 1976): 32.

27. Eliot Freidson, *Profession of Medicine* (New York: Dodd Mead & Co., 1970), p. 67.

28. Marcia Andersen, "Our Expanding Role: Notes on Not Nursing," *Nursing 77* 7, no. 1 (January 1977): 16.

29. M. Lucille Kinlein, *Independent Nursing Practice with Clients* (New York: J. P. Lippincott, 1977), p. 107.

30. Donna L. Wong, "Private Practice—At A Price," *Nursing Outlook* 25, no. 4 (April 1977): 258.

31. Ibid., p. 259.

32. Advertisement for Houston's Methodist Hospital, *Nursing Outlook* 25, no. 4 (April 1977): 217.

33. Joseph Lovett and Rashid Bashohur, "Some Observations on Telemedicine and Its Assessment" (paper presented at the Second International Congress on Technology Assessment, Ann Arbor, Mich., October 26, 1976), p. 13.

34. Kinlein, *Independent Nursing Practice with Clients*, p. 80.

35. *Webster's New Collegiate Dictionary*, (S. V. "Patient.") (1974) p. 840.

36. Maxmen, *Post-Physician Era*, p. 154.

37. Beatrice Thomstad, Nicholas Cunningham, and Barbara H. Kaplan, "Changing the Rules of the Doctor-Nurse Game," *Nursing Outlook* 23, no. 7 (July 1975): 426.

38. Maxmen, *Post-Physician Era*, p. 38.

39. Ibid., pp. 152-153.

40. Sherry R. Arnstein, "Technology Assessment: Opportunities and Obstacles for Health Managers" (paper presented at the Second International Congress on Technology Assessment, Ann Arbor, Mich., October 26, 1976), p. 8.

41. Robert L. Jacobsen, "Does High Academic Achievement Create Problems Later On?" *The Chronicle of Higher Education* 14, no. 13 (May 23, 1977): 4.

42. Mary C. Silva, "Nursing Education in the Computer Age," *Nursing Outlook* 21, no. 2 (February 1973), p. 94.

43. Lynda S. Meadows, "Nursing Education in Crises: A Computer Alternative," *Journal of Nursing Education* 16, no. 5 (May 1977): 13-21.

44. Joseph Newman, ed., *The Computer (How It's Changing Our Lives)*, (U.S. News and World Report, Washington, D.C.: 1972), p. 20.

45. Maxmen, *Post-Physician Era*, p. 83.

46. Peter F. Drucker, *Managing for Results* (New York: Harper & Row, 1964), p. 5.

47. Donald N. Michael, *The Unprepared Society: Planning for a Precarious Future* (New York: Basic Books, 1968), p. 109.

48. Luther B. Christman, in comments at the American Nurses' Association Convention, Atlantic City, N. J., June 9, 1976.

49. E.B. Nyquist, "The Wisest Man Who Had Not the Gift of Foresight" (address given at the Annual Conference of Directors and Faculty Members of Nurse Preparing Programs in New York State, 1961).

50. Gordon I. Swanson, "Career Education: Barriers to Implementation," *American Vocational Journal* 47, no. 3 (March 1972): 81.

51. Claire Fagin, "Can We Bring Order Out of the Chaos in Nursing Education?" *American Journal of Nursing* 76, no. 1 (January 1976): 101.

52. Erline McGriff, "Two Nurses Debate the NYSNA 1985 Proposal," *American Journal of Nursing* 76, no. 6 (June 1976): 932.

53. Carrie Jo Braden and Nancy Herban, *Community Health: A System Approach* (New York: Appleton-Century-Crofts, 1976), p. 127.

54. Christina Maslach, "Burned-Out," *Human Behavior* 5, no. 9 (September 1976): 16.

55. I.M.J. Hotvedt, "Trained Nursing in the Light of Human Progress," *American Journal of Nursing* 14 (1913-14): 265.

56. Freidson, *Profession of Medicine,* p. 76.

57. Ibid., p. 78.

58. William J. Goode, "Encroachment, Charlatanism and the Emerging Profession: Psychology, Sociology and Medicine," *American Sociological Review* 25, no. 6 (1960): 902-914.

59. E.F. Schumacher, "Inflation: Schumacher's View on Why We Cannot Control It," *Futurist* 2, no. 2 (April 1977): 94.

60. Kalisch and Kalisch, "Politics of Nursing," pp. 29-34.

61. Mary Kelly Mullane, "Nursing Care and the Political Arena," *Nursing Outlook* 23, no. 11 (November 1975): 699-701.

62. Jacqueline R. Hott, "The Struggles Inside Nursing's Body Politic," *Nursing Forum* 15, no. 4 (1976): 325-340.

63. Funkhauser, "Probe—Quality of Care," Part I, p. 22.

64. Maxmen, *Post-Physician Era,* p. 94.

65. Ibid., p. 59.

66. Ibid., p. 48.

67. Ibid., p. 59.

68. Ibid., p. 73.

69. Stanley Lesse, "The Preventive Psychiatry of the Future," *Futurist,* 10, no. 5 (October 1976): 229.

70. Maxmen, *Post-Physician Era,* p. 77.

71. Ibid., p. 282.

72. Ibid., pp. 70-71.

73. Ibid., pp. 19-20.

74. Ibid., p. 38.

75. Burt Nanus, "The World of Work: 1980," *Futurist* 5, no. 6 (December 1971): 248.

76. Bennett M. Berger, "The Sociology of Leisure," in *Work and Leisure,* ed. Ervin O. Smigel (New Haven, Conn.: College and University Press, 1963), pp. 32-33.

77. Robert Dubin, "Industrial Workers' Worlds: A Study of Central Life Interests of Industrial Workers," in *Work and Leisure,* ed. E.O. Smigel (New Haven, Conn.: College and University Press, 1963), p. 41.

78. Louis H. Orzack, "Work as a Central Life Interest of Professionals," in *Work and Leisure,* ed. E.O. Smigel (New Haven, Conn.: College and University Press, 1963), p. 53.

79. Edward Gross, "A Functional Approach in Leisure Analysis," in *Work and Leisure,* ed. E.O. Smigel (New Haven, Conn.: College and University Press, 1963), p. 46.

80. Robert Strom, "Education for a Leisure Society," *Futurist* 9, no. 2 (April 1975): 93.

81. James F. Murphy, *Concepts of Leisure* (Englewood Cliffs, N.J.: Prentice-Hall, 1974), p. 35.

82. Charles K. Brightbill, *Educating for Leisure-Centered Living* (Harrisburg, Pa.: Stackpole Books, 1966), p. 148.

83. Ibid., p. 41.

84. Ibid., p. 39.

85. Marshall McLuhan, "Learning a Living," in *The Future of Work,* ed. Fred Best (Englewood Cliffs, N.J.: Prentice-Hall, 1973), p. 103.

Part II
Physical, Social, and Cultural Factors in the Manifestation of Stress

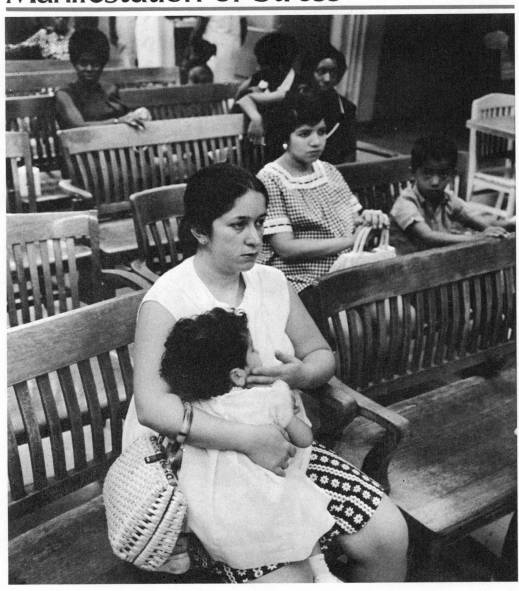

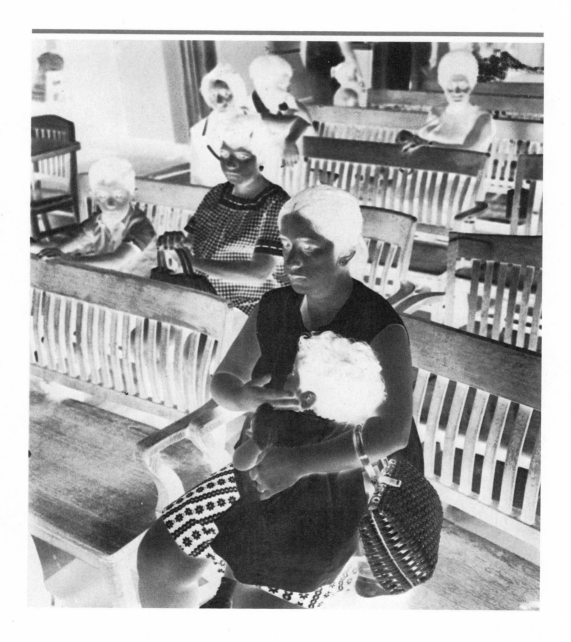

5
Male and Female Response to Stress

IDA M. MARTINSON
STEVEN ANDERSON

According to Hans Selye, a noted authority on stress, "Stress is the nonspecific response of the body to any demand made on it." "Nonspecific" is the key term in this definition and requires elucidation. In some respects, every demand made on our body is unique, that is, specific. Heat, cold, joy, sorrow, muscular exertion, drugs, and hormones each present a particular problem whose solution calls forth highly individualized responses. But all such agents have one thing in common: They bring an increased demand for readjustment, for performance of adaptive functions that reestablish normalcy. This heightened demand is nonspecific, that is, independent of the specific activity that caused the increased requirement. The essence of stress is the demand for activity as such.[1]

Partly through the work of Selye the general reaction to stress has become known as the general adaptation syndrome, which has three classic stages.

The immediate reaction to stress or anticipated stress is called the "alarm reaction." At this time, by some means that have not been determined yet, the hypothalamus is stimulated to release corticotropin-releasing factor (CRF), which is conducted to the anterior pituitary through the hypothalamic-hypophyseal portal vessels. The CRF causes the release of adrenocortiocotropic hormone (ACTH) from the pituitary, which travels through the bloodstream to the adrenal cortex. The ACTH causes the adrenal cortex to release corticoids, which cause thymus shrinkage, atrophy of lymph nodes, inhibition of inflammatory reactions, production of glucose in the liver, and gastrointestinal ulcers if the stress is continued. At the same time, the sympathetic nervous system is more active than usual, releasing norepinephrine from most of its nerve terminals, which causes what is commonly called the "fight or flight" reaction. This consists of dilation of the pupil, vasoconstriction in the nasal, lacrimal, parotid, submaxillary, gastric, and pancreatic glands, copious sweating, increased rate and force of heart beat, vasodilatation of coronary vessels, increased cardiac output and blood pressure, release of glucose from the liver, decreased output of kidney and gallbladder, vasoconstriction of systemic blood vessels in the abdomen and various areas of muscle and skin, with vasodilatation in active areas of muscle and skin, increased coagulation of blood and an increase in blood glucose concentration, increased basal metabolism including oxygen consumption, increased mental activity, and constriction of piloerector muscles. Sympathetic stimulation also causes a general release of epinephrine and norepinephrine from the adrenal medulla. This has the same effects as direct sympathetic stimulation on the various organs of the body except that the effects last about ten times as long since the adrenal medulla releases these substances directly into the bloodstream.

If the stress is continued, a stage of adaptation or resistance occurs. Since no organism can remain in a continuous state of alarm, if adaptation does not take place the organism will die during the alarm reaction within a few hours or days. In contrast to the alarm reaction, in which stores of corticoids in the adrenal cortex are depleted, during the adaptive phase stores of corticoids in the adrenal cortex are replenished. During the alarm phase hemoconcentration, hypochloremia, and tissue catabolism take place but, during the adaptive phase, hemodilution, hyperchloremia, and tissue anabolism are characteristic. The adaptive stage is not accompanied by any great amount of sympathetic stimulation.

If the stress is continued even further the acquired adaptation is eventually lost, and the organism enters the third and last stage of complete exhaustion and death, which may or may not be accompanied by increases in sympathetic nervous system activity.

The reaction to stress that takes place during the general adaptation syndrome can be divided into two basic categories, which help to maintain homeostasis.

Syntoxic reactions allow for tissue tranquilization and passive tolerance of the stress. Corticoids from the adrenal cortex are thought to act mostly in this manner, inhibiting inflammation and taking part in many defensive immune reactions.

On the other hand, a catatoxic response is meant to destroy or in some other way remove the stress, and this type of response is mediated by the sympathetic nervous system and the adrenal medulla, which act to increase blood pressure and pulse rate while putting the nervous system in a general state of alarm.

This general adaptation syndrome is characteristic of many organisms and of both sexes. The differences between sexes begin to appear when the degree to which a person can withstand stress or the types of changes within the environment that cause stress are examined. Information of this sort is not very complete and is often contradictory. Differences in response to stress on the basis of sex are given in Table 5.1.

Selye states at one point that sex hormones have little or nothing to do with the mechanism of stress[2] but states at another time that catatoxic reactions to stress can be mediated by natural steroid hormones of the testes.[3]

Various studies have been done which show that females are less likely to respond to emotionally arousing stimuli (stress) by release of epinephrine, and this appears to be true whether the situation requires a passive or an active response. The fact that males are more likely to respond to a stressful situation with increases in release of epinephrine is in agreement with data showing that males respond in a more aggressive manner than females to stress,[4] which is in part due to larger amounts of circulating androgens.

Gray and Buffery[5] have found evidence which they believe supports the hypothesis that there are two basic systems of emotional behavior involved in reactions to adverse stimuli. First, the "fight or flight" system seems to be an unconditioned response to adverse stimuli that is mediated by structures in the amygdala, stria terminalis, medial hypothalamus, and dorsal longitudinal bundle of Schutz. The second

TABLE 5.1 SEX DIFFERENCES

	Women	Men
Stress	↓ epinephrine	↑ epinephrine
	↑ behavioral inhibition	↓ behavioral inhibition
Normal conditions	↑ circulating estrogens	↑ circulating androgens
	↑ circulating high-density lipoprotein	↓ circulating high-density lipoprotein
Exercise	↓ physical working capacity	↑ physical working capacity
	↓ lung capacity	↑ hemoglobin capacity
	↓ blood volume	↑ energy expenditure (aerobic)

system mediates passive avoidance behavior in response to stress and is controlled by structures in the frontal cortex, medial septal area, and hippocampus.

Contemporary methods of measuring emotional behavior have shown that women are more prone than men to phobias, reactive depression, neuroticism, introversion, and susceptibility to anxiety. There is some evidence that these types of behavior are due to a more highly reactive behavioral inhibition system involving an integrated activity of the latter areas mentioned above. Whether these types of behavior are learned or hormonally mediated is still a controversial issue.

Emotional stress increases coronary disease, ulcers, hypertension, hyperthyroidism, dysmenorrhea, and colitis,[6] and since the percentage of deaths from vascular and hypertensive diseases is greater for men than for women[7] there would seem to be a connection between response to stress, vascular and hypertension problems, and sex.

Transient increases in blood pressure are well correlated with exposure to situations in which the outcome is uncertain. High blood pressure is also correlated with a vigilant attitude, and it has been hypothesized that hypertensive patients are more characteristically "on guard" than are other kinds of patients.[8] Increases in adrenal medullary secretion in response to uncertain outcomes of situations would cause these types of attitudes and would be provoked much more readily in men than in women.

The level of circulating estrogen can also be a factor in the lower incidence of vascular and hypertensive diseases in women. Macrophages of the reticuloendothelial system (RES) play a role in the removal of lipids from the vascular system, and tonic stimulation of the RES by estrogen can facilitate lipid removal from the vascular system. Altered vascular smooth muscle with increases in elastin, collagen, and mucopolysaccharides found in areas of atherosclerotic lesions can be decreased by increases in circulating estrogen levels.[9] It has also been shown that women have greater amounts of circulating high-density lipoprotein, which seems to remove cholesterol from the vascular system, in contrast to men, who have greater amounts of low-density lipoprotein, which carries cholesterol into the arterial wall.[10]

The fact that men are more easily stimulated to increase blood levels of catecholamines may predispose men to the special problems associated with stress ulcers.

Corticosteroids are thought to be permissive rather than causative in relation to ulcerogenesis, but catecholamines including epinephrine have a profound effect on decreasing gastric blood flow. Although a causal relationship has not been proved, it has been frequently observed that erosive gastritis takes place in areas of mucosal ischemia, and it has been postulated that cyclic activation of sympathetic (catecholamine) and parasympathetic inputs to the digestive system, concurrent with stress and nonstress situations, may allow the mucosa to be in an ischemic state after acid secretion.[11]

Histamine has long been a prominent suspect in the search for the major biochemical culprit in ulcerogenesis,[12] and this becomes especially important when considering that catecholamines serve as a releasing factor for histamines, which in turn stimulate acid secretion.

Whether the higher incidence of vascular and hypertensive diseases along with stress ulcers is a result of the differences between the sexes in reaction to stress or more an indication of different amounts of stress in the environments of the two sexes or some combination of the two has not been sufficiently researched to give a conclusive answer.

The differences between males and females in response to physical stress have been researched to a greater degree than other areas of the stress syndrome, and therefore the differences between men and women under physical stress have been well delineated.

"It is well known that physical working capacity is less for females than for males."[13] This ability of men to expend a greater amount of physical energy is mostly due to a more adequate system for supplying oxygen to the skeletal musculature under stress.

When a subject's maximum oxygen intake has been reached, energy must then be delivered anaerobically, leading to increases in blood lactate, which is the by-product of anaerobic energy production. The body tries to fulfill its need for energy aerobically, but at high stress levels the amount of energy released through anaerobic reactions increases more and more. This higher acidity contributes to better utilization of blood oxygen due to the fact that lower pH facilitates dissociation of oxygen from hemoglobin, thereby releasing relatively greater amounts of oxygen under high-acidity conditions. As physical stress is continued still further, lactic acid concentration in the blood increases to a level beyond the limits of the blood bicarbonate buffering capacity, at which point blood pH begins to drop drastically and a state of exhaustion is reached.

Males are also able to expend more energy because more energy is derived from a given amount of foodstuff under aerobic than under anaerobic conditions. Oxidation of 1 mole of glucose yields 38 moles of ATP, which is the energy source of the cell while anaerobic metabolism of 1 mole of glucose yields only 2 moles of ATP.[14]

Lactic acid concentration is the primary determinant of performance capacity, and the concentration of lactic acid that can be tolerated before complete exhaustion ensues varies with age and training. Males and females attain approximately the same maximum values of lactic acid concentration, which shows that women can strain themselves to the same state of physical exhaustion as men, but they are less likely to push themselves to complete exhaustion, possibly for psychological reasons.

If subjects of both sexes are tested at a given work intensity, heart rate, lactic acid concentration, and ventilation, females attain higher values than do males.

The main difference between male and females causing differences in ability to provide oxygen to active tissues is in hemoglobin concentration. Hemoglobin concentration is significantly correlated with speed of movement, strength, and ability to sustain prolonged muscular effort.[15] On the average, adult females have 32 percent lower total body hemoglobin than men, which amounts to a 10 percent lower concentration of hemoglobin in the blood of women as compared to that of men. A lower hemoglobin concentration is in accordance with the fact that females have a maximum oxygen concentration that is 10 percent lower than that of males and that oxygen capacity is 12 percent lower for women than for men after 16 years of age.

Total, vital, and residual lung capacities are 26 percent lower on the average for women than for men, but these differences are probably a result of differences in body size and do not affect differences in providing oxygen to active tissues.

Difference in blood volume is another parameter affecting delivery of oxygen to the tissues. Mean blood volume is 20 percent less for women than for men, and since a large quantity of blood is necessary to attain a high minute volume pumped from the heart, which also enhances provision of oxygen to the tissues, men have a relative advantage in this respect also. At high levels of stress adult males have slightly lower heart rates than women, which is in part due to a larger stroke volume for men than for women.

Maximum oxygen consumption for males increases roughly linearly with increases in body weight, but above a weight of about 48 kg (105.6 lb) females have a relatively lower maximum oxygen consumption, which is reflected in the differences in hemoglobin concentration since maximum oxygen consumption per unit of total hemoglobin is the same for males and females.

In both males and females, it has been noted for some time that a behavioral syndrome is associated with adrenocortical dysfunction. Although noted clinically at an early date, it was not until the early 1930s and 1940s that real attention was directed toward exploring the relationship between behavior and the adrenal function. This area remained important during the 1950s and gradually became even more significant as it became increasingly apparent that regulation of adrenocortical function rests, in part, in the brain.

Although much attention has been directed toward clinical instances of alteration of adrenal function and behavior, e.g., cyclothymic patients, psychiatric cases, electroencephalogram tracing abnormalities, convulsiveness, and fear, much of this work has been reproduced and extended in animal studies.

Recent findings indicate that the mechanism connecting psychosocial conditions and adrenal function is so complex that a complete understanding of it will be achieved only when the workings of the brain are more fully elucidated. Presently there is much evidence that steroids (adrenocortical as well as reproductive) and brain biogenic amines are involved in the mechanism. Input to the mechanism may originate either centrally (limbic), peripherally, or from a combination of the two, with the resulting effects often depending on the previous state of the organism.

Fortunately, each time an individual, whether male or female, is exposed to a stressor, there is a tendency to learn the nature and degree of activity required to resolve the situation, and one develops greater facility for handling the demands with which one is faced. For instance, muscles develop greater capacity by usage, and the antibody system becomes more efficient in a crisis when there has been previous exposure to the same or a similar microorganism. In addition, an individual's ability to cope with multiple stressors simultaneously is developed by frequent but mild situations in which one is bombarded by several stimuli at once. An individual, whether male or female, becomes less vulnerable to the stressor or similar stressors and is less apt to exceed the limits of the steady state when adjustments are called for. Consequently, intensification of the stress state can be a positive factor in the process of living.

Male and female response to stress is a complex phenomenon, and there is much left to learn. It is an area worthy of nursing research.

NOTES

1. Hans Selye, "Implications of the Stress Concept," *New York State Journal of Medicine* October 1975, pp. 2139-2145.

2. Hans Selye, *The Stress of Life* (New York: McGraw-Hill Book Co., 1976).

3. Hans Selye, "Forty Years of Stress Research: Principal Remaining Problems and Misconceptions," *Canadian Medical Association Journal* 115, no. 1 (July 1976): 53-56.

4. J.A. Gray, "Sex Differences in Emotional Behavior in Mammals Including Man: Endocrine Bases." *Acta Psychologica* 35 (1971): 29-46.

5. J.A. Gray and A.W.H. Buffery, "Sex Differences in Emotional and Cognitive Behavior in Mammals Including Man: Adaptive and Neural Bases," *Acta Psychologica* 35 (1971): 89-111.

6. H.B. Webb, "Emotional Factors and Heart Disease," Letter to the Editor, *Journal of the American Medical Association* 235, no. 19 (May 1976): 2081.

7. J. Stamler et al., "Socioeconomic Factors in the Epidemiology of Hypertensive Diseases," in *The Epidemiology of Hypertension,* ed. J. Stamler et al., (New York: Grune & Stratton, 1967), pp. 289-313.

8. A.M. Ostfeld and R.B. Shekelle, "Psychological Variables and Blood Pressures," in *The Epidemiology of Hypertension,* ed. J. Stamler et al. (New York: Grune & Stratton, 1967), pp. 321-331.

9. B.M. Altura, "Importance of Sex and Estrogens in Amelioration of Lethal Circulatory Stress Reactions: Relationship to Microcirculatory and Reticuloendothelial System Function," *Advances in Experimental Medicine and Biology* 67 (1976): 289-312.

10. A. Leon, Personal communication, Department of Physiological Hygiene, Minneapolis, University of Minnesota, 1977.

11. F.G. Moody et al., "Stress and the Acute Gastric Mucosal Lesion," *American Journal of Digestive Diseases* no. 1 (February 1976): 148-154.

12. Ibid.

13. P.-O. Åstrand and E. Munksgaard, *Experimental Studies of Physical Working Capacity in Relation to Sex and Age* (Copenhagen: 1952).

14. L.E. Morehouse and A.T. Miller, Jr., *Physiology of Exercise,* 4th ed. (Saint Louis: C. V. Mosby Co., 1963).

15. H. Cullumbine et al, "Influence of Age, Sex, Physique and Muscular Development on Physical Fitness," *Journal of Applied Physiology* 2 (1950): 488.

6
Female Sexuality

ROSEMARY HUERTER

There are few areas in women's lives where they have not been stressed. There are also few areas where women have been under more severe or sustained stress than the area of sexuality. Historically a woman's sexuality was bound up with her economic worth. A virgin was more desirable for marriage, not because of moral or religious scruples so much as the notion of the virgin as "undamaged goods."

These stresses may be related in part to the menstrual and childbearing functions of women. They may also be related to the supposed weakness of the female. Whatever the reasons, societies have maintained four characteristics related to sexual behavior control.

The first characteristic is some form of marriage. Marriage ensures several things. One is the continuation of the race. Although different cultures have held differing views of children being born to unmarried mothers, and sometimes this has been encouraged, the usual view is of some kind of family bond for the upbringing of the child. In addition to this there is the assurance of access to sexual partners; marriage takes certain people out of the arena of sexual competition and establishes kinship and the obligation of kinship.

A second characteristic of societies is the agreement that forced sex is prohibited in one's own group. It was permissible for conquering armies to rape the conquered, for masters to rape slaves, or simply for members of one tribe to rape women of another tribe. In some of the biblical stories that tell of revenge for rape, the rapist was of the same tribe as the woman. This characteristic has become less important in our present society. Statistics are increasingly revealing that women are being raped by people they know, at least people they know casually.

A third characteristic of sexual behavior control is the existence of taboos related to the eligibility of sexual partners. The incest taboo has been fairly universal throughout history. Some primitive tribes allowed marriage only within the group; others allowed marriage only outside the group. Today there are still religious groups that look with disfavor on any exogamous relationship, particularly in marriage. Only within the past decade has the idea of interracial marriage been considered tenable in most parts of the United States.

A final characteristic of control in the area of sexual behavior is the existence of some form of exception to most rules. Because it was recognized that inflexibility breeds trouble, there were always methods of circumventing the rules. Exceptions to the incest taboo in ancient Egypt are well known. This may have been for the sake of keeping wealth in the family, but it still represents an exception. In our society, divorce is one method of breaking the ties of kinship and its obligations. The time-honored custom of kissing under the mistletoe is a way of allowing more intimacy between men and women than they might otherwise enjoy.

Although all four characteristics supposedly apply to both men and women, there has been more pressure on women to conform than on men. The famous "double standard," which still regulates much of our sexual thought and ideals, is a perfect example of this. Men were encouraged to become sexually experienced, whereas women were expected to wait for marriage. A man who had many sexual partners was thought to be a great guy and was looked up to by his peers. A woman who had many sexual partners was considered "fast," "loose," or a whore. Although the women's movement has been instrumental in breaking down some of these barriers and prejudices, the conditioning that most women have received from parents and society will remain with them for a long time. The final equalizing of the sexes with regard to sexual expectations will come only through a concerted effort made by both men and women.

In the past women were generally told about their sexuality by men. They were taught to distrust their own feelings and ideas and to look to men for answers to their sexual problems. Even when women began to enter the professions that related to women's sexuality, e.g., medicine, anthropology, and sociology, women were trained by males, and often repeated what they were taught by these male teachers. Fortunately, this is changing. Women are beginning to say, "I know something too; in fact, when it comes to my body and my sexuality, I know more than any man could possibly know."

It is hoped that this chapter is an affirmation of this budding attitude and a reinforcement for women that they do indeed "know something too"!

WHAT DETERMINES A PERSON'S SEXUALITY?

How do women get to be women? Some parts of the answer to this are obvious; others are a little more subtle. There are six things that determine whether we are female or male: (1) the chromosomes we get from our parents, specifically the X or Y we get from our fathers; (2) the gonadal structure we develop in utero; (3) the hormonal activity and output of our bodies; (4) hormonal spurts at puberty; (5) sex assignment and rearing; and (6) how we feel about being female or male.

At the time of conception we receive the chromosomes from our parents. The mother contributes an X chromosome, whereas the father contributes either an X or a Y chromosome. If the father gives an X chromosome, the child will be a girl; if he gives a Y chromosome, the child will be a boy. For the first six weeks there is no further sexual differentiation. About six weeks after conception, if the chromosomal structure is an XY, the conceptus will begin to develop testosterone, and the sexual differentiation of a male will occur. If the chromosomal structure is an XX, no testosterone will be produced, and the gonadal structure of a female will develop. If the chromosomal structure is that of a male, but for some reason testosterone is not produced, the differentiation will not occur and gonadal female structures will continue to develop.

After the initial development of gonadal structures between the sixth and twelfth weeks there appears to be little or no additional sexual differentiation. This is regarded as one critical period in the development of the sexuality of a person.

The interrelationship of the six factors that make us either male or female is understood relatively well. Whether one is more causally dominant is not as well understood. There appears to be a considerable body of evidence that the lack of testosterone in a conceptus that is genetically male will result in the lack of gonadal development appropriate to a male. The tissue masses that eventually differentiate into clitoris/penis, ovaries/testes, and labia/scrotum are present in both female and male conceptus. Whether estrogen is necessary for female differentiation is not clear, but if there is no testosterone present the fetus will develop as a female, regardless of the chromosomal structure.[1]

At some point in early childhood, probably before the age of 2 years, further differentiation of female and male occurs. By the age of 2, children know whether they are "boy" or "girl." Their understanding of what this means is still undeveloped, and their sexual identity will continually be modified and added to. The first two years of extrauterine life will be crucial in the development of a sexual identity. Thus, the sex assignment, and rearing of the child in accordance with the sex assigned, will be of prime importance in these early years. Researchers who have dealt with gender-identity disorders have estimated that, when the genitalia are not clearly differentiated and the sex of the child is unclear, if a sex reassignment is to be made it should be done before the age of 18 months.[2] A child reared for two years as a boy and then declared a girl (or vice versa) will have not only his/her confusion to deal with, but that of parents and other family members. The earlier a sex reassignment is completed, the better is the chance that the child will adapt satisfactorily. This author, however, knows of a case in which a girl decided much later that she had always felt like a boy and underwent a sex change in late childhood. The change was made successfully. This is not to be confused with the changes undergone by a transsexual.

A final factor that determines whether we are female or male is how we ourselves feel about being the sex we are. Children who are loved and wanted as either the girl or boy that they are will probably grow up feeling comfortable with their sex. The parent who wants a girl and gets a boy, or vice versa, may be instrumental in making the child feel that there would be something inherently better in being the other sex. Something so fundamental and basic as our sexual selves, if not accepted by persons significant to us in our early childhood, will likely have serious repercussions in our adulthood life and practices.

PHYSIOLOGY OF SEXUAL STIMULATION

Basic to an understanding of sexuality and sexual functioning is an understanding of the sexual response cycle. Masters and Johnson in their research on the physiology of sexual stimulation identified four phases: excitement, plateau, orgasm, and resolution. Both females and males experience all four phases, but the patterns differ. Masters and Johnson also identified three patterns of orgasm for women and one pattern for men.[3] The four phases will be discussed briefly.

Excitement develops from any source of physical or psychic stimuli. If stimulation is adequate, the intensity increases rapidly.

Plateau is a consolidation period that follows the excitement phase if stimula- is continued. Sexual tension becomes intensified and reaches a level at which orgasm is experienced. Both the excitement and the plateau phases can be interrupted or terminated altogether by distracting stimuli.

Orgasm is the involuntary climax of sexual tension. It involves only a short period of time in the cycle, usually not more than a few seconds. It usually cannot be prolonged, although some women have a pattern of peaking and declining, with multiple orgasms occurring from one cycle of excitement and plateau. Once orgasm has begun there is no way to stop it. As mentioned previously, Masters and Johnson identified three patterns of orgasm for women. In the "minimal" type, the feelings are not very intense, the peak of the orgasm is low, and resolution requires a moderate amount of time, about 20 minutes. The second is a multiple type, in which the peak of feelings is higher than in the minimal type, and the peak repeats itself. Resolution is more prolonged than in the minimal type. The third type of orgasm is one in which there is a high intensity of feeling and a rapid resolution of these feelings.[4]

Resolution is the phase during which changes occur that restore the preexcitement status. Some women may be restimulated and again begin the excitement phase immediately. Males have a refractory period, however, and cannot be restimulated until the resolution phase has been completed. In general the resolution phase lasts as long as the excitement phase. Sexual tension dissipates slowly.

Sexual response is a total-body response and not just a reaction of the genitals. In fact, as the saying goes, "The brain is the primary sex organ." As yet no research has been done on the effects of the sexual cycle on the brain. Much research has been carried out on the effects of sexual stimulation on the rest of the body. The following chart gives some general idea of the physiologic changes that occur during each phase.

FEMALE	MALE
EXCITEMENT	**EXCITEMENT**
Genital	*Genital*
1. swelling of clitoral glans	1. rapid erection of penis (may come and go)
2. elongation of the clitoral shaft	
3. enlargement of the clitoral shaft	2. tensing and thickening of scrotal skin
4. vaginal lubrication	3. elevation of scrotal sac; testes elevated toward perineum
5. vaginal expansion, both length and width	4. shortening of spermatic cords
6. vaginal vasocongestion	
7. possibly uterine elevation	
8. changes in labia in effort to open vaginal introitus	

(Cont.)

FEMALE	MALE
EXCITEMENT	**EXCITEMENT**
Extragenital	*Extragenital*
1. nipple erection	1. nipple erection
2. increase in breast size	2. tensing of abdominal and inter-costal muscles
3. engorgement of areola	
4. "sex flush"—redness and rash over breast and epigastrium	
5. increase in heart rate and blood pressure	
PLATEAU	**PLATEAU**
Genital	*Genital*
1. retraction of clitoris against symphysis, under clitoral hood	1. increase in penile circumference at coronal ridge
2. vasocongestion of outer third of vagina and labia minora	2. deepening of color at corona
3. further increase in depth and width of vagina	3. increase in testicular size, some-times as much as 50%
4. full elevation of uterus	4. testes elevated closer to perineum (indicative of impending ejaculation)
5. vaginal tenting due to cervical rise	5. secretion from Cowper's gland; con-tains active spermatozoa
6. engorgement of labia majora	
7. color change in labia minora, from red to wine colored	
8. some secretion from Bartholin's gland	
Extragenital	*Extragenital*
1. continued nipple erection and turgidity	1. sometimes nipple erection and turgidity
2. sex flush possibly over whole body	2. sex flush, late in phase, occasionally
3. muscle contraction—facial, abdominal, intercostal (both voluntary and involuntary)	3. further voluntary and involuntary contractions
4. occasionally, voluntary rectal contractions to increase stimula-tion	4. hyperventilation late in phase; pulse rate increased to 100-175; blood pressure elevated, usually higher than in female
5. hyperventilation; pulse rate in-creased to 100-175; increased blood pressure	

(Cont.)

FEMALE	MALE
ORGASM *Genital* 1. cervical contractions, called orgasmic platform 2. contractions of uterus, starting at fundus and spreading downward	ORGASM *Genital* 1. expulsive contractions of entire length of penile urethra 2. contractions of secondary organs such as the vas deferens, epididymes, seminal vesicles, and prostate 3. closure of internal bladder sphincter
Extragenital 1. sex flush intensified 2. involuntary spasms and contractions of muscle groups 3. increase in respiratory rate 4. rapid heart beat, possibly an increase 5. high blood pressure, possibly an increase	*Extragenital* 1. sex flush in some men 2. occasionally "goose bumps"; spasms of various muscle groups, especially rectal sphincter 3. increase in respiratory and heart rate similar to female 4. blood pressure elevation more pronounced
RESOLUTION *Genital* 1. return of clitoris to normal position, 5-10 seconds after cervical contractions cease 2. return of other genital structures to normal in 10-30 minutes	RESOLUTION *Genital* 1. superimposition of refractory period (unable to restimulate to excitement) on resolution phase; may be as short as 10 minutes, but appears to definitely exist 2. rapid loss of vasocongestion of penis; detumescence to 1.5 times normal size
Extragenital 1. rapid loss of sex flush 2. slower return to normal of vital signs 3. some persistence of myotonia 4. widespread film of perspiration	*Extragenital* 1. return of vital signs to normal 2. occasionally sweating of palms of hands and soles of feet

FEMALE SEXUALITY AND MYTH

Some time ago the author presented a workshop to a group of professional nurses. One concern was to discover their knowledge level. As a preparation for this workshop, a list of myths about sexuality was developed. [To the author's surprise (and horror) it was relatively easy to gather a large number.] The result was a document entitled "The Ninety-Nine Most Cherished Myths in Sexuality." While many researchers have made inroads into the area of myth, there are still many misconceptions. Sometimes it seems that we dispel one myth only to have it replaced by another. An example of this is the outmoded Victorian idea that women do not enjoy sex, and submit to it only for the sake of having children. We replace that idea with the notion that all women must enjoy sex, have sex all the time, and furthermore have multiple orgasms, and we are no further ahead than we were 50 years ago. Some of the more prevalent myths attached to female sexuality are as follows:

☐ *Myth 1.* Women should satisfy men in sexual encounters, since women's needs are secondary to those of men. A slightly more current version of this is that each partner should be concerned with the sexual satisfaction of the other and that sexual pleasure is the responsibility of the partner.

Somehow this myth has survived a great deal of exploration. The original version implies that a woman's sexuality is just a cut below a man's. His feelings must be tended to; his needs must be met. If a woman's needs happen to be met and her feelings tended to, that is fine. But the man is the more important partner.

Sometimes the consequences of a woman violating the norm presented by this myth are serious. She may be accused of being unfeminine, selfish, and even castrating.

Lucy, married at the age of 20, believed the mores of her generation as taught by her mother. Her husband Bob was a professional man, educated and socially aware. Their marriage continued for nearly 15 years with both of them subscribing to the idea that sexual pleasure was primarily for the man and that Lucy's part in the marriage was to please Bob. When he had repeated extramarital affairs, Lucy blamed herself, saying, "I am not concerned enough about him. I do not satisfy him adequately." She never considered her own satisfaction, or the lack of it, nor did Bob ever give it any thought. In her quest to find an answer Lucy attended a seminar conducted by the author. During this seminar it was suggested that each partner in a relationship was entitled to some pleasure and consideration and that each was responsible for her or his own pleasure. A consequence of this was that each partner had a right to ask for certain things, and each had the right to refuse certain things that were not pleasurable for her or him. Most important, it was stressed that women were not responsible for their partner's pleasure or lack of it.

Lucy had never heard such ideas proposed before, but, the more she thought about them, the more they seemed to apply to her. She readily acknowledged that living by the ideals she had been taught had not resulted in happiness for herself. Nor had this life style resulted in happiness for her husband. She had always blamed herself for everything that was wrong in the marriage, particularly in the sexual area. Also, Bob had obliged her by blaming her. She decided to make some changes in her life. If Bob could be part of this change, she would be happy; if not, she would have to find some other way to work the situation out.

She began by telling Bob about the seminar and what it had meant to her. He agreed intellectually that it would be acceptable to make some changes. She initiated this by telling him during lovemaking the things he did that she liked. He responded with astonishment at first, then with anger. "After fifteen years are you telling me how to do it?" he demanded.

"No," she told him, "after fifteen years I'm telling you what things you do that I like."

Her next step was to ask him to continue a particular activity that she found pleasurable. He had frequently asked the same from her and had never thought that it was anything but the way it should be. Her change in this regard left him unsettled and wondering if he had been inadequate during the previous years of the marriage. He was unable to ask her directly about his adequacy, and her sensing of his need for verbal reassurance on this point did little to allay his worry. Finally, one night Lucy initiated sexual activity. Bob failed to achieve an erection, blamed Lucy for this, and then proceeded to tell her how wonderful she had always been and how she had changed. It took them many months to work this out, and there are still parts that are unresolved. Lucy has made it clear to Bob that she will no longer settle for his half-hearted attempts to satisfy her or for his assumption that their sexual activity is primarily for his pleasure. He is trying to change, but there are still times when both think they would do better to separate and start over with someone else.

Possibly the most positive outcome of this has been that, when Bob had another extramarital affair, Lucy was able to say that he was responsible for his own behavior, that if he was unhappy about something in their relationship she would be willing to work with him on it, but that she would not be blamed for his unfaithfulness.

The current version of the myth, that each partner should be concerned with the other and is responsible for the other, is more subtle and on the surface looks good. Yet in such a situation someone nearly always comes out second. Lovemaking is such an intensely personal experience that concentration on self is inevitable. If the partners adhere to the creed that each should concentrate on the other, the person with the better skills will be more successful. In general women have been taught to be more concerned about others, and men are socialized to be more self-concerned. It's not difficult to imagine who concentrates harder on the other person.

□ *Myth 2.* Women are slower to arouse sexually than men.

This is a very old myth. There are still books available that tell adolescent girls that boys will become sexually aroused while girls in the same situation will remain calm and cool. In fact, it will take a great deal of stimulation for girls to become aroused sexually. The same books indicate either directly or by implication that "holding the line" or "giving in" is the responsibility of the girl.

There are two things wrong with this myth. One is that the girl who is easily aroused is led to feel that she is unusual, perhaps abnormal. The second is that there are enormous variations in both men and women, and within the same person over a period of time. Some women, because of adverse experiences that they may have had, need hours to be aroused. Some men may have had experiences that have lead to impotence and cannot be aroused at all. Variation in the individual may be such that what is arousing one day may make little or no difference the next. Very few people, female or male, go through life with only one pattern of arousal.

Ellen and Fred had been married six months when they came to see the author about a "problem." According to both of them in separate assessment sessions, Ellen was swift to arouse, often climaxed before Fred, and seemed to be aroused sexually more frequently than Fred. When questioned, both said that Ellen never discontinued intercourse after orgasm but was happy to continue until Fred had climaxed. She enjoyed intercourse even after her climax and was never in any hurry for Fred to finish. When asked what they thought the real problem was, neither could identify it. Nonetheless, they had been having intercourse less and less frequently, and they were not as satisfied as they had been at the beginning of the marriage.

Further discussion sessions finally revealed that Fred believed a "real woman" should not be so easily aroused, that if she was easily aroused she should wait for the man to become aroused, and in fact hold back until he was ready. His reading, his locker-room buddies, and hints from his father had led him to believe that women could be satisfied sexually only if the man worked hard at it. There was something unusual, if not pathologic, about a woman who was so easily aroused as Ellen. When it became apparent to Fred that this was his expectation and he was able to understand that there are wide variations in both sexes, he and Ellen were able to work out the problem.

☐ *Myth 3.* Women who are raped ask for it, and secretly every woman wants to be raped.

Probably no one knows how such a myth came to be. The linking of sex and violence is not new to our generation or culture. Susan Brownmiller, in her book *Against Our Will: Men, Women and Rape*, has explored the history of rape thoroughly. She concludes that wars, pogroms, riots, and revolutions have always been an excuse for men to rape women. Although she further explores many cases of rape, there seems to be little evidence that women actually want to be raped.[5]

During a class the author taught on sex and the law, one student devised and carried out a project on rape. His major emphasis was on the treatment of the victim by the police and the experience from a legal point of view. He interviewed several rape victims and asked a variety of questions designed to assess the victim's perception of the experience.

The structure of the interviews was not geared to this myth, but two of the victims alluded to it. "No one asks to be raped," one woman stated. "I was minding my own business, coming home from work. It wasn't even dark, and the clothes I was wearing weren't seductive. I was just there. If I had been old, or ugly, or even crippled, he would have still raped me.

Another victim stated: "The sexual act itself was no big thing. It was nothing unusual. People always think it is something special and that all girls fantasize about being raped. It wasn't like that at all. The actual intercourse just made the whole thing more humiliating."[6]

This myth is all the more incredible since no one who is robbed or mugged is ever asked if they want to be robbed or mugged. Rape is the only crime in which the victim is under fire rather than the offender. Rape is basically not a sexual act but an act of violence. Most women do not want acts of violence committed against them.

☐ *Myth 4.* When people engage in lovemaking, men automatically know what to do and do not need directions from the partner.

This myth makes about as much sense as saying that people are born knowing how to walk. It can be easily observed that children learn how to walk only through trial and error, and usually with the help of some person or object.

There is no validity to the assertion that one person can know "instinctively" what another person likes or dislikes, still less that anyone can know what feels good to another. Living with this myth is often damaging and ends with one of the partners feeling put upon. If the man thinks he knows what the woman likes and acts accordingly, she may feel strange if she doesn't like it. After all, he is supposed to know these things. On the other hand, if the woman tells the man that he is doing something she doesn't like, he may feel that he has failed, since he is supposed to know. Some things feel good to one person and not to another. Some things feel good to a person at one point in life but not so good later. People are not known for their ability to read each other's minds with any degree of accuracy. Clear communication between partners about sexuality, sexual performance, and sexual likes is essential to a happy relationship.

Marian complained that Chad had no sensitivity to her sexual needs. He wanted to use "funny" positions and liked to manipulate her breasts during lovemaking, especially in the early stages of excitement. She found the positions tolerable but got almost no stimulation from breast manipulation and in fact usually found it distracting. The author asked her if she had ever mentioned this fact to Chad. "Of course not," was her reply. "He ought to be able to figure that out. I squirm enough. Besides, men ought to know."

Chad and Marian had been sexually active with each other for six months of their eight-month relationship. They discussed with the author other aspects of their relationship: where they went together, what kind of books each read, what kind of gifts were exchanged, if any, and what kind of food they ate. Marian liked Chinese; Chad preferred Italian. The ensuing conversation went something like this:

MARIAN: In fact, I fixed him a big meal of spaghetti and clam sauce just last night.

INTERVIEWER: And did he like that?

M: He loved it. It's his favorite meal.

I: How do you know it's his favorite meal?

M: He told me so.

I: You mean you didn't just know that?

M: Of course not. How would I know such a thing?

Marian seemed to hear her own words. Finally, a look of wonder and amusement crossed her face. "Is that what you were trying to tell me?" she asked. "We don't know what other people like unless they tell us?"

She started telling Chad what she liked and what was not pleasant to her. She also stopped trying to convey her message nonverbally through squirming. Their relationship and sexual experience have improved immensely.

□ *Myth 5.* Children, especially little girls, should not be told about sex. It just puts ideas into their heads.

Of all the myths pertaining to human and female sexuality the author believes that this one is the most dangerous and damaging. In classes and seminars women repeatedly tell of the pain and anguish they experienced as a result of not being prepared for menstrual periods and not knowing about male sexual development, penile erections, the sexual feelings that girls experience, or having babies. Children are constantly exposed to books, magazines, newspapers, and television. The amount of material in these media that is directly connected with sexuality is staggering. Children probably do not even need these stimuli to be curious about sex and interested in the subject.

At the age of 5, Mona crawled out on the roof and looked at her mother taking a bath. She asked, "Is that where I sucked as a baby?" Her mother was angry and told her to get down from the roof immediately. In relating this story some 40 years later, Mona was convinced that concern for her safety was less important to her mother than the question she had asked. The fact that her mother had never answered the question, had never discussed any aspect of sexuality with her, and still acts as though sex and sexuality do not exist has reinforced Mona's original feeling: Sex is bad; don't talk about it.

If children do not learn about sexuality from the media, they are likely to hear about it from their peers, and such information is not always accurate.

When Sharon was 10, she had a friend who was 12. The friend, Wilma, showed Sharon a sanitary napkin one day and tried to explain how it was used. "But why do they bother?" Sharon asked.

"Because they bleed," Wilma told her.

Sharon tried to think where the blood came from. She was aware that there were two openings but did not know about the vagina. Finally she asked, "Why do they bleed? Where does the blood come from?"

"Oh, they scratch themselves with their fingernails somehow. And then they bleed," was Wilma's knowing response.

Children are full of curiosity about all of their world, and the world of sexuality is no exception. Wynne still laughs when she remembers her young niece asking if Wynne could have a uterine transplant to enable her to have babies after a hysterectomy. If you can get a new heart, why not a new uterus?

Many parents believe that the sexual education of children is the prerogative of the schools, whereas the schools say that it is the responsibility of the parents. The ideal situation is neither but rather a cooperative plan whereby both parents and schools take the resonsibility of educating the child for this important aspect of life.

Even when there are attempts at education on the part of the schools, there may be serious gaps in the curriculum. A very small survey of sex education in junior and senior high schools was conducted by one of the students in the author's class. Obviously the sample was restricted and may not be representative of all schools in the area or country. Nonetheless, the student's findings may be significant, even with the restrictions in sample. The basic questions she wanted to research were: What are students taught in schools about sexuality and when are they taught it? What do students like about the suitability of the topic for their age? If a particular topic pertaining to sexuality is not included in the curriculum, do students think it should be?

The questionnaire was answered by 25 juniors and seniors in one high school. The topics included were menstruation, intercourse, conception, contraception, abortion, and masturbation.

All students in this sample thought that all the topics should be covered somewhere in the school sex education curriculum. However, less than 20 percent had received any information about abortion, and less than 10 percent had learned about masturbation from the school curriculum. All students in the sample had been given some explanation about the menstrual cycle and the resultant ability to conceive, but only about 50 percent had received any information about intercourse from the school curriculum. About 30 percent had been given information about contraceptives.

Where information had been given on any topic, the age varied from seventh grade (age 12 to 13 years) for menstruation to twelfth grade (age 17 to 18 years) for information about contraception. Considering that many girls begin their periods earlier than the age of 12 and that by the junior year in high school (eleventh grade) a considerable number of both males and females are sexually active, this would appear to be inadequate. Students need information about menses before the period starts, not a year later. By the time most students in this sample had received information from school programs, the need for the information as a preparation for an event was long past. The students recognized this and pointed it out to the investigator.[7]

The age of menarche has dropped in the past generation. Age 12 or 13 might have been early enough for parents or schools to begin discussion of menses 20 years ago. Today there is a likelihood that at least one girl in the 11-year age group will have started her periods. Once she has, there is little basis for the expectation that the other girls in her circle of friends will remain ignorant of the fact. Even if they did, what purpose would be served? If menstruation is a normal function, as people like to say it is, there are more reasonable ways to educate little girls about it. An ideal setting would be a household in which having menstrual periods is such a part of the routine that girls (and boys) would always know about them. Girls would then be prepared, and the onset of menses would not be a worry nor a shock to them.

☐ *Myth 6.* Women are not interested in sex following a hysterectomy or menopause.

For many women the opposite is true. Once the possibility of pregnancy is eliminated a woman can often be more relaxed and interested in sexual intercourse than she was previously. Part of the unspoken basis for this myth comes from the idea that women are sexual primarily in order to bear children, and, when they are no longer able to bear children, they are not interested (should not be interested) in sex.

Also, women have been led to believe that having a hysterectomy will automatically lead to a decreased hormonal output, and this in turn will cause a lessened sex drive. Although a total hysterectomy involving removal of ovaries, fallopian tubes, and uterus will result in loss of hormones, in many instances an estrogen replacement therapy can be used. Many hysterectomies are not total, and the hormonal level previous to surgery is maintained.

Menopause is the gradually decreasing functioning of the ovarian hormone and occurs simultaneously with other changes that are apt to begin at about the late forties and early fifties. The danger of this myth is that rather than each person being considered individually, an artificial norm is created and everyone is expected to conform to it. Such expectations create pressures on women to be something other than what they are and end by stifling women's self-expression and spontaneity.

When Polly first became aware that her periods were changing, she expected that her interest in sex would diminish. Her mother had never discussed the menopause with her, and she had no idea what to expect. The accompanying physical phenomena of menopause bothered her a great deal. She found that many nights she was unable to sleep. She was often irritable, and she found herself identifying with victims of tragedy, even though she did not know the people involved. Once, for example, she read a short news item about a Kansas family who had been left homeless by a tornado. Polly cried nearly half an hour over this newspaper article, although she did not know the Kansas family. Such behavior was completely foreign to her usual cheerfulness.

However, her interest in sex continued and, as she became aware that she had been released from the concerns about pregnancy that she had experienced earlier in her marriage, sexual activity and enjoyment increased. Her relationship with her husband was strengthened by this, and she was given support from him during those periods when she was unable to sleep or felt depressed over other people's troubles.

STRESSES PLACED ON FEMALE SEXUALITY

As mentioned earlier in this chapter, all societies have had ways of regulating sexual behavior. These regulations pertained to both men and women, but emphasis has often been on conformity by women, while men have had more freedom to violate these restrictions.

There are many who would argue that the double standard is dead, but it is alive and well in America. One has only to read "Dear Abby" and many other newspaper articles to see evidences of it. Not too long ago on the radio a news item began, "Today a 55-year-old grandmother was arrested for. . . . " No one ever states that a man who has been arrested is a grandfather. Infrequently his marital status is mentioned or possibly the number of children.

We are becoming more aware that female sexuality involves a great deal more than mere childbearing functions. Obviously we haven't discovered sex in our generation, but we may be in the process of rediscovering it. A study initiated in 1890 was recently published in *Psychology Today*.[8] This study indicated that not all Victorian women were repressed and hated sex. Nor did all of them have unwanted and unlimited hordes of children. Many women cited in the study used some form of birth control and apparently found it effective, since many of them had fewer children than women in similar circumstances in the early 1970s.

In this section, some of the specific problems women face in their sexual lives will be discussed.

One of the major stresses placed on a woman's sexuality is the attitude that sex is mostly for men. Women are still socialized to believe that men are "out for just one thing," and that, of course, is sex. Sex will not do a woman any good except to give her a reputation (usually bad) or a bunch of children. Neither of these things is very desirable.

Vicki's mother made frequent reference to the "bestiality" of men. Vicki determined never to have to submit to such demands, decided she would never marry, and further cut herself off from the necessity of relating to men sexually by entering a religious group. When she discovered that this way of life did not completely protect her either from her own feelings or from the advances of men, she became profoundly depressed. She left the religious group and then a year later rejoined it. She repeated this pattern of behavior once more and was finally advised that her destiny lay elsewhere. The last time the author saw her she was still fighting the attitudes her mother had instilled in her.

A second problem women encounter is that they are raised to be sexually dependent on men. They must learn all the "womanly skills" and then await the time when the prince will come and arouse the sleeping beauty within them. If he never comes, a woman often believes it was because she was not good enough. If he comes and she does not like something he does, she dare not rebel. After all, he might go elsewhere, to another woman, to divorce, or, worse yet, to playing poker with his buddies. Thus, women believe that they must endure much for the sake of having a man to satisfy their sexual needs. If the man does go somewhere else, whatever will a woman do?

One of women's needs is to become sexually autonomous. This may include developing the freedom to say no when they do not want sex; it may mean initiating specific sexual acts and relationships; or it may mean finding ways of satisfying their sexual needs through masturbation or other means. It certainly means getting to know themselves and their sexual needs and being able to say what these needs are.

In one of the author's classes a series of films on some means of sexual satisfaction other than intercourse was shown. After the film on masturbation, most of the women said that they did not engage in this activity. Some of them had at one time but had discontinued the practice when they had developed a sexual relationship with a man. One of them said, "Why should I bother to do that when I have a man to take care of me? I resent having to take care of myself." Yet when questioned whether they thought their partners masturbated, and if so what they thought about it, all of them said they assumed their partners masturbated at least occasionally, and it seemed acceptable to them.

Still another problem that faces women is that of guilt. Women more than men are still socialized to believe that sex is wrong. Lois, a woman now in her mid-forties, relates that, in her childhood she had such a strong feeling that sex was wrong, she believed it was sinful even in marriage. "I was raised a Catholic, and I really thought that after having sex my mother confessed before going to communion." Neither parent ever said this directly; it was simply an impression Lois had. She never thought her father confessed this.

Rarely do parents say directly that sex is wrong or bad. The nonverbal message gets through, however, and children are often confused by it. This is particularly true if there is a double message involved. If sex is beautiful, why don't parents want their children to know about it? On the other hand, if sex is dirty, why the constant admonition to save it for someone you love? These attitudes cannot fail to have effects on people for many years. Old conditioning comes back to haunt even those who consider themselves enlightened or liberated. Some of the best literature on the market about sexuality still refers to sexual jokes as "dirty."

Another problem is the attitude toward intercourse during the menstrual period. In the past many religions and cultures prohibited intercourse during menses. But why does the proscription remain? Men who do not have intercourse during their partner's period state that it is because menses is messy. This is a strange and interesting response; the implication seems to be that semen is not messy or—what is worse—if semen is messy that is just too bad.

When a woman is having a period she is often experiencing physiologic changes that are not particularly pleasant or reassuring. She may feel sluggish or bloated due to hormonal changes or concerned about odors that might be generated due to menses. If during these times a woman's outside resources fail her or reinforce her feeling of undesirability and questionable cleanliness (messiness), no wonder she becomes hard to live with.

Another problem women encounter is lack of information. In teaching classes in human sexuality, the author has observed that many women are still not adequately prepared for their first period, either by their mothers or through the schools. If there is no open communication between mother and daughter about menstruation, one can be sure that it is all downhill from there on. A mother who does not discuss menstruation with her daughter will not discuss male sexual development, wet dreams, necking, petting, intercourse, orgasm, conception, delivery, birth control, or masturbation. Daughters are forced to seek other avenues of information.

These other avenues may be satisfactory, but often they are not. Peer groups are usually the first source, and they are usually notoriously inadequate as far as facts are concerned.

Adulthood may not remedy this problem. In the book *Our Bodies, Ourselves,* many women tell of their experiences with doctors.[9] Presumably obstetricians and gynecologists are highly knowledgeable about female sexuality and female sexual functioning. After all, they deal with this every day of their professional lives. Yet this has not been the experience of many women. They have found that these doctors are cold, impersonal, sometimes ignorant of all but the most basic anatomic and physiologic facts, and often unsympathetic with the problems of their clients. The author's experience in counseling echoes this. Only in recent years has there been material on human and female sexuality incorporated into medical school curricula.

Other sources of information include school programs, reading, and experience. In recent years lectures, seminars, and workshops about sexuality have become widespread for professional groups and often for other groups as well. These can be a tremendous help to people but cannot meet everyone's needs.

At one workshop where the author conducted a small group, during an opening exercise each participant told a little about herself or himself and what each hoped to get from the experience. One man stated that he came mostly out of curiosity. He was a Canadian, and nothing of this sort was available in Canada. He wanted to know what went on at such a workshop. Whether he learned anything and whether he was disappointed we never learned. At the first break he disappeared and never returned.

Books can be of real benefit, but there are two problems in their use. One is accuracy of content. For a person well versed in the field of sexuality inaccuracies may be easy to spot. For the vast majority, however, glaring falsehoods may not be noticed. A second problem with books is the interpretation. For example, think of the many interpretations given to that very sexual book, the Bible. There are few ancient books that discuss sex as freely as this one, but centuries of interpretation and reinterpretation have now given it the reputation of being repressive of sex. One of the favorite passages of the antihomosexuals is from the Book of Genesis. Lot, visited by two angels, is beseiged by male inhabitants of Sodom. The implication seems clear that the natives of Sodom want the visitors in order to "abuse" them. Lot refuses and gives them instead his daughter (a virgin of course). No thought of pity ever seems to be given to the poor girl who could be subjected to gang rape at her father's whim. People use the story to "prove" that homosexuality is sinful. It might be just as easy to use the story as an example of hospitality. It seems probable that some 40 centuries later there is no complete certainty about what the story was initially intended to convey.

Women have another problem with their sexuality. They are often raised to believe some funny things about themselves. Two important examples of this are the attitudes they learn about erotic literature and about masturbation. These attitudes may be a result of the idea discussed earlier that sex is mostly for men. Pornography is supposedly a male preserve, for only men are sexually aroused by pictures of nude women. Nude men would be offensive to women, so the theory goes. Reading a book with erotic content would be of no use to a woman; such matters are only for men. Yet erotic literature can be helpful to both men and women, as far as arousal is concerned. Apart from the exploitative nature of pornography as in movies or "girlie" magazines (would magazines featuring pictures of nude males be called "boyie" magazines?), if it is arousing, it can be helpful. Erotic literature is sometimes a help in achieving orgasm also, by helping people concentrate on sexual matters and reducing distractions.

Masturbation is another area that remains a seemingly male prerogative. At puberty, if women are told about periods and conception, they are rarely ever told about the clitoris and its function in sexual pleasure. Since the penis is visible and boys learn early how good it feels to stroke and handle the penis, most males discover masturbation on their own, early in life. Most women, on the other hand, do not discover masturbation until much later, some not until they are well into adulthood. Unless they read about it, their discovery, too, is accidental. While most parents try to discourage both sexes from masturbating, the usual attitude is that "boys will be boys, but girls should not."

Karen told about an experience that occurred at the age of 4. Her mother was horrified to find her fingering her genitals in the bathtub. "I don't ever want you to do that again," she said. "Promise me you won't." Karen promised, not knowing for sure what she had been doing that was so terrible and not knowing what she was really promising. Twenty years later she was still confused.

All too often parents refer to masturbation as "that," as though the activity is so terrible that it cannot even be named. Many women are confused by the proscription, not knowing just what is so terrible about their genitals.

Adela was raised by strict parents and had little information about her sexuality. Although she had no remembrance of any prohibition against masturbation, she assumed it was placed on her at an early age. She never remembered masturbating as a child. She grew to adulthood repressed and unsure of herself and remained sexually inactive until well into her thirties. When she was 36 she had the opportunity to do some nude solitary swimming. After several weeks of this she discovered that whenever she swam by the inlet stream of the pool the quick rush of water was especially pleasant. She experimented with the water on various parts of her body, including her genitals, and had her first orgasm this way. She described the experience as overwhelming, and she began to cry. She had read enough to know intellectually what was happening to her, but nothing had prepared her for the emotional response she felt. Later when she was no longer able to use the pool she experimented with other forms of water, such as the hose, the shower, and the bathtub. She finds this to be her most intense orgasmic response.

Still another problem women have is to see their concerns as unique, as never having been experienced by another person. This comes in part from a mistrust of other women and a consequent inability for women to open up to each other. When Corrine was first asked to do a self sexual history in one of the author's classes, she went about it in a half-hearted way. After several days of fighting with herself she finally wrote as much as she dared. The idea of writing about her sexual self was very threatening. Even verbally sharing her sexual past or present feelings with others seemed incomprehensible to her. When she ventured to say this timidly in the group, she found her feelings echoed by most women there. Most of them had complied with the assignment because they were accustomed to having someone tell them to do an assignment, and they obeyed.

When women start to discuss their sexual past with other women, they frequently find a commonality not previously suspected. In one group, Denise said that there were a couple of things she was unable to talk about; in fact, she was unable to write them down. No one pressed her for any details or even hints about what these experiences were. Instead, those who felt comfortable started to talk about their experiences, and soon the rest joined in with, "Oh yes, that happened to me too." About halfway through the group session Denise interrupted another woman to say, "I can't believe this. Why did I ever think it was such a big deal? At least four of you have had the same experience I did." And she proceeded to tell the entire story to the group. For the first time in her life Denise was able to put her past sexual life and experience into the perspective of a common bond with other women.

A further difficulty with women's sexual experience is the tendency to see the problems as unique to women. Women do not see them in the context of human problems. Many times women are embarrassed about their bodies; they think that they have too much of one thing and not enough of another. But they seldom connect these feelings with the anxiety of the man who measures his penis every day or flexes his muscles before a mirror. Nor do they often see their concern about being preorgasmic or turned off by certain acts as being related to a man's frustration if he is too tired to have an erection or is not interested in cunnilingus. Nearly all sexual problems are human problems and are not specific to either sex.

What, then, can women do to alleviate some of these stressors on their sexuality? Women need to become comfortable with their sexuality. They need to know themselves as sexual persons and to value the sexual part of themselves as much as they would the ability to fly an airplane, dance gracefully, bake a lemon meringue pie, or sculpt a statue. Most of the foregoing discussion has pointed to the fact that women's socialization is not aimed at these goals. It is, in fact, aimed at preventing them from finding any large measure of comfort or value in their sexuality. However, there are some things that women can do.

The first step is to write your sexual history. Begin with childhood: What thoughts and ideas did you have about sex then, what attitudes and ideas did your parents convey to you, what kind of childhood sexual play did you engage in, who were your friends and what did they contribute to your concepts of sexuality? Try to remember what your mother told you in preparation for your menstrual periods and dating or any other talks you might have had with her. Move from there to your first experiences with dating, kissing, necking, petting, intercourse, and masturbation. Recall any same-sex experiences as well as opposite-sex encounters. Try to remember not only the experience but your feelings at the time. Bring yourself up to date with your sexual experiences: going steady, engagement, marriage, honeymoon, divorce, widowhood, remarriage—whatever is appropriate to your life circumstances. This exercise helps you see where you are now and gives you some insight into why you are at this particular place.

In writing her self sexual history, Donna realized that her unwillingness to become close to any woman was connected with her attendance at a slumber party some years before. Many of the girls were just entering adolescence and were aware that they would soon be dating and kissing boys. During the slumber party most of the girls practiced hugging and kissing each other in an attempt to see what it felt like to kiss another person romantically. Donna participated in this activity but felt so guilty about it that she soon withdrew from this group of friends and never developed any other friends among the girls at school. In exploring this experience she was able to acknowledge that her greatest fear was that she was a lesbian. She married when she was very young in an attempt to prove to herself that she was heterosexual. Once she learned how common the experience was she was able to relax and become friends with other women.

It is important to write the history rather than to just think about it. There is something salutary about seeing your own history written by your own hand. And once the basic history is complete additions can be made as recollections occur.

Remnants of the past shape the present attitudes and behavior of many of us. Many of the half-remembered bits of information, parental prohibitions, and repressions from other authority figures still affect us. We often do not take the time to look at these attitudes from the vantage point of adulthood. Consequently, we go through life with ideas and attitudes that are left over from our childhood. Only by examining these ideas are we able to determine which ones are appropriate in adult life and which need to be replaced by more mature concepts. Carrying this load of childhood ideas is a great waste of energy.

The second step is taking time to know yourself sexually. This may mean locking everybody out of your room for an hour a day while you get in touch with your body. It may mean experimenting with new positions or behaviors in lovemaking. It may mean masturbating with a new object or motion. It may mean just starting to masturbate. It may mean abstaining from intercourse for a time. We need to overcome the early conditioning to let everybody else come first and, if there's any time left over, then do something nice for ourselves. When we take care of ourselves, when we tell the world by our behavior that we are valuable and worth taking care of, others will respect this and take care of us too.

Jill's mother, Bette, made herself a slave to everyone else. If Bette needed something and one of the children wanted something, Bette would always go without. The result was an unhappy woman with selfish children and a pushy husband. "She was always giving up something for someone," Jill recalls. "As a result she never had any of the things she wanted. And she continually told us how much she had sacrificed for us. Now that we are all grown wouldn't you think we would repay her for all those 'sacrifices'?" None of the children ever visited her or took her a gift. Jill often forgot her mother's birthday and had not sent her a Mother's Day card for three years. The children never expected Bette to want anything and took her at her own evaluation, which was "I am not worth anything; I am not worthy of any consideration."

In the area of sexuality specifically, women need to learn to say no when they don't want sex and to initiate it when they do. It is all part of the pattern of taking care of themselves.

The third step is to actively work toward incorporating a degree of positive regard for your sexuality. If your past has been mainly negative toward your sexual self (and that is true of most women), the time to start changing this is yesterday. Read about the experiences of others, talk to other women, and, more than that, trust your own experience. If you feel unhappy or put off by a given situation or behavior, do not try to pretend that those feelings do not exist or that these feelings are wrong. They are your feelings, and you have a right to them. If you want to do something about the situation or feeling, do it—not because your next-door neighbor tells you that you must or because you read a book that said you should, but because you want to, and for no other reason. Every person has a right to a fulfilling, happy sexual life. But you will not have such a life by doing what comes naturally, in most cases. It has to be worked for, and the achievement is up to you.

NOTES

1. Nancy Fugate Woods, *Human Sexuality in Health and Illness* (St. Louis: C. V. Mosby Co., 1975), chap. 2.

2. John Money and Anke Arhardt, *Man and Woman, Boy and Girl* (Baltimore: Johns Hopkins Press, 1972), p. 13.

3. William Masters and Virginia Johnson, *Human Sexual Response* (Boston: Little, Brown & Co., 1966), chap. 1.

4. Ibid.

5. Susan Brownmiller, *Against Our Will: Men, Women and Rape* (New York: Simon and Schuster, 1975), chaps. 4, 5.

6. Scott Johnson, *Three Perspectives on Rape,* unpublished manuscript, 1976.

7. Gail Horner, *Sex Education in the School System,* unpublished clinical study, 1976.

8. Jody Gaylin, "Those Sexy Victorians," *Psychology Today,* December 1976, pp. 137-141.

9. Boston's Women's Health Book Collective, *Our Bodies, Ourselves* (New York: Simon and Schuster, 1975), p. 15.

7
Childbearing

Its Dilemmas*

SHARON SCHINDLER RISING

"Who controls a woman's body: Doctors? Lovers? Drugs? Women?" Thus reads the provocative cover of a recent addition to the growing library of books directed toward issues of women. This book, *Vaginal Politics*, seeks to raise women's consciousness about what is possible in health care, for it is only through consumer pressure that our illness-oriented medical care system will change its focus to that of health/wellness care, treating "patients" as people and not as conditions.[1]

Perhaps in no area of human need has there been such exploitation as in the needs of women regarding their femaleness: childbearing, abortion, contraception and sterilization, rape, and gynecologic problems necessitating surgery and causing disfigurement. Women have not had the benefit of even basic information on which to base crucial decisions about their own lives or, if such knowledge was present, have had to struggle against great odds to find responsiveness in the system. There is no question that the rising tide of consumerism is a threat to the male-dominated medical care system. It is precisely this surge of activism that makes women and women's health issues such an exciting avenue for exploration.

A chapter dealing with childbearing concerns could be endless. But the discussion in this chapter is confined primarily to an overview of the most pressing concerns surrounding childbearing, placed in a decision-making theoretical model. This is followed by an in-depth exploration of an area that has received little attention in our care systems: the preparation of parents for parenthood.

THE ISSUE

Is childbearing a crisis? How often this has been claimed—and yet studies demonstrate varied results. There are many definitions of crisis; for example a turning point with potential for growth, a state of dis-ease, or a state when usual behavioral patterns are inadequate and new ones are called for. The decisions surrounding childbearing certainly fall within these definitions for most women/couples. Within a family, the state of organization of the family unit at the time of the crisis is crucial. How severe or sustained that emotional disruption is for the woman and her family is dependent on many variables: Does she want to be pregnant? Now? Is

---

*Parts of this chapter have been revised from S.S. Rising, "Preparation for Parenthood," in J.J. Sciarra, *Gynecology and Obstetrics* (Hagerstown, Maryland: Harper and Row, 1978).

there enough money? Now? Is there a support system? Does that system (father/couple) want to be pregnant? Now? If not, is abortion a viable option? Is adoption?

These issues probably come together most forcefully for care givers in the pregnancy counseling situation. It is here that one sees intense joy, intense grief, and extreme ambivalence. "A baby, yes; now, no" is the ambivalence expressed by many women who struggle with issues of their autonomy, need for control, and emergence of personal essence, for having a baby is a lifetime decision, one that demands ongoing energy and investment. It is not a decision that can or should be made lightly. Whelan's book, *A Baby . . . Maybe,* clearly describes the conflicts inherent in making that decision.[2]

Women's "Coming Out"

The deluge of books directed toward, and written by women is astounding. Women welcome the insights gained by sharing in them and feel the anger engendered by the truths expounded in them. Female nurses share in the corporate embarassment over the inadequate, degrading system in which most women receive their medical care. As caregivers they also worry about the pressures that will be placed on the system of which they are a part by the response of consumers to the latest revelations. Being women and health care providers at times places them at opposite ends of the pole. That creative tension can lead to many new insights in both spheres.

The women's movement has helped women to feel their personal power. As the initial surges of freedom have passed, some of the either/or dichotomy has also faded. It is now possible to talk of motherhood *and* career, marriage *and* freedom. A book entitled *Living with Contradictions: A Married Feminist* explores some of the discrepancies that are possible and resolvable for today's feminist. McBride states, "Press the button and I feel guilty about anything."[3] There is a constant pull in two directions: toward tradition and toward feminist ideology. Today's woman must learn to live with contradictions.

Coming to terms with self is essential if one is to survive healthily today. Part of that process is the recognition of one's self-worth as a person—apart from titles, occupation, or roles. It is in this context that the recognition of personal power has such meaning. As a woman comes to respect herself, she can also respect others in a way that is most powerful to the interpersonal relationship. Carl Rogers talks of how issues are confronted openly, children are reared with respect, and each partner has freedom to pursue a life direction, make career choices, and engage in life's activities in his/her own way.[4] The emphasis for women on assertiveness has been a strong force for encouraging women to feel their power and to successfully negotiate their many relationships. Healthy avenues for the expression of anger have also demonstrated to women the validity of their anger and the ability of their significant people to respond meaningfully to that expression.

WHY THE CHANGE

One of the most monumental advances in recent years has been the development of "effective" contraception. As recently as the early 1960s some states still had not made the dispensing of birth control methods legal. As long as a woman had no control over her fertility she really had little control over the direction of her life. Even though there still is no ideal method of birth control, women do have the option of using methods with high reliability. In reviewing the field of birth control it is puzzling why more advances haven't been made in controlling male fertility. A strong hunch is that part of the reason must be due to the predominance of men in medical research leadership positions.

Women must deal with their anger over the "dumping" of responsibility for birth control. It is the female who has had to deal with the side effects of the pill and intrauterine devices. It is the female, primarily, who has had to deal with the emotions surrounding sterilization and abortion. It is no wonder that an increasing number of women are returning to the earlier methods of birth control: foam and condom and diaphragm, as well as the evolving natural family planning methods. And women are electing these methods partly because of the joint responsibility required.

Society and Change

Several social changes have given each woman "more options, more chance for dignity, more possibility of discovering her own self-worth."[5] Rogers has outlined the following changes:[6]

1. Greatly improved methods of contraception. As discussed above, this has had enormous impact. Years ago wives were expendable because there seemed to be no other alternative; death often came at an earlier age, the result of repeated childbearing.

2. Lengthened life span of men and women. This longer expectancy gives new significance to relationships. More effort is needed to keep pace with the ever-changing elements that affect relationships.

3. Increasing social acceptance of divorce. The increased liberalization of attitudes means that women don't necessarily have to feel bound to an undesirable marriage.

4. Family mobility. With the transiency of the family increasing, there tends to be less contact with an extended family.

5. Availability and acceptance of women working outside the home. This factor has made women more independent and has increased the potential for contact with other men.

6. Increased sexual freedom. More women are sexually experienced before entering a marriage contract. This can have a profound effect on the marriage itself.

One thing is certain. With this amount of change occurring within society, new patterns must be developed for dealing with the process of living in today's world. Old patterns aren't adequate; there are few prototypes. A woman's mother has lived a generation removed—perhaps completely removed—from the perplexing issues facing today's young woman. It is only with great difficulty that values are claimed and goals established.

DECISIONS

How often have we heard, "Just tell me what to do and I'll do it"? Why is it so difficult to make decisions? Clearly, the more that is at stake, the more difficult it is to make the decision. Considering the magnitude of the decisions surrounding childbearing it is understandable that there is enormous ambivalence and indecision present. It is a truism that no woman really decides to get pregnant; it just happens.

How does one make "good" decisions? There is no absolute answer, but guidelines have been developed. Janis and Mann have listed seven criteria to help to ensure high-quality decisions:[7]

The decision maker, to the best of his/her ability:

1. Thoroughly canvasses a wide range of alternative courses of action

2. Surveys the full range of objectives to be fulfilled and the values implicated by the choice

3. Carefully weighs possible positive and negative consequences that could flow from each alternative

4. Searches for new information relevant to further evaluation of alternatives

5. Takes into account new information received about alternatives

6. Reexamines positive and negative consequences of all known alternatives before making a final choice

7. Makes detailed provisions for implementing chosen course

There is likely to be intense conflict whenever one must make a decision of great magnitude in the face of uncertainties. The decision is likely to be postponed. The person may experience hesitation, vacillation, and signs of acute stress, which may include apprehension, a desire to escape, and self-blame for allowing such a predicament to occur. Usually the intensity of symptoms experienced is dependent on the perceived magnitude of losses anticipated from the choice made. In general, it is felt that a moderate amount of stress actually leads to better decision making than either mild or severe stress. Some stress is needed to prod the person into thoughtful decision making, but too much stress may lead to panic.

When a person is faced with a decisional conflict, one with simultaneous opposing tendencies to accept or reject a given course of action, the consequence of each alternative course can be divided into four main categories:[8] (1) utilitarian gains and losses for self, (2) utilitarian gains and losses for significant others, (3) self-approval or disapproval, and (4) approval or disapproval from significant others. A very helpful tool, the balance sheet grid, has been developed by Janis and Mann to aid this process. A modification of this grid is shown in Figure 7.1.

Types of Anticipation	Alternative Courses of Action			
Examples from Conflict with Pregnancy	Alternate 1: Continue with Pregnancy		Alternate 2: Terminate Pregnancy	
	+	—	+	—
A. Gains or losses for self				
1. Career				
2. Income				
3. Effect on Health				
4. Age				
B. Gains or losses for significant others				
1. Prestige				
2. Income				
3. Family stability				
C. Self-Approval or disapproval				
1. Moral considerations				
2. Body image, sexuality				
3. Goals, aspirations				
4. Self-esteem				
5. Growth potential				
D. Social Approval or disapproval				
1. From significant other				
2. From extended family				
3. From close friends				
4. National expectations				

Fig. 7.1: Schematic balance sheet grid for conceptualizing decisional conflict.

Adapted from Janis and Mann.[9]

Identifying as many alternatives as possible and then carefully analyzing each, such as is required by this type of grid, will help to ensure that a thoughtful decision is made. The clearer one is about the problem area the clearer the many alternatives will be. The more alternatives outlined, the less chance that the person will feel boxed in with no choices available. Probably one of our most serious problems with living today is that we fail to realize all of the alternatives that are available. How often have we said, "She just seems to have her blinders on"?

To further elaborate on the example used in the grid it may be helpful to consider some of the material in Gail Sheehy's book, *Passages*.[10] Many of the conflicts in section A of the grid, "Gains and losses for self," are present in the state she describes as the Catch-30 transition. She sees that point (the transition from the 20s to the 30s) as a time of great change, turmoil, and crisis. Many who thought they knew what they wanted in the 20s find themselves tearing that up and striking out into new territory. Suddenly, they want to get married or want a child, or, if they have those, they are questioning both. Some literature has been exploring the postponement of childbearing until careers are established, the increasing number of couples who have one child or no children, the many older women who decide to be solo parents, and the large number of teenage parents who are electing to keep their children. Liberalization of the abortion option has also changed the alternative column for many women.

Sheehy also describes five women's life patterns that have roots in history:[11]

Care-giver: woman marries early in 20s or before and who at that time sees herself only in a domestic role

Either-or: woman in 20s who feels required to choose between children and love or work and accomplishment. There are 2 types:

Nurturer who defers achievement: postpones career but intends to pick it up later

Achiever who defers nurturing: postpones motherhood and perhaps marriage until professional preparation completed.

Integrator: woman who tries to combine marriage, career, and motherhood all in her 20s.

Never-married woman: these women include paranurturers and office wives.

Transient: women who wander sexually, occupationally, and geographically.

There is no question that a woman's basic choices when she is in the late teens and 20s have a profound effect on her subsequent decisions regarding herself, her childbearing, and her relationships.

DECISION FOR PREGNANCY

Why do people actually decide to have babies? Many don't know, often because there really was no decision. "If you start believing that normal women have babies because they love children, you may be knee-deep in guilt before the doctor confirms you are pregnant."[12]

Many women and couples find that the satisfaction in their marriage or significant relationship is far from that romantically envisioned. They have grown farther apart and experienced communication that has become routine and shallow. Some of these couples decide that a child will fill the gap. This solution may work well for these couples throughout the child-rearing years, but the crisis returns when the last child leaves home. The divorce rate among middle-aged and older couples is startling and undoubtedly is related to unresolved problems in the early relationship of the couple. Ironically, studies show that marital satisfaction is at a high before the advent of the first child, when it falls dramatically and doesn't again peak until the children have left home and married.[13]

Some women struggle with a sense of worthlessness and a lack of self-confidence. For so many years the stereotype for success included marriage and children; it was the "thing" for a woman to do. With the growing strength of the women's movement, this image has been seriously questioned. Such stereotypes are so ingrained in most individuals that they are largely unaware of their biases. Motherhood has been a sure way to say to the world, "I can produce; I am fertile; I can do what I was made to do." Children are a credential. Much of the identity of a woman with this bias is gained through identifying with her offspring. This often leads to an unhealthy relationship between mother and child, most aptly characterized by the hovering, oversolicitous mother whose children, in turn, tend to become demanding and unlikeable.

Many couples now postpone pregnancy until their relationship has matured. This provides time for husband and wife to become established in their respective careers. As the couples mature, their ability to provide a stable home increases. Many couples elect to live together for various periods before entering into a formal arrangement. There is little evidence in the literature as to the influence that the latter life style has on the ability to parent. It seems only fair to say that the more stable the relationship, the more problems and concerns the couple has had time to work out and the more established each partner is in terms of her/his own identity, the greater the readiness of the couple to assume the tasks of parenting.

There is a well-recognized trend toward smaller families. This shift is partly in response to world overpopulation and the raising of the national and international consciousness. A decrease in population is seen as essential for survival. Also, there seems to be a change in the orientation toward family. Previously, the family was the focus for activity of its members. Children were essential for basic tasks necessary to keep the family alive. Transportation was not rapid, convenient, or readily available, and the family members relied on each other for entertainment and enrichment. Roles were clearly defined and family oriented.

Improvements in technology have led very quickly to changes in life style and to a shift in the original roles and family patterns. Making a living is considerably easier today, and there is more leisure time and money. The telephone, automobile, radio, and television promote instant communication. The movement toward urban areas has had an impact on the closeness of the family. Members have become more aware of their wants and needs, as individuals increasingly seek outside sources for gratification. A new loneliness and alienation have developed; some members have begun to look to nonfamily groups for significant relationships to fulfill basic needs.

The Human Potential Movement is extremely popular because it responds to a demonstrated need for personal growth. Glasser has described the phenomenon in terms of a major societal shift from a "civilized society" to an "identity society."[14] He sees the civilized society, existent since 10,000 B.C., as oriented toward power and security and directed by outside influences. The identity society is inwardly directed and focused on love and a sense of worth. It is more individual oriented than family oriented.

This change has led couples to reevaluate the pattern of large families and has encouraged many to consider having no children or having only one or two. Studies show that children in smaller families tend to be more intelligent than those in large families. The ability of the parents to continue to develop their own relationships is enhanced by the fewer demands of the smaller family circle.

Many couples choose to have children because they genuinely enjoy them and want to share in their development and growth. These couples see their children as contributing to their increased appreciation of life and its wonder. They covet the privilege of sharing values and life experiences with the children. Children complete their family unit. These couples have a mature relationship and are ready to extend their personal and dual boundaries.

The Solo Parent

There are many unmarried, or solo, parents who struggle with parenthood. One group consists of adolescents who decline marriage but desire to have and keep their babies. Although these teenagers are usually a part of extended families, which may become "parents," the responsibility for child care is often assumed by the parent. When one views the maturational crisis of adolescence and imposes the crisis of pregnancy and parenthood, the responses needed seem almost overwhelming.

A recent newspaper article points to the alarming increase in the number of births, especially in the white teenage population. This study, from the National Center for Health Statistics, calls this a "puzzling" trend in light of the fact that birth rates among older women have dropped sharply and because of the availability of cheap, effective contraceptive devices as well as legal abortions, which have widely been available to the teenager. The rate of out-of-wedlock pregnancy among girls aged 15 to 17 has nearly doubled in the decade from 1966 to 1975. During this time, the birth rate among 18- to 19-year-olds dropped by 29 percent, and for all women in childbearing ages (15 to 44) the drop was 27 percent. Some of the possible attributable causes are increased sexual activity and increased social acceptance of unmarried pregnancy. It does seem, however, that although contraception is being used more, the pattern followed by teenagers today is the same as in previous years, that is, having sex, becoming pregnant, and then going on to use contraception.[15] Intense support for these teenagers by those especially interested and prepared is essential.

Many single women are becoming parents either through their own pregnancy or by adoption. These women tend to be in their 20s and early 30s, secure in a career but wanting the experience of rearing a child. They may live in a commune to give the child exposure to men. Another special group consists of parents (or parents-to-be) who are separated, divorced, or widowed. This is a traumatic situation, especially when it occurs during pregnancy or the early postpartum period. In such cases, the relationship with the new child may be severely impaired. Solo-parent groups have been formed in an attempt to give special support to those in this situation.

There is a definite difference in needs between a group of solo parents and a group of married couples. It is probably best to have single parents share together as a group to facilitate meeting their particular needs. One such group spent almost two hours dealing with concerns relating to their own mothers. Other concerns include dealing with society, ensuring income adequacy for basic needs, and providing positive male influence in child rearing. Group experience may be especially important for these women to give a support base and assist them in developing an assertive manner to deal with the complexities of their life.

PARENTS-TO-BE

Much of this chapter has dealt specifically with the concerns of women surrounding their own femaleness. It would be possible to discuss parenting simply in light of the woman herself, but that would be talking about a situation that is less than ideal for both the mother and the children in the family. Therefore, in the following sections, pregnancy is discussed in terms of the parents. If one of the parents is absent, the adjustments within the childbearing-child-rearing experience are often much more acute and the need for a firm support base is even more imperative. When pregnancy occurs, parents are faced with many decisions; probably the most crucial are the steps that they must take to move themselves toward parenthood. Unfortunately, most parents have had little prior preparation for the kinds of responsibilities they must undertake when they become parents.

They may begin by reviewing their own experiences as a child with parents, including what they liked and what they wish to avoid repeating. This information should be shared because the parents often come from different backgrounds. They may consider their experiences of child care, e.g., caring for younger siblings, baby-sitting, or caring for children of relatives and friends. They should consider their ability to relate to children and their experience with newborns. Since infants tend to be sheltered, most people have had little experience in caring for them. If at all possible during this preparatory time, parents should have some contact with infants, preferably with newborns. This will help to put into perspective their images of the kind of child they will be bringing home from the hospital. If they are imagining the six-month Gerber baby they may be very disappointed with their new offspring.

Together they may read some books on care of infants and share their attitudes on it. If they can begin to agree on what aspects are most important, they will begin to feel united in their movement toward parenthood. Some couples even get an animal on which to test their emotions and discipline techniques. A dog, especially, will help the parents to learn some of the responsibility that comes with caring for another living being.

Perhaps the most important thing for a couple to do during pregnancy is to reassess their relationship as a couple. They should affirm activities that are important to them and that they enjoy doing together. These should be planned into their "parent schedule." They should also consider activities that are crucial to their survival as individuals. There must be continued provision for these activities in their new schedule. Contracting with each other for specific aspects of their day-to-day life may help them retain their individual identities and their relationship as a couple. Adjustments will have to be made, but they will be less threatening if provisions have been made to retain the most important aspects of the parents' individual and shared lives.

It is especially important for the woman to reaffirm her self-worth and to recognize her needs as legitimate. Otherwise, she may find herself in the trap of always responding to everyone else and neglecting her own wants and needs. After the baby comes, her wants and needs may be difficult to sort out as she responds to the many demands of her baby and family.

During this time the couple may begin looking for other couples who are also experiencing pregnancy. At one time, communities were relatively insulated from the rest of the world, and women and men shared ideas in a personal, helping way. Today we have mass-media communication with essentially nonpersonal input. Also, the ease of travel and the movement to urban areas have contributed to a lack of community milieu for many young couples.

Alienation and lack of support can be rather frightening for a couple working through changing goals, new roles, and anxiety about labor, delivery, and parenthood. They have no background against which they can compare their dreams and fantasies and no objective sounding board.

THE NEW FAMILY UNIT

One day, with the onset of labor, the anticipation of having a new child clearly becomes reality. Besides feeling the concern for safety that they have related to labor, the couple realize that the reality of the newborn is soon to be on them. As the mother goes through labor she is also laboring psychologically to achieve a proper relationship with a new, nonparasitic person. It is not a simple jump from being pregnant, to having delivered, to needing to start nurturing a new being. In fact, if labor progresses too rapidly the mother may find that she has not done the necessary psychological work of labor prior to delivery and may have to take considerable time after delivery to work through the process of delivering.

If it is a first child, the couple have not had to widen their circle to consider another dependent being. They still may be trying to determine who they are as a couple. The younger they are, the more probable it is that they are still working through self-identity. If this is their second or later pregnancy, they may be coping with such questions as, "Can we afford another?" "Do we have enough love, enough time, and enough of ourselves to give?" "Have we prepared our children adequately?" Feelings of confidence and self-doubt, anxiety and excited anticipation race through them at the time of birth.

Integration within a family involves an understanding and a melding of all characteristics into a whole, perhaps not always a harmonious whole, but one that is unique. Each member contributes unique characteristics to the larger unit, i.e., the family image. There is a certain openness during the first hour or two after delivery that may never occur again during the postpartum period. The mother tends to be very alert and almost oversensitive, and the baby, if she/he is not medicated, is usually crying and sucking in response to stimuli. This is a crucial time for all members of the triad to begin to get familiar with each other. Barring any unusual problems the baby should be kept with the parents, if they desire, and should be kept warm, preferably under the covers next to the mother's body. There the child is more likely to be content and to enjoy a continuation of the contact stimulation felt in utero.[16] Ideally, other children in the family would also be present during this immediate bonding time. Since that practice is not common, there is nothing in the literature indicating what the effect is on children who are present and available during and around the time of birth, but one would surmise that sibling rivalry would be decreased if children felt they were an integral part of the experience and felt little or no separation from their mother and father.

A variety of behaviors is displayed by couples during these first few minutes. It is important that they have time with each other and the child. Claiming behavior is common to all animals and is essential if subsequent attachment is to occur. This early encounter forms the basis for their subsequent interactions and is critical in setting the tone. A father who is encouraged and becomes involved at this point is much less likely to feel like an outsider than a father who is excluded from any meaningful participation with his wife and new child.

During this early postpartum period, it is crucial that the couple identify their needs as clearly as possible. Studies have shown that a mother is not really ready to care for her infant until her needs for restoration have been met. The mother and father must be clearly attuned to the needs of each other or these needs will be overlooked in trying to meet the demands of their infant. One good practice is to go out together as a couple, perhaps for a meal, before leaving the hospital. If the couple has left the birthing place early, a delightful substitute might be for another couple to come over and assume the responsibilities for child care, thus freeing the new parents to enjoy some time alone. Support from professionals helps them to place added legitimacy on their needs as individuals and as a couple.

Postpartum Period

The first few weeks at home with the new baby are critical. The mother is tired and probably overwhelmed with her new responsibilities. If she is breast feeding, she may be wondering if the baby is getting enough milk. What can be done if the baby has cried for a half an hour and she has tried everything to quiet the child, or when she has been up for the fifth time in the night and may be tempted to abandon the demanding infant? When the father goes back to work, the mother often feels trapped at home and tries to rationalize her feelings of ambivalence. She may be experiencing an abrupt change from a very active work or career life to a life of domesticity. She may miss her old contacts and her old sense of achievement and may begin to wonder why she decided to have a child. She must be helped to see her achievement in her new mothering role.

The mother must receive positive, nurturing input during this period in order to be able to give to the new baby and to her family. She may feel that everything is going out of her: the baby, the placenta, the lochial flow, her breast milk, her tears. She must have replacement of that output through love, care, affirmation, understanding, and encouragement. Physically and psychologically her body is experiencing enormous changes. There is no organ that even begins to match the outstanding involutional feat of the uterus, which shrinks 1,000 grams in a period of only six weeks.

PARENTING PREPARATION

There is no question as to the value of the programs for preparation for childbirth. These programs are couple oriented and usually have about six sessions devoted to discussion and exercising. The topics discussed include conception and the menstrual cycle, physiologic and psychologic changes during pregnancy, stages of labor, analgesia and anesthesia, and delivery techniques. Some programs include material on breast preparation and feeding. The exercises emphasize relaxation with specific concentration techniques as well as various types of abdominal and chest breathing.

These classes fill a void in helping couples prepare for childbirth but give them little help in adjusting to and caring for their child. Most hospitals have a series of demonstrations designed to help mothers with bathing and feeding infants as well as with birth control. Frequently, fathers are not present, and no special effort is made to include them. Follow-up studies indicate that these efforts seems to have little effect on the mother's ability to cope at home. What, then, needs to be done?

A Comprehensive Program

Most couples who are expecting a baby are beset with many questions relating to the conduct of pregnancy, to concerns about parenthood, and to their relationship as a couple. A formal parent preparation program starts with opportunities for group contact in both the first and second trimesters. Early in the program the parents' primary focus is not labor and delivery; this freedom provides an ideal atmosphere for promoting group cohesion and discussing issues of parenthood. Some of these issues are ambivalence of pregnancy, adjusting career to motherhood, changing sexual feelings, the couple's binding into the pregnancy, and anxieties about competence as a parent.

These groups should be small (four to six couples) and should be relatively unstructured to allow for a sharing of joys and concerns by the group members. The leader should be viewed as a facilitator rather than a lecturer or teacher. Occasionally, resource people in family life education might be used to advantage. Phone numbers may be exchanged to facilitate continuing informal contact by group members. These contacts may help to establish the couple's support base, which will be invaluable during the early stages of child rearing. Parenthood is much more difficult when faced alone.

The third trimester is usually the period for intense concentration on preparation for labor and delivery. Attendance at some formal series of classes should be strongly encouraged. Besides presenting information and providing an opportunity for learning relaxation and breathing methods, these classes should emphasize the couple's innate resources for dealing with labor, delivery, and early parenting. A couple should also be helped to develop realistic expectations for their birth experience, for subsequent satisfaction is very dependent on how closely these expectations were met.

Support Group Concept

Human beings are social beings. Much of their lifetime is spent in interaction. One of the primary reasons for marriage and family life is to provide an opportunity for close sharing and support. However, neither a husband nor a wife can totally meet the needs of the other. Contact with a larger group is vital to a couple's relationship and to the health of each individual.

Gendlin has made some predictions relating to continued development of interaction. He believes that individuals must be encouraged to focus on their own experience as the most honest, valid way of coping with life. He believes that in the future, children will be taught in school how to listen and to share meaningfully with each other. Ordinary people must be taught how to provide a therapeutic process for each other. He sees the need for social programs that build opportunity for intimate human interaction. In addition, he believes that one cannot effectively deal with only one part of a person; he or she is a total being that needs to be viewed in the entire life situation.[17]

A support group concept is employed at the University of Minnesota. A group of couples whose babies are due within the same month meets together weekly to share feelings and concerns about childbearing and parenthood. The groups are formed four to six weeks before due dates; ideally, they will have met together occasionally since the first trimester.

These weekly meetings provide couples with an organized opportunity to discuss questions with a professional and also to gain considerable support from other group members struggling with similar concerns. Topics usually explored include dreams, concerns about death, continuance of the relationship of the couple, separation from the baby, coping with grandparents, division of household/baby responsibilities, resumption of career by the mother, and managing early labor. As soon as some couples become parents, they give a full report to the group; some have given reports on the same day as delivery. Besides giving the waiting couples firsthand data with which to compare their images, this approach gives the delivered couple an opportunity to begin analyzing their own experience, which is essential to their successful progression as parents.

As couples in the group move beyond the childbearing event, the concerns begin to center on early childrearing, breast and bottle feeding, handling of crying, getting out of the house, and coping with fatigue. Babies are brought to the group sessions, and couples have an opportunity to watch each other handle crying infants and perform feeding and cleansing routines. It seems especially helpful to fathers to watch other fathers engaged in these activities. Members of the group also have the satisfaction of seeing their own baby claimed by a larger community; this is a very important affirmation.

Participation in support groups should continue for at least two months after delivery. Many studies show that the new family is more crisis prone during these early months. It is wise to have co-group leadership that includes someone knowledgeable in childrearing. In our institution, leadership is usually shared by a nurse-midwife and a pediatric nurse practitioner, both of whom have had special preparation in group facilitation. Experienced parents can also add an important dimension to these groups.

A study was done of couples' perceptions of the support received while participating in one of these groups. These data included an articulation of the following components of support: the opportunity to share experiences with group members, receiving assistance and information from group members, receiving positive feedback and pleasant attitudes and feelings, and sharing problems and feelings with other group members.[18]

A formal format for early childrearing classes could include a variety of topics dealing with caretaking activities of the newborn, mother-father relationship issues, changing roles, babysitters, and infant stimulation. Several excellent media resources are available that could supplement content presentation.

GETTING PERSPECTIVE

Is the advent of the first child really a crisis for the family? Studies vary in their findings but clearly show that it is a crisis for many families. Le Masters interviewed 46 married, middle-class, well-educated couples. Eighty-three percent of those couples indicated "extensive" or "severe" crisis in adjusting to the first child. Among these couples, 92 percent of the pregnancies were either "planned" or "desired." One of the strongest findings was that these couples seemed to have completely romanticized pregnancy.[19]

In another study conducted by Dyer, the percentage of couples indicating "extensive" and "severe" crisis totaled 53 percent, but a definite correlation was found with strength of family organization. Mothers and fathers were asked about their experiences, problems, and reactions in adjusting to their first child. Mothers responded as follows:[20]

1.	Tiredness and exhaustion	87%
2.	Loss of sleep	87%
3.	Feelings of neglecting husband	67%
4.	Feelings of inadequacy	58%
5.	Inability to keep up with housework	35%
6.	Difficulty in adjusting to being tied down and home and curtailing outside activities	35%

Fathers reported as follows:

1.	Loss of sleep	50%
2.	Adjustment to new responsibilities and routines	50%
3.	Upset schedules and daily routines	50%
4.	Ignorance of great amount of time and work required	—
5.	Financial worries	—

There are tremendous adjustments to be made by new parents; it is hoped that an increasing number will have the opportunity for more extensive preparation for their new role.

Recently, a workshop entitled "Parenthood: Full or Flat" was held. The response to the title was interesting. Did it mean pregnant and then delivered? Did it mean a house full of children and then an empty nest with all having left home? It could have meant either, but the focus was on how to make parenting a full, enriching experience rather than a flat, depressing one. Part of the key probably is to make good prepregnancy counseling available to couples who want to have a better handle on the meaning of parenthood for them. This seems to be one of the best ways out of the loneliness and alienation that is felt by much of our society. Our sense of ourselves is best experienced through meaningful relationships with others: "We cannot be loving, amusing, exciting, generous, forgiving, in isolation. Only the potential exists until there is someone present to be loved, to be amused, to be excited, to be grateful, to be forgiven. It is the response which this intimate other makes to us that validates our self-image."[21]

One tool that has been used to help individuals and couples focus on their needs for intimacy has the structure shown in Figure 7.2.

| Dimension | Time Spent (%) | | How to Spend Time (%) | | | | |
	Now	Would Like	Alone	With Significant Other	With Friends	Feels Okay	Needs Change
Sexual							
Intellectual							
Emotional							
Social							
Cultural							
Spiritual							
Recreational							
Vocational							
Family							

(Total time available in a week: 100 hours)

Fig. 7.2. Dimensions of intimacy.
Adapted from Clinebell and Clinebell.[22]

Included in the tool are dimensions of life in which each of us experiences interest and need. In some we may desire more intimacy than in others. Each person is encouraged to think about his/her needs in each area and to mark the approximate percentage of time currently spent in each area and the percentage of time desired. The next step focuses on how the person would like to spend that time, i.e., alone, with significant others, or with friends. An additional step looks at whether the person judges the dimension overall to "feel okay" or whether it "needs work." This exercise should help individuals and couples to sort out where they are and where they would like to go.

Another mechanism is for the significant unit to participate periodically in enrichment groups: marriage, family, sex-related, sexuality. These programs are oriented toward "growth rather than problems . . . development rather than symptom relief."[23] These groups have a preventive approach and seek to stimulate insight and communication.

CONCLUSION

The factors to weigh, the decisions to make, and the dilemmas to resolve all contribute to the complexity and stress of the childbearing issue for women today. There are many, and they are difficult to resolve. Our changing society has provided a dynamic climate in which to live. But the pace is almost breathtaking. When is there time to engage in thoughtful decision making? Who has time to listen and reflect? Where are those caring people who are needed for the support base so essential for survival today?

It is not only possible but important for self-fulfillment to approach living intentionally by taking control of life rather than letting it be in control. This intentionality has several characteristics:

1. Valuing yourself, developing self-esteem through quality interpersonal relationships, acknowledging differing wants and needs

2. Taking charge of your own destiny

3. Consciously balancing expectations of society with your own wants, needs, and values

4. Deciding your future by setting goals, strategizing, looking ahead, and being accountable

5. Acting in a proactive, rather than reactive, fashion

6. Constantly reflecting on your experience, and repeating the cycle

As women become clearer about their needs and are therefore better able to articulate them, there may be a surprising response from other women and from men. Slowly there is a response building to some of these needs: daycare facilities, pregnancy benefits, part-time benefits, the Equal Rights Amendment, and equal pay for equal work. As women find other opportunities both available and satisfying there may not be as great a need to have a baby because it is "the thing to do" or "the only way to achieve some status." And for those women who do decide to have children, it need not be such a stressful experience; in fact, it can be an exciting and rewarding one.

NOTES

1. Ellen Frankfort, *Vaginal Politics* (New York: Bantam Books, 1972).
2. E.M. Whelan, *A Baby . . . Maybe* (New York: Bobbs-Merrill Co., 1975).

3. A.B. McBride, *Living with Contradictions: A Married Feminist* (New York: Harper and Row, 1976).

4. Carl Rogers, *On Personal Power* (New York: Delacorte Press, 1977).

5. Ibid., p. 45.

6. Ibid., pp. 43-44.

7. I. Janis and L. Mann, *Decision Making* (New York: Free Press, 1977).

8. Ibid., p. 137.

9. Janis and Mann, *Decision Making*, p. 138.

10. Gail Sheehy, *Passages* (New York: E. P. Dutton & Co., 1974).

11. Ibid., p. 242.

12. A.B. McBride, *The Growth and Development of Mothers* (New York: Harper and Row Row, 1973).

13. A. Campbell, "American Way of Mating: Marriage Si, Children Only Maybe," *Psychology Today*, May 1975, pp. 37-43.

14. W. Glasser, *The Identity Society* (New York: Harper and Row, 1972).

15. "Birth Rate for Teens Soaring, Alarming," *Minneapolis Tribune* Section B (September 25, 1977): 3.

16. S.S. Rising, "Fourth Stage of Labor: Family Integration," *American Journal of Nursing*, May 1974, pp. 870-874.

17. E.T. Gendlin, "A Short Summary and Some Long Predictions," *New Directions in Client-Centered Therapy*, ed. J.T. Hart and J.M. Tomlinson (Boston: Houghton-Mifflin, 1970).

18. K. Lindquist and M. Meyer, "Childbearing and Childrearing Support Group: Verbal Interaction and Support" (Plan B Paper, University of Minnesota, 1976).

19. E.E. Le Masters, "Parenthood as Crisis" *Crisis Intervention*, ed. H.J. Parad (New York: Family Service Association of America, 1965), pp. 111-117.

20. E. Dyer, "Parenthood as Crisis: A Re-Study," *Crisis Intervention*, ed. H.J. Parad (New York: Family Service Association of America, 1965): 312-323.

21. G.P. Fullerton, *Survival in Marriage* (New York: Holt, Rinehart and Winston, 1972).

22. H. Clinebell and C. Clinebell, *The Intimate Marriage* (New York: Harper and Row, 1970).

23. R. Fowler and D. Schultz, "Total Family Enrichment: A Systems Approach," *Theological Markings 5*, no. 2 (Winter 1975): 31-37.

8
Communication Patterns of Women and Nurses

MARIE LOLAND MENIKHEIM

INFLUENCE OF SOCIETAL STATUS ON COMMUNICATION PATTERNS

Positions that individuals occupy in society are sociologically defined as social statuses. Statuses provide a basis for social identity. Each status has rights, obligations, and prestige, which constitute a social role. A social role is the pattern of behaviors expected with a particular status position in society.[1]

A social role is attached to sex status, just as roles are attached to all positions in society. Sex status is considered an "ascribed status," along with race and age.[2] This type of status is assigned at birth and is independent of skill, effort, and ability. Nonetheless, virtually every society has formed a complex set of explicit and implicit rules for proper behavior based on sex differences. Different cultural expectations for male and female social roles are taught and reinforced from birth.

This socialization determines in large part identity development and sex concept. In general, socialization is considered training for a social environment or culture.[3] Brim more specifically defines socialization as "the process by which individuals acquire the knowledge, skills and dispositions that enable them to participate as more or less effective members of groups and society."[4]

Socialization is a reciprocal process. Culture provides the framework of societal standards. As the individual learns and demonstrates appropriate behaviors consistent with societal standards, the framework is strengthened. The individual, in turn, is rewarded for behavior that conforms to these societal standards.

Infants are given behavioral reinforcement consistently for appropriate behavior. Parents treat infant boys and girls differently as they talk to them, play with them, and handle them. Youngsters observe their parents and other adults, imagining themselves in the role of the adult. Children learn to differentiate between men and women and identify a sex role preference. Schooling, peer groups, and various media further influence sex role formation. Children then begin to live out sex role behavior, ultimately internalizing it.

The sex status ascribed to men continues to be superior to the sex status ascribed to women in American society. Men and masculine characteristics are more highly valued. Even as young children, boys prefer their social role to that of girls. Some girls wish they were boys.[5]

The culturally determined social roles based on unequal sex status determine in large part the interaction patterns between men and women in American society. The value system and behavior are interactive. Communication patterns reflect this paternalistic orientation with its authority/subordinate parameters.

Communication patterns also reflect sex role stereotypes, i.e., consensual beliefs about the different characteristics of men and women. Broverman et al. found that stereotypes continue to be persistent and pervasive in American society. Female traits are regarded as less socially desirable than male traits and less mentally healthy.[6] Table 8.1 identifies current stereotypic behaviors based on sex role as described by Broverman et al.[7] and Bardwick and Donavan.[8]

TABLE 8.1. STEREOTYPICAL CHARACTERISTICS OF MALES AND FEMALES

Males	Females
independent	dependent, passive, fragile
aggressive	nonaggressive
competitive	noncompetitive
task oriented	interpersonally oriented
outwardly oriented	inner oriented
assertive	passive
self-disciplined	other-disciplined
stoic	empathic
objective	subjective
innovative	conforming
analytic minded	intuitive
unsentimental	sensitive

Adapted from Broverman et al.[7] and Bardwick and Donavan.[8]

Despite the apparent value on maleness, American society proclaims equality for both sexes. Consequently, there is conflict between the ideal and the reality of sexual equality. Although men and women are told they are equals, the American system does not provide equal reinforcement or support for women's advancement. The values and norms revolving about the social role related to sex status for women are contradictory and ambiguous. Behaviors appropriate to the feminine stereotype may be incompatible with behaviors appropriate to equality.

Communication patterns between men and women reflect this conflict in roles. As the inconsistencies in role increase, communication patterns reflect the stress of the role conflict.

Individuals occupy several statuses in society at one time. Thus far, this chapter has discussed sex status, an ascribed status in American society. Individuals also occupy statuses that are classified as achieved. "Achieved statuses" are not assigned at birth; they are chosen and earned. There may be special educational preparation necessary for their attainment. The social roles of wife, mother, and nurse are role-achieved statuses. As the statuses occupied by a person multiply, the roles associated with them often contradict each other. Communication patterns of women that conflict between ascribed (sex) and achieved (wife, mother, and nurse) roles are uncertain and often unclear. The communication style is further influenced by this additional conflict.

Communication patterns are further affected by the institutional inconsistencies relative to the equality value. In American society attributes associated with leadership in organizations are considered masculine. Attributes associated with most professional roles are also considered masculine. The behaviors associated with the role of a professional woman and those appropriate to the social role of the female in society can be mutually exclusive, further complicating woman's concept of herself.

The further women move from stereotypical behaviors associated with sex status, the more conflict occurs in their communication patterns with others.

COMMUNICATION PATTERNS OF MEN AND WOMEN

Differences have been found in language which reflect male and female roles in American society. The linguist assumes that there is a system in the language and that the data gathered about it can be studied, analyzed, and described. Sapir and Whorf in their widely credited linguistic relativity theory discuss language as the articulation of the particular notions which define a culture.[9]

The English language reinforces the male authority role and the female subordinate role. In a classic work Otto Jespersen[10] described English as the "most positively and expressly masculine" of languages.

> The Bible regards Eve as merely an offshoot from Adam's rib—and English follows suit by the use of many Adam's rib words. The scientific name for both sexes of our species is the word for only one of them, *Homo* "man" in Latin; our species is also referred to as *human* (derived from Homo) or *mankind*, two other words which similarly serve to make women invisible. The average person is always masculine (as in *the man in the street*) and so is the hypothetical person in riddles and in examination questions (If a man can walk ten miles in seven minutes, how many miles can he walk in twelve minutes?).[11]

Male identity is considered the norm. It is men who retain their name in marriage. It is male identity that is recognized. Consider "Four score and seven years ago our *fathers* brought forth upon this continent a new nation, conceived in liberty and dedicated to the proposition that all *men* are created equal" (italics added). Miller and Swift[12] found words associated with masculinity and femininity reflecting the stereotypic bias. "Sissy" from the word "sister" indicates timidity whereas "buddy" from "brother" indicates friendship or closeness. Furthermore, male identity is associated with high-ranking job categories. The personal pronoun "he" is automatically applied to bank presidents, physicians, and heads of state. This linguistic sexism permeates everday activity. It influences the thoughts and communication patterns of even small children.

Studies of language patterns show that women and men speak differently. Kraemer[13] identifies differences in women's interactions which indicate subordination or uncertainty.

Illustration is often given in national cartoons to the American male coming home after work who demands, "When's dinner, Honey!", and the woman who responds questioningly, "Five o'clock?" Lower volume and higher pitch are associated with women's speech habits. Women use more adjectives and nouns, whereas men use more verbs.[14] Women use a relatively large number of questions. Males use more declarative statements.[15]

Lakoff[16] identifies a particular communication form among women: "tag-questioning." A tag-question turns a declarative sentence into a question. For example: "Mary is here, isn't she?" "The weather is the worst ever, isn't it?" "It [a tag] is midway between an outright statement and a yes-no question: It is less assertive than the former, but more confident than the latter."[17] Tag-questions avoid conflict. They also limit commitment on the part of the speaker.

Jespersen[18] was the first to note a syntactic looseness about women's speech. Women are more prone to jump from one idea to another, not completing sentences during conversations. Women refer more to others in their speech, whereas men are more involved with themselves.[19] Men show great interest in action, movement, and doing, while women focus more on feeling states and expressions.[20]

Baird[21] found that studies of sex differences in verbal interaction patterns in groups (1950-1975) generated results that parallel sex role expectations; Table 8.2 illustrates identified differences in interaction patterns.

This chapter has focused on communication patterns of women in relation to men as determined by position in society (status) and socialization into role. The marginality of women is reflected in the dominant "maleness" of the language. The subordination of women to men is further exemplified in society's expectations of the ways in which women should speak and the ways in which women are spoken to. One of the most consistent findings produced by studies of sex differences in communication is that women tend to conform more to group norms than do men.[22] Females' conformity is maximized in mixed groups, where they often express concern about disagreements and wish to maintain good personal relationships. As women conform to fulfill societal role expectations, their behavior is reinforced and societal values strengthened.

COMMUNICATION PATTERNS INDICATING STRESS AND CONFLICT

Many women today are dissatisfied with their sex status in society. The implicit programming of sex stereotypic roles through socialization is being questioned. The conservative model of sex role evolution, which rigidly adheres to male dominance based on survival needs, is being disputed. Cross-cultural studies indicate that a variety of sex roles is appropriate, thereby challenging basic assumptions about what is "right" and "natural" for men and women in American society. Maccoby

TABLE 8.2. DIFFERENCES IN INTERACTION PATTERNS BETWEEN MALES AND FEMALES IN GROUP COMMUNICATION

Males	Females
initiate interaction	respond to interaction
give more information	express warmth, helpfulness
task/goal dimension	social-oriented dimension
use more words	participate less as men
talk more often	talk more
interrupt more often	withdraw from unpleasant interaction
demonstrate positive attitudes	communicate negative attitudes
objective	opinionated

Adapted from Baird.[21]

and Jacklen [23] indicate that many of the popular beliefs about the psychological characteristics of the two sexes have little or no basis in fact.

New, alternative models have been proposed which focus on differential access of men and women to scarce resources and commodities as determinants of sex role. The demographic limitations placed on women give males greater access to means of production, ownership, and control.[24]

Women wish to change the social role associated with their sex status in society. There is, however, great pressure on women from society to conform to the norms. As differences in values and beliefs are expressed, conflict results. A conflict exists whenever incompatible activities occur.[25] Communication patterns in conflict often represent exaggerated forms of day-to-day communication styles. Women under stress may therefore respond to conflict helplessly. Out of fear of the authority figure, a woman may hesitate and respond apologetically for her position. She may express behaviors considered "childlike." These behaviors, which may include pouting and crying, may have been dependent responses to conflict during childhood.

The polarized response of power is also seen. As women learn that control is established through authoritarian means, they may unconsciously role-model this behavior during "conflict." Aggressiveness is also seen in women acting out in rage against society. Aggression may be indirect or passive. Women respond to conflict with confusing communication. There are incongruences between verbal and nonverbal patterns. Women may use qualifying statements such as those beginning with "yes, but" or "it depends." Women who are unable to express anger in conflict may feel guilt. Women who are dissatisfied may suppress their anger, misplacing it and thereby punishing themselves. Guilt is frustration turned inward.[26]

NURSING AS AN OCCUPATIONAL ROLE
REFLECTING FEMALE SEX STATUS AND
COMMUNICATION STYLE

Nursing is said to be a profession that supports the sex status of women in American society. Nursing has come to be viewed as an extension of the sex role. Mauksch[27] studied personality traits common to nurses before, during, and after educational preparation. Generally, the nurse was found to be an individual who genuinely wants to help people, who is very conscious of what others think of her, and who is compliant. The nurse is fearful of making mistakes. This fear manifests itself in what Mauksch describes as "blame avoidance." Blame avoidance is characterized by a fear of being wrong which is so strong that the person can *never* be responsible for a wrong act; the individual *always* has to be right. There is an extreme desire to be safe and correct.

The authority/subordinate relationship between physicians and nurses reinforces the male/female societal role. Society sees the physician role as most important. The doctor's influence, even control, can be seen in the Nightingale Pledge and the Nurse Practice Act. Duberman[28] discusses nursing as a sex-stereotyped occupation along with elementary teaching, social work, and librarianship. Like men and women, occupations hold status, and nursing has consistently been labeled as inferior to medicine. Some studies indicated means by which these status inequalities are communicated. Goffmann discusses interaction rituals associated with status.

"Doctors had the right to saunter into the nurses' station, lounge on the station's dispensing counter, and engage in joking with other nurses. Other ranks participated in this informal interaction with doctors, but only doctors had initiated it."[29] If interactions occur between persons of equal status, they are guided by symmetric familiarity. In interactions occurring between persons of unequal status, the relations are asymmetric.

Paternalism, self-sacrifice, and self-dedication are qualities Leininger identifies with nursing. Traditionally, nurses have been socialized to be quiet and humble in the presence of father-like authority figures, and their behavior revealed signs of respect, attention, and reverence to them.[30]

The phrase "doctor's orders" says a great deal about the type of communication patterns that exist. Consider the following anecdote in which a nurse noted that a physician prescribed Librium for a patient. After thanking the doctor for the drug orders, the nurse commented, "Oh Doctor, I forgot to tell you that the night nurse reported that Mrs. M. was nauseated after each Librium. Did you want to write a new order?"

"Yes, thanks, Trudy. I did want to change the order."[31]

This doctor-nurse game situation reflects how a nurse can indirectly demonstrate knowledge without threatening the physician's authority. According to Hoekelman, the most important rule of the game is that open disagreement between the players must be avoided at all costs.[32] How distant are these communication patterns from those of the wife who informs her husband of the need to buy a washer for the sink after identifying a dripping faucet or the secretary who validates with her boss regarding contracts to be countersigned. The nurse cared for the physician as the wife cared for her husband and as the secretary cared for her boss.

Nursing leaders have also represented superiors with authoritarian roles. A nurse responded to a nurse educator, nurse supervisor, or nurse director as she did to a physician/administrator. Seldom did a nurse question the decision of a nurse leader since the leader was perceived as possessing great intelligence and knowledge.

This model of authority continues as Ura, Ozimek, and Walsh identify the strong authoritarianism that characterizes nursing service today: "Authoritarianism is a vestige of the developments of nursing from the military hospital model. . . . Militarism is a curse upon nursing that endures."[33]

In communication patterns among nurses this authoritarian frame is also visible. The behaviors that relate to the need to be correct in situations are often present in conflict situations. For example, a great deal of time is spent by nurse faculty members in criticizing and fault finding, even scapegoating, among themselves. In attempting to do the best for clients, patients, and students in the communities, hospitals, and colleges, nurses often negate one another and themselves.

Patterns of communication between nurses and patients reflect this authority/subordinate role. The care recipient has been a passive, dependent model. It has been relatively easy for nurses, having been conditioned as women, to relate to that passive model and to discourage independence and autonomy in clients.[34] The nurse often evades direct questions from the patient. There is often a compulsory pretense regarding the patient's condition. This communication style indirectly negates the nurse's understanding of the patient's condition from the patient's perspective. It encourages the patient to seek answers from the doctor. Like the tag-question discussed earlier, it negates commitment on the part of the speaker, in this case the nurse. In a recent study[35] 261 medical-surgical patients ranked 49 events related to the experience of hospitalization from most to least stressful. Important stressful events as expressed by the patients were related to a lack of communication of information by the nurse or a lack of communication in a meaningful way.[36]

Just as women in American society are questioning their position in the culture, so nurses are questioning the highly authoritarian behavior of physicians and nurses in the leadership positions of their profession. Conflicts are coming into being as the concepts of authority are challenged. Nurses often respond to conflicts either submissively or aggressively.

ALTERNATIVE COMMUNICATION PATTERNS: STRATEGIES FOR CHANGE

A need exists for women to recognize that, in learning to be women in our society, a constraining image has been accepted and internalized. Once this is recognized, old roles can be unlearned and new roles accepted. As the underlying assumptions that influence sex role behavior continue to be exposed as myths rather than realities, the social role can be identified. Relearning will gradually occur. Attitudes will slowly change.

As an example of a communication pattern that reflects these differences, the statement "There is nothing to be done about the situation" is made into a question: "What can be done about the situation?" The question is then rephrased as a statement: "This is what can be done about the situation."

The process of developing new communication patterns can be awkward, even painful. Old ways are predictable and comfortable to everyone. Motivation for change develops within oneself. Although the steps to change may appear complex and strange, they may not be as difficult as they seem.

Change can be as simple as a practical relaxation exercise. For example, once you recognize feeling tense in a communication and begin to feel helpless, tell yourself to relax. Take a deep breath and hold it. Hold it for 5 seconds and then let your breath out slowly. Deliberately relax your muscles as you let your breath out. Continue your conversation. Nine times out of ten the person with whom you are communicating will not even notice your silence and if so will more than likely attribute it to interest in the conversation.

Recently the need for changes in communication patterns has been reinforced by consciousness-raising groups. These groups help women to increase their awareness of their sex role in society. What is unconscious becomes conscious as common experiences are shared. This new insight often causes emotional responses in the member. Feelings of anger, frustration, sadness, fear, and even rage are not uncommon. Once the person recognizes the discrepancy between the real and the assumptive world there is strong incentive to change.

Many present psychosocial theories encourage relearning of communication patterns. Approaches toward more egalitarian communication patterns are presented within these frameworks. The human potential movement shifts emphasis from continuous criticism of self to recognition of personal strengths and development of individual potential. The concept of personal power and its impact on making choices and responsible decisions is also stressed by Rogers.[37] He asserts that there is a natural tendency toward complete development in human beings, an underlying flow of movement toward a constructive fulfillment of their inherent possibilities. Facilitating self-ownership by the client, placing the locus of decision making on the client, and placing responsibility for the effects of these decisions on the client form the politics of Rogers' client-centered approach.[38] Rather than focusing on what one should have and blaming others for what one does not have, emphasis is placed on assessing one's position and then taking responsibility for changing it.

The values-clarification approach encourages individuals to personally and consciously choose beliefs and establish certain behavioral patterns to act on these beliefs.[39] Assertiveness training focuses on speaking for oneself, taking responsibility for one's actions. It fosters the emergence of new communication styles based on honest, direct, open communication.[40] A discussion of assertive techniques is presented in Chapter 3.

Transactional analysis emphasizes equality-oriented communication patterns (transactions). The parent/childlike nature of most learned human interaction is identified, and adult/adult (egalitarian) patterns are encouraged.[41] Behavior modification addresses specific patterns of communication, reinforcing appropriate patterns and extinguishing patterns seen as negative to individual development.[42]

Once a woman realizes the authoritarian/subordinate nature of language and has learned methods by which a more equal communication pattern can be established, she is able to act on her new beliefs and practice a new communication style. The communication style, if egalitarian, will conflict within the established norms of almost every group with which the woman has contact. Equal communication patterns create imbalance in aggressive/submissive language styles.

An egalitarian communication style redefines external and internal expectations of a relationship. It facilitates a collegial, cooperative perspective. Communication becomes more direct and lateral rather than horizontal as prevails in authority/subordinate relationships. As the communication style is practiced consistently, the imbalance creates uneasiness and stress. Equal communication patterns challenge the powerful position in authority/subordinate relationships. No person, group, or institution gives up power easily. Much work and struggle are involved in this type of pervasive change. A sociologist has identified major changes in life that affect large areas of the assumptive world as *psycho-social* transitions."[43] Such situations are seen as turning points for better or worse in psychosocial adjustment.

There is great pressure to accept and submit to societal norms of communication once an individual identifies the consequences of a true commitment to an egalitarian communication style. To make a satisfactory adjustment, an individual must give up one view of herself and her assumptive world and acquire another. Parkes[44] states that avoidance and depression are the two most common alternatives to the acceptance of reality. It is interesting to consider the commonality of these behaviors among many women in society today.

Communication in conflict situations is particularly difficult for women. It has also been found to be difficult for nurses as a group. Kramer encourages a reorientation of nurses toward conflict, advocating the learning of appropriate skills for the management of constructive conflict.[45]

Similarly, there is a great challenge to act out these new communication patterns. Research indicates that conflict, if faced reasonably, contributes to rather than detracts from growth.[46] There is great potential for all relationships as the dyad-group-institution is broadened to include the feminine perspective. The feminine perspective is not the same as the masculine perspective. It is not less than or more than the male contribution; it is a different contribution.

> The cry within the sciences to open up what one can see by admitting
> as data that which one feels, to place emphasis on the whole of the ex-
> perience instead of the measurable parts is a rejection of the limitations
> of a scientific, masculine reality and an acceptance of the need for the
> addition of the holistic feminine. In addition to knowing, it is necessary
> to feel—to know love and tenderness and fire and rage and passion.[47]

As attitudes change the caring orientation of nursing will be seen as equal to the cure orientation of medicine. Nursing is different than, rather than less than, medicine. As all personal characteristics are accepted in communication, the affective orientation of women will be reinforced. Conflict patterns will move from competitive situations to cooperative ones. The indirect communications system described by Stein as the doctor-nurse game will become more open and direct.[48] This collaborative effort is prevalent in true interdisciplinary functioning in rehabilitative centers today. The "win-lose" orientation of the authority-subordinate relationship can be changed to a "win-win" situation if all members' perspectives are taken seriously.

NOTES

1. C.S. Stoll, *Female and Male* (Dubuque, Iowa: W.M.C. Brown, 1974).

2. Ibid.

3. *Webster's 7th New Collegiate Dicitionary*, S.V. "Socialization."

4. O.G. Brim, Jr., "Socialization Through the Life Cycle," in *Socialization After Childhood*, ed. O.G. Brim and S. Wheeler (New York: John Wiley and Sons, 1966).

5. David B. Lynn, "The Process of Learning Parental and Sex Role Identification, *Journal of Marriage and the Family* 28 (1966): 446-470.

6. I.K. Broverman et al., "Sex-Role Stereotypes: A Current Appraisal," *Journal of Social Issues* 28 (1972): 59-78.

7. Ibid.

8. T. Bardwick and E. Donavan, "Ambivalence: The Socialization of Women," in *Women in Sexist Society*, ed. V. Gornick and B.K. Moran (New York: Basic Books, 1971), pp. 225-241.

9. E. Sapir and B.L. Whorf, "Language and Thinking," in *Reading About Language*, ed. Charlton Laird and R.M. Gorell (New York: Harcourt, Brace, Jovanovich, 1970), pp. 18-20.

10. Otto Jespersen, *The Growth and Structure of the English Language* (New York: D. Appleton, 1923).

11. Peter Farb, *Word Play* (New York: Alfred A. Knopf, 1975), p. 160.

12. C. Miller and K. Swift, "One Small Step for Mankind," *New York Times Magazine*, April 16, 1972.

13. C. Kraemer, "Women's Speech: Separate but Unequal?" *Quarterly Journal of Speech* 60, no. 1 (February 1974): 14-24.

14. D.W. Warshay, "Sex Differences in Language Style," in *Toward a Sociology of Women*, ed. Constantina Safilios and C. Rothchild (New York: John Wiley and Sons, 1972) p. 3-9.

15. Kraemer, "Women's Speech."

16. R. Lakoff, "Language and Women's Place," *Language in Society* 2 (April 1973): 45-79.

17. Ibid.

18. Jespersen, *English Language*.

19. Warshay, "Sex Differences."

20. N. Barrch, "Sex-typed Language: The Production of Grammatical Cases," *Acta Sociologia* 14, no. 1-2, (Winter 1971): 24-42.

21. J.E. Baird, Sex Differences in Group Communication: A Review of Relevant Research," *Quarterly Journal of Speech* 62, no. 1 (April 1976): 179-192.

22. Ibid.

23. E.E. Maccoby and C.N. Jacklen, *The Psychology of Sex Differences* (Stanford, Calif.: Stanford University Press, 1974).

24. C.A.H. Caine and T.A. Caine, "The Evolution of Male Dominance" (paper submitted to the Department of Women's Studies, University of Minnesota, January 6, 1976).

25. M. Deutsch, "Conflicts: Productive and Destructive," *Journal of Social Issues* 25, 1969: 7-43.

26. Leo Madow, *Anger* (New York: Charles Scribner's Sons, 1972), p. 6.

27. H.O. Mauksch, *The Nurse: A Study in Self and Role Perception* (Dissertation, University of Chicago, 1966).

28. Lucile Duberman, *Gender and Sex in Society* (New York: Praeger Publishers, 1975).

29. Ervin Goffmann, *Interaction Ritual* (New York: Anchor Books, 1967), pp. 47-95.

30. Madeline Leininger, *Nursing and Anthropology: Two Worlds to Blend* (New York: John Wiley and Sons, 1970), p. 67.

31. F. Lewis, "The Nurse as Lackey: A Sociological Perspective," *Supervisor Nurse*, April 1976, pp. 24-27.

32. R.A. Hoekelman, "Nurse-Physician Relationships," *American Journal of Nursing*, July 1975, p. 1151.

33. Helen Yura, Dorothy Ozimek, and Mary B. Walsh, *Nursing Leadership: Theory and Process* (New York: Appleton-Century-Crofts, 1976).

34. W.S. Heide, "Nursing and Women's Liberation: A Parallel," *American Journal of Nursing*, May 1973, p. 826.

35. B.S. Valicer and M.W. Bohannon, "A Hospital Stress Rating Scale," *Nursing Research* 24, no. 5 (September/October 1975): 352-359.

36. Ibid.

37. C. Rogers, *On Personal Power Inner Strength and Its Revolutionary Impact* (New York: Delacorte Press, 1977).

38. Ibid. p. 14.

39. S.B. Simon, L.W. Howe, and H. Kirschenbaum, *Values Clarification* (New York: Hart Publishing Co., 1972).

40. R. E. Alberti and M. L. Emmons, *Your Perfect Right: A Guide to Assertive Behavior* (St. Luis Obispo, Calif.: Impact, 1970).

41. T.A. Harris, *I'm OK, You're OK* (New York, Avon Books, 1967).

42. A.R. Sherman, *Behavior Modification Theory and Practice* (Monterey, Calif.: Brooks Kole, 1973).

43. C.M. Parkes, "Psycho-Social Transitions," *Social Science and Medicine* 5 (1971): 101-115.

44. Ibid., p. 110.

45. M.S. Kramer, "Conflict: The Cutting Edge of Growth," *Journal of Nursing Ad* October 1976, pp. 19-25.

46. R.D. Nye, *Conflict Among Humans* (New York: Springer Verlag, 1973).

47. J. Bardwick, "Androgyney and Humanistic Goals or Goodbye Cardboard People," in *The American Female: Who Will She Be*, ed. M.L. McBee and K.A. Blake (Beverly Hills, Calif.: Glencoe Press, 1974), p. 63.

48. Leonard J. Stein, "Male and Female: The Doctor-Nurse Game," *Archives of General Psychiatry*, June 1967, pp. 699-703.

9

The Stress of Sexism on the Mental Health of Women

DIANE K. KJERVIK

The mental health of women has been jeopardized by the sexist orientation in our society, a society that has taught women to believe that they are inferior to men. Women are often able to overturn the effects of sexism, at least in part, and to become more assertive, autonomous individuals. Stages through which women pass in confronting sexism are discussed in this chapter along with methods that therapists can use to facilitate this process.

SEXISM: DEFINITION AND MANIFESTATIONS

In order to understand the status of women in this society, the concept of *sexism* must be clarified. Sexism, according to Shortridge, is "a belief that the human sexes have a distinctive make-up that determines their respective lives, usually involving the idea that one sex is superior and has the right to rule the other."[1] Shortridge also includes the political and societal support of such an asserted right in her definition. This concept is similar to the concept of caste, according to which, by birthright, persons' roles within society are fixed. Sexism exists in educational, economic, religious, legal, and political arenas of this society. Less apparent to the public is the sexism that exists in the health care field, specifically in the mental health care system.

Women are cast into societal roles at birth. Women, as a group (and there are always a few exceptions to the rule), are taught in school and in their families to be passive, nurturant, and expressive of emotion, whereas males are reinforced for aggressive, emotionless, and rational behavior. Girls learn to look to boys or men for the answers rather than within themselves. They grow up being encouraged to marry a lawyer rather than to become a lawyer. We know about this sex role socialization process, and some of us know that women earn 57 percent of what men earn according to the government's latest figures. This percentage has been steadily declining since 1960, when women were earning 61 percent of male salaries (median income for year-round, full-time workers).[2] As a sidelight, male nurses earn one-third higher salaries than female nurses on the average.[3] In that money is a kind of power, one can see that women are disadvantaged economically.

Also, in religious, legal, and political areas women are underrepresented in leadership roles. It is interesting that female achievement in occupational, economic, and educational realms between 1940 and 1965 declined to below the pre-1940 levels. Before 1940, women were not equally represented.[4] One could speculate that the declining status of women has been an impetus to the resurgence of the women's movement in the 1960s.

Despite the efforts of the women's movement, sexism holds fast in many facets of our society. Recent evidence points to a lack of progress for women in higher educational administration. Two surveys have found that colleges and universities have not achieved equality for women administrators, in either salaries or number of positions held; in fact, women were found to be grossly underrepresented.[5]

The abortion rights of poor women are threatened by recent congressional action limiting federal funds to pay for abortions. The Supreme Court ruled in December 1976 that companies do not have to pay for pregnancy-related disability benefits (General Electric v. Gilbert), which means that working women must choose between their jobs and motherhood if they suffer disabilities such as severe varicose veins that prohibit walking following labor and delivery.

On the other hand, progress toward equality continues in other places. Married couples, as of June 1977, may maintain individual credit accounts if they so choose. A recall election was held in Madison, Wisconsin, which resulted in the removal of a judge from office for ruling as "normal" the behavior of an adolescent boy who allegedly raped a 16-year-old girl. A nurse who was discharged from the navy in 1967 because she was pregnant will be allowed reinstatment at her old rank and will receive ten years of back pay.[6]

It is not the purpose of this chapter to examine why or how the discrimination against women evolved but rather to focus on one way that sexism is maintained, i.e., by beliefs about the mental health of males and females, respectively.

WOMEN AND MENTAL HEALTH

John Stuart Mill, the great nineteenth century philosopher, acknowledged in his essay entitled "On the Subjection of Women" the importance of the subversion of the mind to the maintenance of the second-class status of women: "All men, except the most brutish, desire to have, in the woman most nearly connected with them, not a forced slave but a willing one, not a slave merely, but a favourite [sic]. They have therefore put everything in practice to enslave their minds."[7] Mill goes on to say that the enslavement of a female's mind occurs as a result of males conveying to females that meekness, submissiveness, and resignation of their will into male hands is essential to sexual attractiveness.[8] Wherever one's identity is so wrapped up in one's sexual attractiveness, as in our society, this form of mental enslavement as described by Mill contributes to keeping women in a submissive, dependent position in relation to men.

Work done by a psychologist in Colorado, Anne Wilson-Schaef, tends to support the idea that women need to seek male (specifically white male) approval. She relates this need for approval to the "original sin of being born female," which she believes every woman carries with her.[9] If males like what a woman does, she can eliminate some of the pain of this original sin that is inherently a part of her femaleness. Thus, a woman can save herself only by being saved by someone else!

Alexandra Symonds, a psychoanalyst, describes women clients who are very successful professionally yet have great dependency needs on the personal level. She notes the difficulty in working with these women because of their deep sense of inferiority and repulsion about their femaleness. These clients believe that they need a man so that they can value themselves.[10]

The effect of this need for validation from others is a tremendous lessening of a woman's self-esteem. In the author's practice as a psychotherapist, she finds that often female patients do not have a negative or poor opinion of themselves; rather, they have no self-concept. When asked what they need or want, they answer that "my father wants me to be . . . " or "my sister thinks I am . . . " They draw a blank on self-evaluations.

One of the author's clients stated that she felt unreal, not human. Part of this nonperson feeling she connected to the possibility of not having a male lover. On the other hand, she felt worthless when she cared for a man, as if her self was abnegated. This conflict manifested a very weak, if not absent, sense of self. Her relationships with females were no better. She distrusted other women and was jealous of any woman her male friend was near. She could not accept these jealous and nonperson feelings and, probably as a result of this, was extremely anxious and suffered from asthmatic attacks. Despite these limitations she was a successful artist. This client was much like Symond's clients who displayed extreme dependency on the personal level. At one point, the client acknowledged her wish to be mothered and admitted that she clung to her "sick role" in an effort to maintain the therapy relationship. The deep dependency need is described by Horney as "having the center of gravity outside oneself."[11]

Another of the author's clients was trying to decide whether to stay in an unsatisfying relationship with a man. One of her primary wishes was to be taken care of by him, and her chief complaint was that he was too dependent on her. She put it this way: "If he needs me that much, he isn't a man." The belief that males and females have distinctly different psychological needs and abilities led this client into a rigid way of viewing herself and her partner. Mental health is often seen as the ability to move flexibly from one stage of development to the next or from one role to another without major conflictual problems. This client's stereotyping held her to a rigid expectation of herself and her friend. It did not allow her to grow beyond the assigned behavior.

These women in therapy acted out, in a sense, attitudes toward females that are present in society. Studies have shown that negative opinions of females prevail generally in our society, among both women and men. Broverman et al. showed that, regardless of the respondent's age, sex, religion, educational level, or marital status, males and females were described differently—men having characteristics in the "competence" realm, and women having characteristics in the "warmth and expressiveness" realm.[12] Very significantly, the male characteristics were more often valued than the female characteristics.

Statistics relating to psychiatric diagnosis, treatment, and prognosis reveal further differences based on sex. Women are more often treated for mental illness;

Chesler's study showed that around 60 percent of the total patient population was female.[13] Brandon found that women are more often admitted to psychiatric hospitals and once there stay longer than men.[14] Fabrikant found similar evidence when he looked at psychotherapy that therapists themselves had received: Female therapists had had more treatment than male therapists and spent more time in psychotherapy. Female patients were found to have been in therapy over twice as long as male patients.[15] Fabrikant's evidence was gathered from the patients' own reports and might have been influenced by the possibility that it is more acceptable for women to be in a sick role in society than it is for men.

Ineichen reports that women, more often than men, are afflicted with neuroses.[16] Seiden states that more women are judged to be clinically depressed than men.[17] Chesler discovered that females are more often labeled depressed, frigid, paranoid, neurotic, suicidal, and anxious. Men's symptoms are alcoholism, drug addiction, personality disorders, and brain diseases.[18] Think of why these diagnostic differences might exist. Notice that the symptoms attributed to women are considered more treatable than the male symptoms. Treatability means, of course, the opportunity to become dependent on a therapist. Since the vast majority of psychotherapists are male, this means another kind of dependence on males in a form different from dependence on a husband or a father.

A 1976 study showed that the use of mood-altering drugs is a major problem for the mental health of women. Women consume 70 percent of prescribed tranquilizers and 72 percent of prescribed antidepressants.[19] This again supports women in their passive patient roles. Thomas Szasz calls the conglomerate of female symptoms "dread of happiness" indicators—part of a slave psychology or, as the author sees it, the psychology of oppression.[20] A question that could be posed is: Do the symptoms really vary or are people placed in slots according to their sex?

A study published in 1976 supports the latter contention by demonstrating that children were apt to be referred to mental health professionals when they demonstrated behavior inappropriate to their sex. That is, when boys were passive or girls were aggressive they were often judged to be in need of psychiatric help.[21]

The judgments in the Feinblatt study were made by graduate students in one of the mental health training programs. What becomes apparent, then, is the importance of the beliefs of the mental health professionals themselves in making supposedly objective decisions about diagnosis and treatment plans. A study conducted by Broverman et al. and published in 1970 showed that mental health professionals considered mental health to be a different phenomenon for males than for females. Mentally healthy males were considered the same as mentally healthy adults, but mentally healthy females were given a separate description. Mature, mentally healthy females were considered to be different from healthy males or adults by being "more submissive. less independent, less adventurous, more easily influenced, less aggressive, less competitive, more excitable in minor crises, having their feelings hurt more easily, being more emotional, more conceited about their appearance, less objective and disliking math and science."[22] The beliefs of these clinicians (psychiatrists, psychologists, and psychiatric social workers) were in agreement with generally held beliefs about the characteristics that are socially desirable for a male or female. Also, there was no significant difference between male and female clinicians in holding these beliefs. The results of this study pointed to a double standard of mental health for males and females, whereby a woman might have to give up her femininity in order to be considered mentally healthy. One wonders then, what route a therapist will take in guiding her or his female client to mental health—a road to femininity or a road to adulthood? Psychotherapists are very influential, not only with individual clients but also in directing societal notions of mental health. The Broverman study indicates a subtle form of sexism being supported by mental health professionals.

The ramifications of this double standard of mental health are great. If females cannot achieve adulthood without losing their femininity, is it any wonder that our language reflects such a situation? For example, women of any age are referred to as girls, and, not surprisingly, masculine pronouns are used generically, to mean everyone. Occasionally reference is made to an individual having to decide whether *he* will have an abortion.[23] Adult males typify normalcy—females are deviations from the norm—and our language reflects this. The problem with the use of "man" for everyone is that authors often switch from the generic to the specific in very confusing ways, especially if the reader is a woman. For example, Swami Ajaya in *Yoga Psychology* discusses the process of meditation by mentioning that people often try to find happiness in external objects, which only provide temporary solice—examples of external objects being a football game, an ice cream cone, or a girl. People are always stated to be "man," of course. Later he says that meditation leads to enriched relationships with other people: "Seeing people less as objects to satisfy your desires allows you to notice things about them which previously went unobserved." However, seeing women as objects seems to be something this swami continues to do after years of meditation.[24]

Is it surprising that women fear success so often, as Matina Horner's studies have found?[25] Studies conducted after Horner's showed that when females feared success it was because they feared social rejection, whereas when males feared success it was the value of success itself that the males questioned.[26] These studies indicating that females fear social rejection if they are successful tend to support Wilson-Schaef's idea of the female need for approval, an approval that begins to seem impossible to find. Approval by males then loses its impact. It becomes meaningless in view of a double standard of mental health. If a woman is commended for aspects of her femininity, then her adulthood is challenged and vice versa. This kind of conflict could lead to emotional problems, and, with women who choose a contemporary sex role behavior, this is apparently what happens. Powell and Reznikoff found that women with contemporary sex role orientations have more symptoms of psychological problems than those who are oriented to traditional roles. They speculated that the reason for this difference is a conflict between personal needs and cultural role expectations within the women with contemporary orientations.[27]

The double standard of mental health also affects treatment plans. A good example of this is an article by Dr. J. Houck entitled "The Intractable Female Patient."[28] Behavioral problems in this type of patient are depression, anxiety, and dependency needs. The treatment suggested is, among other things, that the patient's attention be firmly fixed on home, family, and adult obligations. The husband must also be worked with because "he is obliged to modify lifelong attitudes of passivity and diffidence and to assume a posture of strength and resolution—especially toward his wife."[29] She will resist, of course, and test the husband to see if he means it, "but she is often aware at last that she really hopes she will not win."[30] This physician has taken a prevalent societal attitude that women enjoy being pushed around and has manufactured a psychotherapeutic regimen based on it. Szasz possibly would refer to this as a victimization and dehumanization process that happens to persons who deviate from the norm.[31] It is doubtful that a male would be subjected to this kind of treatment since the diagnosis is in terms of female intractability.

A replication of the Broverman study was published in 1975 which showed that male counselors in training (not female trainees) held differential standards of mental health.[32] A 1974 study showed that female therapists were more accepting of new roles for women than were male therapists.[33] The latter study by Brown and Hellinger in Canada included psychiatric nurses, although their educational backgrounds were not identified. Psychiatric nurses were the most accepting of new roles for women, but Brown and Hellinger were not certain whether this was because of their profession or the fact that most of the nurses were female.

A study that focused on assessments of mental health by psychiatric-mental health nurses prepared at the master's level showed less sex role stereotyping than that found by Broverman in 1970. In fact, these nurses rated ideals of mental health higher for females than males on some traditionally male characteristics such as self-confidence and higher overall on both male and female valued qualities.[34] This was a primarily female clinician population, and some authors believe that female clinicians might hold less sexist attitudes than male therapists.[35] The Kjervik and Palta study indicates the possibility that a different kind of sex role stereotyping is occurring, i.e., that in which females are expected to achieve higher levels of behavior than males in order to be considered "healthy" by clinicians. This could be indicative of attitude change, possibly a swing away from old sexist ideals to new beliefs.[36]

Expecting more from females could have the beneficial effect of the self-fulfilling prophecy: If you expect little, you often get little in return. Women so often look to external persons for encouragement or validation that, if they get this from a psychiatric nurse, they may respond favorably, by meeting higher standards. On the other hand, being expected to leave a comfortable status in a traditional female role for a more demanding role as combination career woman and homemaker might be a problem.

The research that has been presented indicates that a change in attitude with regard to women's roles in society is possibly occurring. Traits that have been labeled masculine such as aggressiveness and leadership are being seen more often as proper for women as well as for men. Traditional female qualities such as expression of tender feelings are becoming more acceptable for men. In this sense, a kind of androgyny is evolving, not in which males and females are the same any more than individual persons are carbon copies of one another, but in which males and females can choose from among a variety of behaviors and not feel compelled to act passively or aggressively if they do not want to.

This change has become apparent in our language. Politicians are now more careful to say "women" instead of "girls," and many curricula in the human service areas are substituting the concept of humankind or humanity for mankind. Simone de Beauvoir in her book *The Second Sex* talks about the "otherness" of the female.[37] The male is the subject—he is the doer—whereas the female is the object—she has things done to her or watches the male being active. It is hoped that changing language usage will bring the female into the subject category and out of her role as "the other." If our language acknowledges both female and male counterparts, women will learn to think of themselves as responsible, important adults.

As women have been considered "others" in society, so, too, have they been thought of as "others" in their roles as health care givers. Anne Davis reported during the American Nurses' Association convention in June 1976 that female psychotherapists are stereotypically considered to be quiet, practical, nurturant earth mothers.[38] Chesler notes that there are many more male therapists than female therapists in the two leading mental health groups—psychiatry and psychology.[39] These evidences of sexism may be removed as the public and health care givers learn that female clinicians often have attitudes that are less sexist than those of their male colleagues.

UNDOING THE SEXISM IN MENTAL HEALTH

The major aspects of the concept of mental health that have been alluded to thus far and that are pertinent to this section are the following: (1) a sense of self, (2) a sense of control or authority over one's own self, (3) communication of one's needs and desires to others, and (4) valuing oneself. Women have learned that others are more important than they are and that they exist to serve others rather than to develop themselves. This is detrimental to reaching a mentally healthy state. As one client said, "My happiness comes when others are happy." Pleasing herself, for herself only, did not occur to her. When the author was a child she was told that pleasing herself was selfish and to be avoided. Selfishness could be restated as self-assertiveness and then not seen in such a negative light. Total other-directedness leads to not knowing oneself. Males, by the way, suffer from the impact of sexism as well. They must affiliate with individuals on an unequal basis, i.e., with women who cannot state a need or desire clearly and thus look totally to males for support, placing a great burden on the males.

Four stages through which women pass in undoing their own sexist attitudes will now be discussed. These ideas are based both on the author's work with clients and contact with other women who were at various stages and on her own growth and change as well.

Stage 1: Making Connections

This stage could be likened to a honeymoon; i.e., one that is pleasant. The "Ah ha" reaction is predominant, and the woman is delighted to see that things that made her feel uncomfortable in her past now make sense. She may have wondered why masculine pronouns are used for everyone, why female nudity and rape are more common than male nudity and rape, and why physicians are mostly male. Now these odd occurrences fall together and manifest a pattern. The woman also experiences a sense of diminished guilt, which is refreshing. Whereas she felt guilt for being uncomfortable about these things and receiving strange looks at parties for mentioning them, she can now comment on them and know that others (persons sympathetic to the women's movement) are with her. The extent of her exposure to feminist ideas and feminist persons will determine the length of time spent in this stage and following stages.

Stage 2: Anger

Because enlightenment alone does not remove the problem, the woman begins to be irritated. She thinks, "It makes so much sense. Why don't others want to change their behaviors? Anything this obvious should be easy to remedy. It's so logically wrong." She begins to show others the errors of their ways. She may give men dirty looks for opening doors for her or make sure that, when a man touches her, she touches him back (and in the same place) or insist that she be addressed as Ms. rather than Miss or Mrs. This is the time when she joins a consciousness-raising group, which serves to increase her anger and outrage as she listens to the numerous injustices suffered by her "sisters." She begins to experience the problem of sexism as overwhelming, and she may at this point enter therapy (usually with a female therapist) to handle the growing anger. Some clients project fear onto the therapist, expressing their concern that the therapist might be overwhelmed by their anger.

Stage 3: Action

After the woman discovers that her anger can be expressed without destroying herself or others, she begins working (usually with a feminist group) to undo sexist practices. She attends lectures on legislative effectiveness and assertiveness and begins to practice these. She takes a less hostile approach than in the previous stage and therefore expects to be effective in changing others' behaviors. Change does not come as quickly as she expects, because her expectations continue to be based on what she now thinks is logically right and just treatment for women. Since sexism defies her newly acquired sense of right and wrong, her expectations are not met and she becomes hopeless and depressed.

Stage 4: Balance

As the woman shares her hopelessness with others in therapy or women's groups, she learns that these feelings have been experienced by others, and she learns that she can reach out for support from other women and receive it. This point is extremely important because her previous socialization has taught her not to trust other women (they might take her man away from her). She learns the necessity of delaying gratification because attitude change does not happen in a few weeks. However, she does not lose her commitment to the cause. Within women's groups she learns to work for small, objective changes, one at a time. The author worked on an "action" with a local women's group to enable nurse-midwives to have their names on the birth certificates of the babies they delivered. A great sense of satisfaction was experienced by the author when a favorable decision was made by the State Department of Health. The woman learns patience with others who are in previous stages or who have not even reached stage 1. Part of her patience comes from the realization that what is logical, right, and just will not happen right away because the feelings that support sexism (inferiority vs. superiority) are not based on logic—*they just are*.

Therapist's Role in Undoing Sexism

When a woman has not reached the first stage of undoing her own sexist beliefs, the therapist may be faced with an extremely difficult task, i.e., dealing with a woman who genuinely believes that she is inferior to men. An extreme example of a woman in this position is one who is being battered by her male companion. A less extreme example is the "happy homemaker" who probably would not come into therapy for herself but might appear because of her concern with another family member. The ethical question for the therapist is whether to begin pointing out the realities of sexism in order to foster the onset of stage 1.

In these cases, the therapist can question the happiness or satisfaction that is expressed by the woman. She may ask, "If you're so happy, what about these problems in your family?" Then if the client retorts, "I just want to learn how to please my husband," the therapist can ask what she thinks pleases him. Often a double-binding situation is discovered in which the husband directs the wife to do her own thing, stand up to him, be intelligent, and express her desires. He also expects her to do what he tells her to do, e.g., make his meals and clean the house. The treatment in this instance would be the same as dealing with any double-binding communication, i.e., increasing the awareness of the dysfunctional pattern and/or changing the relationship rules through the use of therapeutic double binds.[40],[41]

Dealing with these women is similar to being faced with someone who denies the reality of a death. Change is needed, but the woman isn't ready for it. She would have to give up too much of herself. As in working with denial, the therapist would not hit the problem head on, thus reinforcing the defensiveness. Rather, it would be important to follow the immediate concerns of the woman and to role-model attention giving. Assuming that she will learn behavior displayed by the therapist, the woman will learn to attend more accutely to herself. Battered women may need direction (rather than support) such as, "No one deserves to be hit or pushed around."

The therapist's role is one of teaching new attitudes through role modeling. Respecting the woman (having an idea of what has led to her current behavior) while not agreeing with the values that she expresses is important for the therapist for use in dealing with the woman's other relationships, e.g., with unruly children or a difficult husband. As in dealing with a suicidal patient, the therapist should show the woman alternative choices for action. Exaggeration of the existing situation can be used as a paradoxical strategy to change the problematic behavior. Watzlawick might refer to this strategy as prescribing the symptom.[42] For instance, the therapist may direct the client to "elaborate on the feeling about yourself when you are waiting on your husband. What is that like for you?" She may discover that "waiting on" is not always fun and that there is a tiny bit of resentment for the giving without receiving.

During stage 1, the woman probably will not seek out therapy for sexism-related concerns. The enlightenment is rewarding. When she becomes angry in stage 2, the feelings might become overwhelming so that rage needs to be expressed.

Wilson-Schaef provides a "rage room" where women can vent this anger by hitting or destroying items of their choice without having to clean up their messes.[43] It is useful not to allow the woman to vent all her anger, because anger is a form of energy that is basic to the action stage. During the third stage, the woman may want to develop assertiveness skills, which the therapist can facilitate. Along with assertiveness, the woman needs to learn more about what she wants and needs so that she knows what to assert. This builds her sense of self. When she becomes hopeless during stage 3, the therapist should provide a supportive atmosphere of listening and responding to the woman's concerns. Reminding her that change will take a long time will help her to begin to put the desired changes in a reality-centered perspective. Helping her to see that being assertive about what she wants does not guarantee getting what she wants will again teach her the limitations of reality. This reality is the boundary between herself and other's selves. Again, this will help her to develop her self-concept.

FEMINIST-ORIENTED COUNSELING

In the practice of psychotherapy, a new interest in feminist-oriented therapy has evolved. According to Williams, feminist therapy gears itself to the following goals:[44]

1. To support women who are struggling to become assertive

2. To increase women's sense of power, self-esteem, and autonomy

3. To help women lessen self-defeating feelings in roles they currently play

4. To help women see that they have choices in their patterns of living

5. To give women insights into the connection between their own behaviors and societal structures that nurture these behaviors

6. To acknowledge the therapist's socialization as a woman, which might lead to a kind of motherly "overprotectiveness"

The goals direct the therapist as well as the client. For example, goal 6 is the expectation that the therapist will be aware of her own conditioning within society which affects her ongoing behavior in therapy. Reynolds discusses what she considers to be distinctive elements of the feminist perspective in counseling. One element is the assumption that all women are oppressed, and another is that women are distinct human persons who are not extensions of other persons. To this end, the therapist must identify her own oppression and empathize with the oppression of her clients. Reynolds recommends that her clients attend consciousness-raising groups, women's support groups, or assertiveness training groups so that they will begin to believe that change can be made. She also recommends bibliotherapy with feminist-oriented books if the client enjoys reading.[45]

Both Reynolds and Williams emphasize the importance of the therapist's self-knowledge and appreciation of her own oppression. It is useful for the therapist to review her past in order to decipher any sexist messages that were taught her. One such message might be that girls should grow up to marry men who are stronger and more intelligent than they are. This overlooks several possibilities for a woman: that she may choose a man of equal intelligence or strength, that she may choose a female partner, or that she may choose no one at all, to mention a few. The therapist must examine her feelings about these various possibilities for life styles. Some therapists and educators have noticed a change in their attitudes toward their clients after they have begun to conceive of their students or clients as women rather than girls. Kronsky also believes that the feminist-oriented therapist should be aware of the subjective experience of being caught in a double-binding kind of situation in the male-dominated society. She concludes that in this sense, the feminist-oriented therapist may have to be a female.[46] Self-knowledge on the therapist's part, as this is shared with the client, gives the client the message that it is valuable to know oneself and that it is acceptable to develop control over oneself. In this way, the therapist role-models self-appreciation.

Williams discusses the value of role modeling expressions of anger with the depressed woman. The depressed woman often suppresses competitive urges and feels guilty about having these urges. She is basically angry about having to behave "nicely" toward persons who treat her shabbily, usually persons who are perceived as authority figures. The woman needs to learn that expressing angry feelings is acceptable. If the therapist expresses her own anger openly to the patient, the patient learns that it is acceptable for her to do the same. If the therapist does not role-model this anger, the woman is reinforced in believing that she is bad or guilty for feeling hurt or anger, since the authority figure, in this case the therapist, apparently doesn't ever feel anger.[47]

Kronsky suggests that, if a woman is feeling guilty about overidentification with males in her life, a feminist-oriented therapist should attempt to remove the woman's guilt instead of emphasizing an interpretation such as penis envy. Identification with males could be considered normal in a male-dominated society in which males are able to be assertive. The woman in identifying with males is possibly in touch with her wish to become assertive.[48]

Although one of the goals of feminist-oriented therapy is to increase the woman's sense of power over her destiny, the therapist could possibly exacerbate the woman's feeling of inadequacy by reminding her of all the power that she has lying dormant. Wilson-Schaef believes that, if the therapist tells the client how much power she has, it will reinforce society's message that she is too sick, bad, crazy, or stupid to have known this.[49] It seems that a better approach is to build on the woman's statement of concern in the here-and-now situation, as has been described previously.

IMPLICATIONS FOR EDUCATION AND RESEARCH

Educational programs should gear themselves not only to conscious manifestations of sexism, such as those found in textbooks, but also to less obvious forms, such as nonverbal expressions of approval given by teachers to students. In other words, negative attitudes about women should be explored in a discussion of students' feelings about the changing roles of women and men in society in conjunction with provision of facts about the status of women in society.

Research should focus on clinicians' attitudes toward female and male clients, effects of clinicians' attitudes on outcomes of therapy, the status of women's self-concepts, the public's understanding of sexism and its ramifications, and psychotherapeutic or educational practices that are effective in removing sexist attitudes. Both research and education are vital to changing the attitudes in our society from androcentric to androgynous.

CONCLUSION

It is apparent that legal, economic, religious, and health care positions will have to be changed in order to deal with the totality of sexism. And yet it is comforting to accept the system-theory principle that a change in a part will effect a change in the whole. If a change can be made in society's view of the mentally healthy state of women, perhaps changes in other areas of society will follow.

NOTES

1. K. Shortridge, "Women as University Nigger," *University of Michigan Daily Magazine,* April 12, 1970, pp. 4-5, 21.

2. U.S. Department of Commerce, Bureau of the Census, *A Statistical Portrait of Women in the U.S.* (Washington, D.C.: U.S. Government Printing Office, April 1976).

3. W. Chapman *Minneapolis Star,* February 26, 1974, p. 8B.

4. D. Knudsen, "The Declining Status of Women: Popular Myths and the Failure of Functionalist Thought," *Social Forces* 48, no. 2 (December 1969): 183-193.

5. "Women Administrators Found Unequal in Pay Status," *Chronicle of Higher Education* 14, no. 16, (June 1977): 8.

6. *Spokeswoman* 8, no. 1 (July 1977): 7-8.

7. J.S. Mill, "The Subjection of Women," *Essays on Sex Equality,* ed. A. Rossi (Chicago: University of Chicago Press, 1970), p. 141.

8. Ibid., p. 142

9. Anne Wilson-Schaef, Presentation given at Unity Church, St. Paul, Minn. May 3, 1976.

10. Alexandra Symonds, "Neurotic Dependency in Successful Women," *Journal of American Academy of Psychoanalysis* 4, no. 1 (1976): 96-102.

11. Alexandra Symonds, "The Liberated Woman: Healthy and Neurotic," *American Journal of Psychoanalysis* 34, no. 3 (1974).

12. I. Broverman et al., "Sex-Role Stereotypes: A Current Appraisal," *Journal of Social Issues* 8, no. 2 (1972): 59-78.

13. Phyllis Chesler, *Women and Madness* (Garden City, N.Y.: Doubleday and Co., 1972), p. 119.

14. Sydney Brandon, "Psychiatric Illness in Women," *Nursing Mirror* 34, (January 1972): 17-18.

15. Benjamin Fabrikant, "The Psychotherapist and the Female Patient: Perceptions, Misperceptions, and Change," Violet Franks and Vasanti Burtle, eds. (New York: Brunner-Mazel 1974), 94-96.

16. Bernard Ineichen, "Neurotic Wives in a Modern Residential Suburb: A Modern Residential Profile," *Social Science and Medicine,* 9 (1975): 481-487.

17. Anne M. Seiden, "Overview: Research on the Psychology of Women. II. Women in Families, Work and Psychotherapy," *American Journal of Psychiatry* 113, no. 10 (October 1976): 1115.

18. Chesler, *Women and Madness,* p. 40.

19. *Spokeswoman,* p. 12.

20. Chesler, *Woman and Madness,* p. 40.

21. J. Feinblatt, and A. Gold, "Sex Roles and the Psychiatric Referral Process," *Sex Roles: A Journal of Research* 2, no. 2 (June 1976): 109-122.

22. I. Broverman, et al., "Sex-Role Stereotypes and Clinical Judgments of Mental Health," *Journal of Consulting and Clinical Psychology*. 34, no. 1 (1970): 1-7.

23. *Ms.* 3, no. 8 (February 1975): 93.

24. Swami Ajaya, *Yoga Psychology: A Guide to Practical Meditation,* 2 vols. (Glenview, Ill.: Himalayan International Institute of Yoga Science and Philosophy of U.S.A., 1974), vol. 1, pp. 17-23.

25. M. Horner, "Fail: Bright Women," *Psychology Today* 3, no. 6 (November 1969): 36-38.

26. D. Tresemer, "Fear of Success: Popular, but Unproven," *Psychology Toady* 7, no. 1 (March 1974): 82-85.

27. Barbara Powell and M. Reznikoff, "Role Conflict and Symptoms of Psychological Distress in College Educated Women," *Journal of Consulting and Clinical Psychology* 44, no. 3 (1976): 473-479.

28. J. Houck, "The Intractable Female Patient," *American Journal of Psychiatry* 129, no. 1 (July 1972): 27.

29. Ibid., p. 30.

30. Ibid., p. 31.

31. Thomas Szasz quoted in S. Rosner, "The Rights of Mental Patients: The New Massachusetts Law," *Mental Hygiene* 56 (Winter 1972): 117-119.

32. Feinblatt and Gold, "Sex Roles," pp. 109-122.

33. D.R. Brown and M.S. Hellinger, "Therapists' Attitudes toward Women," *Social Work* 20 (July 1975): 266-270.

34. Diane Kjervik and Mari Palta, "Sex-Role Stereotyping in Assessments of Mental Health Made by Psychiatric-Mental Health Nurses," *Nursing Research,* 27, No. 3 (May-June): 166,171.

35. American Psychological Association, *Report of the Task Force on Sex Bias and Sex-Role Stereotyping* (August 1975), p. 8. Washington, D.C.

36. Kjervik and Palta, "Sex-Role Stereotyping."

37. Simone de Beauvoir, *Le Deuxième Sexe* (Paris: Gallimard, 1949).

38. Anne Davis, "Issues in the Mental Health of Women," audiotape, American Nurses' Association Convention, Atlantic City, N.J., June, 1976. On-the-Spot Duplicators, Northridge, Calif.

39. Chesler, *Women and Madness,* pp. 61-65.

40. Paul Watzlawick, *An Anthology of Human Communication* (Palo Alto, Calif.: Science and Behavior Books, 1964), p. 48.

41. Paul Watzlawick, J. Beavin, and D. Jackson, *Pragmatics of Human Communication* (New York: W. W. Norton and Co., 1967), pp. 240-248.

42. Watzlawick, *Human Communication,* pp. 236-240.

43. Wilson-Schaef, Presentation at Unity Church.

44. E.F. Williams, *Notes of a Feminist Therapist* (New York: Praeger Publishers, 1976), pp. 6-10.

45. Phyllis Reynolds, "Counseling from a Feminist Perspective," *Student Counseling Bureau Review* (University of Minnesota) 26, no. 1 (September 1975): 56-60.

46. Betty Kronsky, "Feminism and Psychotheraphy," *Journal of Contemporary Psychotherapy* 3, no. 2 (Spring 1971): 98.

47. Williams, *Feminist Therapist,* p. 109-110.

48. Kronsky, "Feminism and Psychotherapy," p. 97.

49. Wilson-Schaef, Presentation to Unity Church.

10
The Mexican American Woman
Stress Related to Health, Health Beliefs, and Health Practices

MAUREEN JAUREZ
EVANGELINE GRONSETH

ILLNESS AS A STRESSOR TO MEXICAN AMERICAN WOMEN

This chapter provides an example of stress experienced by the Mexican American woman. For her the experience of illness of self or of family member can be a particular stressor. Health-related beliefs and practices as well as factors within the health care delivery system may serve to exacerbate or to alleviate stress.

Health Needs

Illness is reported to be a common experience in the Mexican American population. Mexican Americans have usually been aggregated with other whites in official records, so a review of their health statistics is difficult. Some studies, however, have reported specific health data of the Mexican American population.

In a Colorado study, cited by Moustafa and Weiss, the mean age of death for Spanish-surnamed persons living for more than one year was 56.7 years, in contrast to 67.5 years for all other persons. People with Spanish surnames were more likely to die from rheumatic fever, pneumonia, and influenza than were those of the Anglo population. It was also found that neonatal deaths were three times higher in the Spanish surname group than among the Anglos.[1] Such findings reflect the general health and nutrition of the mother, her prenatal care, and the conditions at or following delivery.

Among the major health needs of Mexican Americans are dental care, tuberculosis detection and treatment, alcoholism treatment, prenatal care and family planning, preventive mental health treatment, and health services for preschoolers and adolescents. Respiratory diseases and back problems are reported to be common among farm workers.

□ *The effects of cultural beliefs on health.* A number of traditional cultural beliefs have been identified by ethnographers in investigations of Mexican Americans in enclaves isolated from Anglo influences. These beliefs include a fatalistic view of illness, with little understanding of preventive medicine; the use of folk health practices, with distrust of scientific health practice; and extensive family involvement in the diagnosis and treatment of an ill member. Illness has been defined both in terms of adequate functioning and in subjective terms. The etiology of a number of diseases is based upon folk concepts rather than upon the "germ theory."

It has been proposed that traditional cultural beliefs form a barrier to effective utilization of scientific health care and negatively influence the health of the Mexican American. For example, Foster has described situations in which gravely ill children have been cared for at home instead of being seen either by the doctor or in the hospital.[2] The physician has been consulted only as a last resort, when the disease has been advanced. It is notable however, that there have been no studies related to the morbidity or mortality of persons using such alternative forms of health care.[3]

□ *Socioeconomic conditions and health.* Many studies of Mexican American health conditions have included sample populations with low incomes. It is questionable to what extent the findings reflect ethnic factors since health conditions are known to directly reflect economic conditions. It is generally accepted that there is an association between illness and low socioeconomic level because of factors such as overcrowded housing and inadequate diet. The high incidence of diabetes in Mexican Americans is possibly related to the high starch diet which frequently accompanies poverty—however, genetic as well as other factors cannot be excluded.[4] The high morbidity and mortality rate prevalent among Mexican Americans does directly relate to their predominantly low socioeconomic level. There are higher rates of death from causes such as pneumonia and premature births, which are often associated with lower socioeconomic conditions.[5] Tuberculosis rates range above national and city averages; however, Mexican Americans are less likely to die of neoplasms, vascular diseases, and heart diseases.[6] Those diseases, associated with aging, are usually less common among poverty populations, which have higher mortality at earlier age levels.[7]

□ *Utilization of scientific health services.* There are few statistics relative to Mexican American utilization of health facilities and hospitals. Reeder and Reeder found Latin American women the least prompt among ethnic groups in seeking early prenatal care.[8] However, they were significantly more regular in clinic attendance. Lindstrom reported no differences in attendance patterns of mothers with children in a clinic facility among low-income whites, blacks, and Mexican Americans.[9]

A 1955 California study found that Mexican Americans have a lower physician-visitation rate per person per year (2.3) than blacks (3.7) or Anglos (5.6), as well as the lowest frequency of hospital admissions per 1,000 persons (16, compared to 82 for blacks and 95 for Anglos). The writers warn that these lower rates may reflect limitations of the survey instrument, problems of communication associated with language barriers, or an unwillingness to admit illness for fear it could lead to investigation by authorities.[10]

Psychiatric facilities have been reported to be underused by Mexican Americans. Jaco related the lower rate of major psychoses to the warm supportive qualities of the subculture.[11] In their investigations of perceptions of mental illness, Karno and Edgerton found that underutilization was accounted for not by different perceptions and definitions of mental illness but by many social and cultural factors.[12]

The factors identified as of most importance were the language barrier, the active mental health role of the general practitioner, the lowered self-esteem induced by the nature of the agency, and lack of facilities in the Mexican American community. Factors of less importance were the open borders that facilitated a return to Mexico, folk medicine, and the Mexican culture.

Morales presented statistics to show that Spanish-surnamed persons in Los Angeles recognized their need for psychiatric services, in that they made more self- and family referrals than did blacks or Anglos.[13] He reported that Mexican Americans were grossly overrepresented in state prisons and jails for illegal drug use and alcoholism, and underrepresented in treatment programs. The seven alcohol-rehabilatative centers closest to the East Los Angeles area were reported to serve few Spanish-surnamed persons and had no bilingual professionals. Their services were rather directed to the more affluent Anglos. Information as to utilization of scientific health services therefore indicates differences in various locations and types of programs.

Sources of Health Knowledge

Numerous health factors have been identified as potential stressors in their relationship to illness. In dealing with the stress of illness, the Mexican American woman can draw upon many sources of health knowledge. Saunders has theorized that ideas concerning illness and treatment for the Spanish-speaking person of the Southwest have come from four sources.[14] Three of these sources are of folk origin, and one belief is derived from scientific theory.

The first source is the folklore medicine of medieval Spain as refined in Mexico. From this source has come the concept of *balance*, an idea based on the Hippocratic doctrine of the four humours: blood, phlegm, black bile, and yellow bile. The humours have qualities of wetness and heat associated with them. A body not in balance possesses an excess of heat and moisture. The purpose of medicine is to restore a balance in the body, through diet, medicines, purging, vomiting, bleeding, and cupping.[15] Other influences from medieval times include the culture of the Celts, who stressed the importance of fire and water to effect healing and restore body balance; the prayers of Christianity; and the Arabs' beliefs concerning the "evil eye."[16]

The second source of health knowledge identified by Saunders has been derived from the cultures of the American Indian tribes. These tribes have added the concepts of soul loss, of possession by spirits, and of witchcraft to the Mexican American concepts of disease.

The third source of health knowledge referred to by Saunders is Anglo folk medicine as practiced in both rural and urban areas. This includes nonprescription drugs and treatments and the use of such practitioners as chiropractors.

Finally, concepts of illness and of treatment have come from the scientific practice of medicine. These concepts require the establishment of objectively verifiable laws of etiology and treatment.[17] They include the use of health professionals, clinics, hospitals, and prescription medications.

Some comparisons can be drawn between the practices of folk and of scientific medicine. First, folk practices are the unique possession of a group, and are transmitted from person to person. They are not subject to scientific evaluation; remedies empirically ineffective will not be used. Scientific health practices are founded on the scientific method of inquiry. Its theories are expected to be continually reexamined in search of more effective health practices. One of the basic tenets is that of the germ theory, which has no meaning in folk medicine. Practitioners of scientific medicine are highly qualified academically. Although the practices of both folk and scientific medicine differ, an interchange between the two exist in which remedies developed by one become a part of the other.[18]

Traditional Views of Health and Illness

There are a number of folk concepts of health and illness that relate to the extent to which illness constitutes a stressor in the traditional culture of Mexican Americans.

☐ *Definitions of health and illness.* The traditional definition of health is composed of several criteria. One criterion, and possibly the most important, is that a person function appropriately for his age and sex role, demonstrating a high level of physical activity. Thus, within the context of normal activity, a person with a sore throat, diarrhea, running nose, or productive cough may not be considered ill. This criterion has been particularly important in the village society in which it has been formulated, since adequate functioning has been imperative for maintenance of the subsistence economy.

A second criterion of health is that an individual have a well-fleshed body and a robust appearance. A fat adult is considered stronger than a slim adult and may therefore be assigned harder work. A thin child may cause much anxiety to his parents.[19]

The final criterion of health is the "feeling state" of the individual. Pain, for instance, may give some indication of illness even when an individual is functioning appropriately. More objective criteria, such as paleness, rashes, and droopy eyes may also be used.[20]

Health is seen to be a situation of balance. Any disruption of the balance between parts of the body, between the individual and society, or between human beings and supernatural beings can produce illness and distress.

One balance identified by several researchers is that of heat and cold. The healthy body is thought to contain a combination of hot and cold components. If an imbalance occurs, illness results. Treatment involves ingestion of food that is classified as "hot" for a cold illness, and "cold" for an essentially hot illness.[21]

Other imbalances that have been identified by Madsen are the dislocation of a bone, the shifting of an organ, foreign objects or evil forces entering the body, immoral behavior, and strife in interpersonal relations.[22]

☐ *Perceptions of illness.* Illness fulfills a variety of functions in traditional Mexican American culture. It may serve to publicize and to punish social offenses. It may provide a means for exempting group members from societal disapproval by affording them a rationale for otherwise unsanctioned behavior, and it may dramatize the evil consequences of cultural change in an attempt to defend the old ways. Illness also serves to ease difficult social situations created by conflicting Anglo and Latin values. Moreover, illness is considered a social as well as a biologic phenomena. While it may be perceived to be the result of the disruption of social relations, it may also be perceived to be the result of scientifically recognized etiologic agents.[23]

Illness is viewed as a particularly unpleasant stressful state, both because of the physical pain and suffering involved and because of the increasing loss of respect for those who are unable to function fully. Adults, and males especially, attempt to continue their usual duties as long as possible, despite illness. This action is attributed to the need for income and to the importance to the male of being considered "macho" or rugged. The younger the child, the less he is expected to bear illness stoically. The adult emphasis on strength and stamina, however, influences attitudes toward sick children. Children are sometimes sent to school with colds, with tonsillitis, or with skin eruptions. Pregnancy is not considered an illness, but rather a delicate state in which duties should be restricted.[24]

☐ *Etiology of illness.* Classification of folk diseases has been accomplished in accordance with disease causation. Good or natural illnesses are reported to result from violation of the balance of the world controlled by God; bewitchment is caused by human adversaries who utilize evil, satanic forces. While treatment for a natural illness involves restoration of the disrupted balance, treatment for bewitchment involves countermagic or removal of the source of harm. An exception is Madsen's finding that the more anglicized Latins use the term "natural disease" to refer to illness resulting from natural phenomena, such as infections or accidents, and "supernatural illnesses" to refer to those caused by God or the devil.[25]

THE WOMAN'S ROLE IN ILLNESS

The Traditional Role

☐ *The curing role.* Traditionally, Mexican American women have taken an active part in the validation, diagnosis, treatment, and prevention of illness in family members and friends. Family and close friends have formed the group that has "validated" the illness of an individual. The latter has customarily presented his symptoms to this group before seeking medical treatment. Following the diagnosis of illness, the group has subsequently relieved him of duties and has supported him, supervising and carrying out the treatment process.

Much has been written about the "curer" in the traditional folk beliefs of Mexican Americans. There is a reported hierarchy of folk curers to whom one can appeal for assistance. This hierarchy begins with the women of the family, including the eldest daughter, the mother, and the grandmother. It extends to the experienced neighbor and progresses to the full-time healer. Mild illness is treated at home by the women relatives; severe illness is referred to those higher in the hierarchy.

The experienced neighbor or the full-time curer may be either male or female. Romano has identified role differences related to the sex of the curers. A woman will assist the grandmother in care of the ill person, while the male will more likely give instructions related to the preparation and dosage of medications. Respected characteristics of the male individual (independence and autonomy) are not necessarily characteristic of a curer.[26]

The term *curandera* is used to refer to folk curers in the upper levels of the hierarchy.[27] These curers are thought to receive their power from God, to maintain relationships with deceased healers, and to be characterized by personal qualities of a deviant nature.

Characteristics of the services of the curer include the maintenance of a warm, intimate contact with the family and the patient. The nature of the illness is often determined by a dream or by an observable sign but with little specific questioning of the patient. Diagnosis is usually familiar to the patient, and treatment is uncomplicated. The *curandera* does not dictate what should be done. Relatives can make suggestions and criticize, and they may reject her advice. She may charge a small fee for service, or she may merely accept a gift as remuneration. The *curandera* has a background similar to that of her clients, is usually well known by them, follows the same social customs, and speaks Spanish.[28]

Another type of folk healer is a *partera*, or midwife. She is usually an older woman and a mother. The *partera* is preferred to a doctor because of her gender, her understanding related to the fears and pains of delivery, and her greater patience in permitting a more natural course of delivery.

The use of folk curers has been reported to have been extensive in the South and in limited geographic areas where the ethnic population has been characterized by a high degree of cultural homogeneity. It is postulated that in such areas "attitudes and beliefs may have influenced behavior with respect to health practices and medical care to such an extent that differences in morbidity, disability, and perhaps even mortality, became apparent."[29]

☐ *Description of five folk illnesses.* Five folk illnesses that are common in Mexican American folk health culture, include *susto, caida de la mollera, mal ojo, empacho,* and *mal puesto.* A study of seventy-five Mexican American housewives in a public housing project in 1966 revealed that 97 percent knew about the five diseases, while 95 percent reported one or more instances of the occurence of these illnesses in themselves, in family members, or in acquaintances. Each of the five illnesses will be described in the following paragraphs.

Mal ojo, or "evil eye," is believed to result from excessive admiration or desire on the part of another. All individuals are susceptible to this disease, but the weaker nature of women and children make them more susceptible to this disease than adult males. The strong glance or attention exposes a person to a power like electricity, which drains the afflicted person of the will to act. Symptoms include headache, fitful sleep, fever, and, for children, crying without cause. Evil eye can be prevented if the potential culprit, after admiring a child, touches him. Recommended treatment is to find the person who has cast the spell and induce him to touch the victim. If this is not possible, treatment consists of a ritual by which the power is drawn out into some other object, such as an egg. Evil eye is not generally interpreted to be a consequence of evil intention, although Madsen has theorized that evil eye is a possible reflection of envy.[30]

Empacho, or "ball in the stomach," can produce illness in both children and adults. The several etiologic factors with which it is associated include undigested food clinging to the wall of the stomach, the involuntary ingestion of foods, the malicious contamination of food by a personal enemy, and constipation. The most common symptom of *empacho* is reportedly stomach pain. Infants may manifest symptoms of diarrhea, vomiting, and fever. Treatment includes the administration of an oral medication, such as a purgative or a mercury derivative, and the therapeutic massage of either the back or the stomach.[31]

Caida de la mollera, or "fallen fontanel" is a disease of the very young. It is thought that infants have a very fragile skull that is in balance with the palate. A blow on the head or a jolt to the suckling infant may precipitate injury to the palate and to the fontanel, with the subsequent interference with the ability to nurse. Diagnosis is effected by the location of a depression over the anterior fontanel. Symptoms include excessive crying, insomnia, digestive upset, and loss of appetite accompanied by high fever. Treatment involves the use of various means to raise the fontanel, such as the application of a poultice over the fontanel; upward pressure on the palata; and holding the child upside down to reposition the fontanel. It has been observed that *mollera caida* occurs when there is dehydration caused by infant diarrhea, and the loss of subcutaneous fluid from the anterior fontanel. There is "confusion as the cause and effect in folk belief; the depressed fontanel and the exaggeration of palatal rugae resulting from fluid loss are assumed to be primary causative factors."[32]

Susto, or "fright sickness," results from a fearful situation, such as an encounter with a ghost, or by the narrow escape from injury inflicted by a vehicle. A part of the self, the spirit, is thought either to leave the body or to become paralyzed inside the body. Rubel states that this illness is the reaction to an inability to fulfill the societal expectations to which one has been accustomed, a manifestation of role helplessness.[33] Symptoms of *susto* include exhaustion, restlessness, loss of appetite, and excessive fear. *Susto* is a very serious disease that, if not recognized and treated, results in death. One cure is effected by placing the person on the floor, followed by sweeping motions with a branch. Prayers and the Apostolic Creed may be recited. The spirit of the person will then be asked to rejoin his body. This treatment usually lasts several days; both the patient and the curer know when the cure has been effected.[34]

Mal puesto is "witchcraft," an unnatural disease. A person can do harm to his enemy by enlisting a witch to put a hex on him. It it thought that the most common type of hex is "image magic," such as poking pins into dolls which represent the intended victims. Motives for witchcraft are related to areas of social friction, such as envy, sexual jealousy, and vengeance. One study found that Mexican American women knew less about this disease than about other folk illnesses. However, it is also suggested that they may refuse to discuss this subject because of embarassment or fear. The diagnosis of *mal puesto* is difficult because it manifests itself in many forms. After treatment for other diseases has failed, *mal puesto* is suspect. Other symptoms, such as those accompanying forms of mental illness, may be signs of bewitchment. Nervousness and insomnia, as well as the deformation of an infant, may also be classified this way. The treatment of witchcraft can be effected by the identification of the witch and by coercing her to undo the hex, or by destruction of the material used for the hex. Knowledge of the hex is gained through the use of spiritualist curers. Amulets and prayers are sold for protection, but are not really believed to be effective as a cure.[35]

Witches are a malevolent source of illness in Mexican American folklore. They are considered to be in league with the devil. Persons who are without sin are not subject to their power. However, it is known that everyone has sinned, and so every Mexican American is thus susceptible.

□ *The concept of disease prevention and health promotion.* Early ethnographic studies of Mexican Americans substantiate findings that health is considered a matter of chance, that there is little a person can do to maintain it. Health and illness are sent by supernatural beings over which man has no control. However, rapid treatment is valued if the potential for illness exists.

□ *Hospitalization as a stressor.* A basic tenet of the cultural interpretation of health behavior is that hospitalization is extremely stressful for Mexican Americans. Good medical care is seen to involve home treatment. Hospitals are viewed as places where people go to die and are considered a synthesis of all of the most objectionable aspects of Anglo medical care.[36] Those aspects include isolation from family and friends, lack of understanding, fear of inability to communicate needs, fear of the unknown, fear of discriminatory treatment, fear of affronts to modesty and dignity, unfamiliar diet, and the inability to meet family responsibilities.

Contemporary Health Care

□ *The combination of folk health and scientific beliefs.* The use of scientific health care is increasing among Mexican Americans, and the manner in which these new beliefs are being integrated with the old has been described in various ways. Martinez and Martin hypothesize that the concurrent beliefs form insular systems.[37] Some diseases are identified as folk illnesses that can be cured solely by folk means. These diseases are completely alien to medical science and are taken as proof of the limited knowledge of physicians. At the same time, other diseases may be recognized as amenable to treatment by a medical doctor. Questionable diseases may be treated by both.

Lindstrom reports that all women, despite belief in folk curers, would ultimately take their children to the doctor if home treatment were ineffective, or if the child appeared to be "really sick."[38] Still another pattern of behavior has been identified by Moustafa and Weiss, in which home remedies and folk curers have been used first; later, the physician is used, while the appeal continues for divine aid.[39] What is important for the Mexican American is the cure, however effected.

Johnson reports that Mexican Americans may not be aware of inconsistencies in their beliefs concerning health and illness and that despite these inconsistencies, the folk and scientific system can exist simultaneously.[40] She recommends that no attempt be made to destroy folk beliefs. Saunders and Hewes recommend that physicians eliminate harmful folk practices and utilize the remainder in ways beneficial to the client.[41] They believe that folk medicine will flourish under the impact of the scientific point of view, because new elements from medical science are continually being added to folk beliefs.

□ *Contact with the scientific health care system.* Today the Mexican American mother is frequently the one who effects contact with the scientific health care system for herself and her children. As major caregiver in the home, she is the one who makes judgments relative to health and appropriate health treatment for family members. She may make minor decisions related to health care and may consult with her husband concerning other decisions. The lack of group support in health care decisions may be very stressful and may even affect the type of care sought by the women. It was found, for instance, that women who were not using a health care facility for their benefit were more likely to be living with their spouses than were those who used the service to their advantage. Apparently, when the spouse was not available for consultation, women turned to the clinic for this role.[41a]

Characteristics of health professionals may evoke feelings of trust, while others may cause stress. Valued characteristics of health professionals include an attitude of caring, an understanding of cultural premises as well as the meaning of role and role expectations, and a knowledge of Spanish. The importance of a friendly, compassionate attitude on the part of health professionals is recognized by a number of investigators.[42] It has been suggested that nurses' actions may be judged more harshly than those of other health professionals, since they perform a role closely related to that of the folk curer.

Factors that contribute to an attitude of mistrust toward health professionals include high fees for service, a lack of knowledge of folk illness, and differences between health professionals and patients. The latter include disparities in social status, in educational level, in language, and in the understanding of roles in illness. The Mexican American may feel that the physician's behavior reflects a feeling of superiority, particularly when his actions differ markedly from those of the folk curer. Self-diagnosis may be denounced as superstition. Submission to a physical examination may invoke feelings of immodesty and embarrassment. Explanations using scientific terminology serve to limit understanding and family participation. Concern over the fee for service may be interpreted as a lack of concern for the individual.

☐ *The relationship of demographic and social factors to health beliefs and practices.* The effects of Anglo culture on health beliefs and practices have been recognized by researchers. With the increasing contact with Anglo culture, there has also been the blending of Anglo health beliefs and practices. Williams found that Mexican Americans had more widely differing health beliefs and practices than did the Anglos of her sample. She typified as being of an "Anglo type" those responses that stressed self-reliance, confidence in professionals, and open discussion between husband and wife. Responses characterized as "traditional" included those indicating family helpfulness, reliance on lay information, and more discussion between female relatives than between husband and wife. The "traditional" responses were seen to reflect a circumscribed environment and role training that emphasized deference to the husband and the importance of being a good wife and mother.[43]

The variety of health beliefs and practices among Mexican American limits generalization about the stress experienced by all Mexican American women in encounters with the scientific health care system. Some differences in the use of the scientific health care system have been related to the social and demographic characteristics of the Mexican American.

Variables identified by Clark that have influenced the relative emphasis placed upon scientific interpretations of disease include age, length of residence outside village Mexico, and educational level. Social class has not been recognized by Clark as a demographic variable influencing health beliefs, perhaps because the group she interviewed was representative of the lower class. However, class affiliation has been recognized by other researchers, in that upper-class descendants of eminent, well-

educated Mexican American families have been shown to manifest medical beliefs
similar to those of the upper-class Anglo. Conversely, the lower class, which has
largely included unskilled workers and migrants, has been shown to lack confidence
in physicians.[44] However, in times of crisis, Madsen reports that Spanish-speaking
persons often turn to folk remedies, whatever their class affiliation.[45]

With the exposure to formal education, Mexican Americans are more likely to believe in scientific health practices. Madsen posits that, while primary school education has had little effect upon changing beliefs in folk medicine, secondary education
has had a considerable effect.[46] McLemore, in an attempt to explore the relationship
between educational level and attitudes to hospitalization among a sample of
Anglos and Mexican Americans, found that there was no significant difference in
attitudes toward hospitalization between the two groups.[47] There was, however, a
significant difference in attitudes at particular education levels. For both the Anglos
and the Mexican Americans, those with more than six years of schooling held more
favorable attitudes toward hospitalization than did those of lower educational levels.

Moustafa and Weiss also report a relationship between health attitudes and practices and age, in addition to rural-urban differences and differences in economic
status. The analysis of rural-urban differences indicates that persons living in metropolitan areas are more influenced by Anglo values than are those living in remote
villages. In his study of concepts of self, Gecas found migrant farm workers to be
more firmly rooted in structural sources of identity stemming from cultural heritage
than were the settled Mexican Americans.[48] He concluded that acculturation was
greater for the settled population.

Differences in the use of preventive health care have been reported among Mexican Americans residing in different parts of the country. For example, Mexican
American women are more likely to seek prenatal care after moving to the North
from Texas. Lindstrom compared thirty families, ten of whom were good users, ten
poor users, and ten nonusers of a Northern neighborhood clinic.[49] The families all
had low incomes, and many had little education. Demographic characteristics of the
group who used the clinic in a comprehensive manner included women as heads of
households, higher than average income within the sample, and socialization outside
of Texas. Age, family size, and command of English were found to be similar for all
three of the groups studied. Contrary to expectations, this study revealed that the
women with less education were better users of the clinic.

In summary, differences within the backgrounds of Mexican American women
can affect the extent to which stress is experienced in interactions with the health
care system.

HEALTH CARE DELIVERY FACTORS
AS STRESSORS

Factors related to the health care delivery system per se may also make its use
stressful or satisfactory to a Mexican American woman. Weaver has suggested that
health care delivery factors are the major determinants of the health care behavior
of Mexican Americans.[50] These factors concern the health care services themselves; their accessibility, availability, and acceptability to Mexican Americans.
Solis, in testimony to a Cabinet Committee Hearing on Mexican American Affairs,

identified deficiencies in health care programs, including excessive costs, insufficient services, lack of facilities, shortages of bilingual manpower, ineffective patterns of delivery through limited hours of service, fragmentation of service, geographic inaccessibility, lack of communication concerning available services, and psychologic barriers to service.[51]

A number of the same factors have been identified by other researchers. Perkins posited that use of a clinic depended upon whether or not the facility was open when the client needed it, whether the client knew about the service, and its cost.[52] Lindstrom found that a reported lack of transportation was related to broken clinic appointments.[53] This sample of Mexican American women was evidently not aware that transportation was provided by the clinic.

The use of Spanish in a health care service not only enhances communication, but helps to create a more acceptable service to the Mexican American. Several researchers have addressed this issue. Solis reported that Mexican American farm workers would shun care by health professionals who neither spoke the language nor recognized cultural traditions.[54] Freeman and Balderrama stated that without communication in Spanish, "delivery of service" was mere fiction.[55] Knoll recommended that staff people speak Spanish and share cultural values with the Mexican American.[56] He also identified the importance of visible services, such as the hospital emergency room.

The need for health professionals to understand and consider the culture of the Mexican American has also been emphasized by a number of researchers. Saunders has suggested that, unless health programs consider the culture of the people whom they serve, the programs would not be readily acceptable.[57]

In an instance where a variety of health care facilities were available, it was found that differences within the health care services offered to the Mexican American contributed to their acceptability. Although Mexican Americans and Anglos stated they preferred the same type of health care, four times as many Mexican Americans received treatment from one facility as did the Anglos. It was suggested that more Mexicans used this facility because of negative experiences with other health providers, and because of the use of the Spanish language in the facility.[58]

A friendly, understanding attitude is a major factor in the use of facilities that provide health care. Murray has conjectured that most Mexican Americans would use health services if the health care personnel would make a greater effort to study and to understand them.[59] Solis has reported that farm workers tend not to heed medical advice if they are not approached with warmth and understanding, and Johnson maintains that "A friendly compassionate attitude on high professional levels can communicate more effectively than any facility in the Spanish language."[60]

IMPLICATIONS FOR THE PRACTICE OF NURSING

In addition to the investigation of factors related to Mexican American health beliefs and health practices in this chapter, there are implications for the present practice of nursing. As indicated earlier in the chapter, there is considerable heterogeneity among Mexican Americans with regard to health practices. Caution must be exercised in the generalization of knowledge from the traditional Mexican American culture to the individual Mexican American woman.

Valued aspects of health care delivery systems have been identified in the literature. For example, skill and friendliness have been evaluated as important characteristics of nurses. The use of the Spanish language by nurses has been particularly valued by the Spanish speakers. Nursing practitioners must adapt nursing practices to the needs and values identified by the Mexican American clients. Williams states: "Nurses must study the people for whom they are caring, so as to understand them and their problems. Otherwise, they will continue operating on their stereotypes and they will not provide the type of care their patients really require."[61]

The present chapter has included a number of critical factors related to the health beliefs and health practices of Mexican Americans in general, and of Mexican American women in particular. These factors need to be considered in further study of the effects of stress in transcultural settings.

NOTES

1. A.T. Moustafa G. Weiss, *Health Status and Practices of Mexican Americans. Mexican American Study Project, Advanced Report II.* Los Angeles, University of California Press, 1968, pp 5-12.

2. M. Foster, "Working with People of Different Cultural Backgrounds," *California's Health (State Department of Public Health)* 13:109, January 15, 1956.

3. Moustafa and Weiss, Op. Cit., p. 46.

4. Ibid., p. 7-11.

5. Ibid., p. 112.

6. C.E. Tejeda, "Mexican American Americans in the North: Chicago. *Bulletin of the National Tuberculosis and Respiratory Disease Association.* 59 pp. 6-7, May 1973.

7. B. Bullough and V. Bullough, *Poverty, Ethnic Identity, and Health Care*, New York, Appleton, 1972, p. 75.

8. S.J. Reeder and L.G. Reeder, "Some Correlates of Prenatal Care Among Low Income Wed and Unwed Women." *American Journal of Obstetrics and Gynecology* 90 p. 1311, December 1964.

9. C.J. Lindstrom, "No Shows: A Problem in Health Care," *Nursing Outlook*, 23 p. 755, December 1975.

10. Moustafa and Weiss, Op. Cit., pp. 16-28.

11. E.G. Jaco, "Mental Health of the Spanish Americans, (In Opler MK (ed): *Culture and Mental Health*, New York, Macmillan, 1959, pp. 467-488.

12. M. Karno and R.B. Edgerton, "Perceptions of Mental Illness in a Mexican American Community," *Archives of General Psychiatry*, 20: pp. 232-238, February 1969.

13. A. Morales, "Mental and Public Health Issues: The Case of the Mexican Americans in Los Angeles," *El Grito*, 3 pp. 3-11, 1969.

14. L. Saunders, "Healing Ways in the Spanish Southwest," In Jaco EG (ed.): *Patients Physicians, and Illness*, Glencoe, Ill., The Free Press, 1958, p. 189.

15. W. Madsen, *The Mexican Americans of South Texas*, New York, Holt, Rienhart and Winston, 1964, pp. 70-71.

16. G.M. Foster, "Relationship Between Spanish and Spanish-American Fold Medicine," *Journal of American Folklore*, 66: pp. 201-217, July 1953.

17. J.A. Sakalys, "The Meaning of Health and Illness," In Mitchel P (ed): *Concepts Basic to Nursing*, New York, McGraw-Hill, 1973, p. 5.

18. L. Saunders, Op. Cit., p. 192.

19. J. Samora, "Conceptions of Health and Disease Among Spanish-Americans," *American Catholic Sociological Review* 23: 320, Winter 1961.

20. L. Saunders, Op. Cit., p. 153.

21. Ibid, pp. 71-72.

22. W. Madsen, Op. Cit.

23. M. Clark, "Social Functions of Mexican American Medical Beliefs," *California's Health*, 16: 155, May 1, 1959.

24. M. Clark, *Health in the Mexican American Culture*, Los Angeles, University of California Press, 1959, pp. 170-171.

25. W. Madsen, Op. Cit., pp. 71-72.

26. V. Romano and I. Octavio, "Charismatic Medicine, Folk-Healing, and Folk-Sainthood," *American Anthropologist*, 67: 1154-1155, October, 1965.

27. Ibid., A.J. Rubel, *Across the Tracks: Mexican Americans in a Texas City*, Austin, University of Texas Press, 1966.

28. W. Madsen, Op. Cit., p. 91.

29. A. Moustafa and G. Weiss, Op. Cit., p. 56.

30. W. Madsen, Op. Cit., p. 76.

31. F.C. Nall and J. Speilberg, "Social and Cultural Factors in the Responses of Mexican Americans to Medical Treatment," *Journal of Health and Human Behavior*, 8: 299-308, December 1967.

32. M. Clark, *Health in the Mexican American Culture*, Op. Cit., pp. 170-171.

33. A.J. Rubel, "The Epidemiology of a Folk Illness: Susto in Hispanic America," *Ethnology*, 3: 268, July 1964.

34. C. Martinez and H.W. Martin, "Folk Diseases Among Urban Mexican Americans: Etilogy, Symptoms, and Treatment," *American Medical Association Journal*, 196: 149, April 11, 1966.

35. Rubel, Op. Cit., pp. 168-171.

36. S. Schulman, "Rural Healthways in New Mexico," *Annals of the New York Academy of Science*, 84: 956, December 8, 1960.

37. C. Martinez and H. Martin, Op. Cit., p. 150.

38. C. Lindstrom, Op. Cit., p. 75.

39. Moustafa and Weiss, Op. Cit., p. 1.

40. C.A. Johnson, "Nursing and Mexican American Folk Medicine," *Nursing Forum*, 3: 111-112, 1964.

41. L. Saunders and G. Hewes, "Folk Medicine and Medical Practice," *Journal of Medical Education*, 28: 46, September 1953.

41a. Clindstrom, Op. Cit., p. 78.

42. F. Solis, "A Clinic for Mexican American Farm Workers," *Bulletin of the National Tuberculosis and Respiratory Disease Association*, 59: 9-11, November 1973.

43. M.A. Williams, "A Comparative Study of Post-surgical Convalescence Among Women of Two Ethnic Groups: Anglo and Mexican American," In Batey MV (ed), *Communicating Nursing Research: The Many Sources of Nursing Knowledge*, Boulder, Colorado, Western Interstate Commission for Higher Education, 1972, pp. 59-73.

44. J.L. Gonzalex, "An Ounce of Prevention May be Worth a Pound of Nothing: A Mexican American Ghetto," *Bulletin of the National Tuberculosis and Respiratory Disease Association*, 59: 14-16, April 1963.

45. Madsen, Op. Cit., pp. 68-69.

46. Ibid., p. 95.

47. S. McLemore, "Ethnic Attitudes Toward Hospitalization: An Illustrative Comparison of Anglos and Mexican Americans," *The Southwestern Social Science Quarterly*, 43: 341- 346, March 1963.

48. V. Gecas, "Self Conceptions of Migrants and Settled Mexican Americans," *Social Science Quarterly*, 54: 579-595, December 1973.

49. C.J. Lindstrom, Op. Cit., p. 758.

50. J.L. Weaver, "American Health Care Behavior: A Critical Review of the Literature," *Social Science Quarterly*, 54: 97, June 1973.

51. Solis, 1967, Op. Cit.

52. M. R. Perkins, "Does Availability of Health Services Ensure Their Use?" *Nursing Outlook*, 22: 496-498, August 1974.

53. Lindstrom, Op. Cit., p. 759.

54. Solis, Op. Cit., pp. 9-11.

55. H.M. Freeman, L. Avila and V. Balderrama, "Chichi, in Paradise: Helping Agencies and the Spanish Speaking, *Public Welfare* 31: 47, Spring 1973.

56. F.R. Knoll, "Casework Services for Mexican Americans," *Social Casework*, 52: 279-284, May 1971.

57. L. Saunders, *Cultural Differences and Medical Care*, New York, Russel Sage Foundation, 1954, p. 177.

58. J.L. Weaver, *Health Care Service Use in Orange County: A Socioeconomic Analysis*, Long Beach, Calif., Center for Political Research, California State University, 1969.

59. M.J. Murray, *A Socio-Cultural Study of 118 Mexican Families Living in a Low-Rent Public Housing Project in San Antonio, Texas*, Washington, D.C., Catholic University Press, 1954.

60. Solis, 1973, Op. Cit.; Johnson, Op. Cit., p. 111.

61. M.A. Williams, "Response to Critique," In Batey MV (ed): *Communicating Nursing Research: The Many Sources of Nursing Knowledge*, Boulder, Colorado, Western Interstate Commission for Higher Education, 1972, p. 80.

11
Health Appraisal of Low-Income Women

Beverly LaBelle McElmurry

> The family lives in abject poverty I never dreamed could exist in this community. No indoor plumbing. Children attend middle class school; cannot adjust; cannot help but smell. One son retarded. Daughter, 11, promiscuous. One child, the result of union between father and daughter, placed in foster home. Cats and dogs in abundance. Mother stated dog had brought in a mangled coon. She roasted it for dinner.*

How would the mother in that home define "health"? The interaction of poverty and states of health is cause for growing concern in the community health field. Health professionals may be limited in dealing with the problem by the gap between their own largely middle-class health values and the health values of the low-income people they serve.

The intent of the research described in this chapter is to provide a nursing perspective of the way in which low-income women view health. This perspective accepts that "a person acts in accordance with his own experience in a particular situation; an examination of this experience is the necessary starting place for helping him to grow."[1]

The author admits certain humanistic assumptions that guide the approach to this chapter, among which are the following:

1. The full health potential of the relationship between a nurse and the recipient of nursing services depends on their interaction as whole human beings.

2. Every person, including the nurse and the client, is a unique interdependent combination of body, mind, emotions, and spirit. It is this unique combination which the nurse looks for when assessing the health status of low-income women.

3. The client and the nurse are colleagues. Such a relationship activates growth and mutual problem solving.

4. Health, for nurse and client, is defined within the context of the life experience of each.

Poverty and the special health promotion and maintainance needs of women have an enduring quality that cautions the humanistic bents of nurse-investigators and dampens the desire to move rapidly into the specifications of nursing practice

---

*From notes of a student. Acknowledgment is given the nursing students who assisted with this study, especially Sue Clark, Pam Miller, and Lois Wilson. The author assumes full responsibility for the work reported in this paper.

interventions for this patient population or to delineate swiftly the outcomes expected from such interventions. The data collection tool used in this study should be further refined. More opportunities to appreciate and respect low-income women are likely to result in more accurate specifications for group-anchored interventions.

The heart of developing clinical nursing in this area is, eventually, to propose nursing interventions that are testable. Such interventions may take the form of models for educational activities with low-income women, but it is premature to propose hypotheses before a valid data base is established, either for an individual or for a group. This line of reasoning led Lefcowitz, in interlinking education, poverty, and health issues, to ask, "What change in health policy—financial and/or structural—will increase utilization among the less educated, given their relatively lower preference for health care?"[2]

To obtain a focus for developing nursing interventions and a set of related or expected patient outcomes, nurses must first comprehend the health status of low-income women and how these women express it.

Time spent with nursing students who cared for rural-area public-aid recipients helped the author to develop preliminary hunches about the indirect ways in which low-income women express their sense of health and well-being. For example, a general or masked depressive state was frequently revealed by the passive-aggressive, manipulative manner in which the women related to those around them. A vicious cycle was evident: Unsatisfied affectional, loving, human-intimacy tendencies left the women less trusting and spontaneous in relating to other people, who then responded negatively to their stiffness and distrust. The press of economic and social situations coupled with low educational achievement left the women with an underdeveloped sense of their physical and psychological selves. Community health and support systems personnel sometimes worsened the cycle by seeming to reject or stigmatize the women as undesirable.

These observations suggested the appropriateness of a more systematic study of low-income women through the development of a health appraisal form. In addition, students might use such a form as a tool for examining nursing practice.

The purpose of this study is to begin the development of tools and methodology with which to describe the reported and perceived health status of low-income, rural, nonfarm women.

REVIEW OF LITERATURE

The literature speaks more directly to the dimensions of poverty than to the health appraisal of low-income women. Chilman cautions that we know only part of what needs to be known about low-income cultures and that "not all the possibly relevant questions have been asked. Moreover, it seems as if research has focused chiefly on the weaknesses of the poor rather than their strengths."[3]

Chilman identifies the following problems of research with low-income or poverty groups: (1) the use of questionnaires when educational levels are so low that literacy is a problem; (2) the difference between statistic and pragmatic significance, (3) moving from group findings to individual diagnosis or predictions, and (4) failure to realize that behavior is complex and multidimensional.

National data on relationships between low income and health states do not provide the necessary data base for nursing practice in the promotion and/or maintenance of health. The data gathered nationally are labeled as health characteristics but are in reality descriptions of illness. The National Center for Health Statistics has reported annual data from health interview and health examination surveys, but the data are essentially reports of illness, such as restricted-activity days, acute conditions, physical visits, and hospital episodes.[4] Other data are more appropriate to the health-related concerns involved in the proposal of nursing interventions for promotion and maintenance of health.

Bergner and Yerby substantiate the need for a data base in their discussion of low-income barriers to the use of health services:

> The poor behaved differently from the middle class and the affluent across a wide spectrum related to health care. Illness is defined differently. There is less accurate health information. The poor are less inclined to take preventive measures, and delay longer in seeking medical care. When they do approach health practitioners, they are more likely to select subprofessionals or the marginal practitioners often found in their neighborhoods.[5]

Many writers suggest that the life of low-income people is improved by raising their educational levels or instituting homemaker and child-care services. Such proposals often come from middle- and upper-class reformers who have never consulted the people whose life style they propose to change. Likewise, many proposals to improve life for low-income people are piecemeal remedies rather than comprehensive plans. Milio, however, demonstrated the supportive role of health personnel in facilitating a group's identification of needed services and in becoming self-directive in designing and implementing its own health services.[6]

Bauer reported many health characteristics that differentiate low-income from higher-income groups.[7] Low-income people have more untreated conditions, a greater number of dental caries, poorer health, more prevalent chronic conditions, higher disability rates, less access to medical and dental care, greater reliance on clinics and emergency units for health care, and more hospital episodes. Bauer also reports that "aid recipients have poorer health than nonrecipients."[8] Pomeroy[9] found that welfare recipients report poorer health for themselves and their children than do nonwelfare people. Criteria for determining "good health" were not, however, developed in Pomeroy's sample.

Komisar[10] notes that the majority of adults on welfare are women. Women are felt to suffer most from a life of poverty.[11] Lesse also believes that American culture creates major stresses for women in the middle years of life.[12]

The author accepts, after a review of the literature, that low-income women present a special concern to those involved in the delivery of health care services. Some evidence indicates a geographic dimension to the problem, since mothers in rural farm and nonfarm areas spend longer continuous periods on public assistance.[13]

Triplett reported the characteristics and perceptions of low-income women as they affected use of preventive health services.[14] Triplett did not focus on the perceived health status of the clients, but she did conclude that low-income women can be expected to talk freely about their health care experiences. In light of Polansky's[15] identification of verbal accessibility as a problem for low-income people, Triplett's study suggests that trained nurse-interviewers can be successful in obtaining interview data from research subjects.

Brinton looked at the value differences between nurses and low-income families, but did not attempt to describe health. Rather, she included among her tools an instrument that compares the importance that nurses and mothers attach to various questions related to health.[16] The questions, however, do not provide a categorization or description of what constitutes a healthy state.

It can be concluded that research literature about low-income women is limited and sketchy. When related to health, it emphasizes, not the presence of a healthy state, but rather its absence.

LaBelle reviewed definitions of the term "health" and concluded that the definition used by a given group (such as nurses) gives direction to the research, service, and educational activities performed by that group.[17] The present inadequate conceptualization of the term "health" demonstrates the need to develop a complex construct. An individual state of health or well-being is characterized by subjective and objective aspects of behavior, which are influenced by physical, emotional, social, and environmental conditions. "A continuing problem," states LaBelle, "is the development of criteria and indices to measure health. The research problem reflects the constantly changing or adaptive components that are a part of health."[18]

METHOD

Low-income, nonhospitalized women receiving public aid were interviewed to determine their status in four dimensions of health: physical, psychological, social, and environmental. Furthermore, the women were asked to identify, in their words, their state of health. Interviews were conducted by student nurses trained in basic techniques by the researcher. The data reported here reflect preliminary work in developing a health assessment interview guide.

TOOL

In the view of Yura and Walsh, the nursing process provides a general framework for examining clinical practice concerns and should be related to research endeavors.[19] Consistent with this outlook and with this author's earlier definition of health, the tool developed was used to obtain information about physical, psychological, social, and environmental variables.

Examples from the interviewer's assessment guide are included here. Figure 11.1 shows major categories within each variable, as well as the type of question asked in each category. Figure 11.2 illustrates the nurse's conclusion and intervention record following assessment of health data. In essence, a patient health problem becomes a nursing concern if it is expected to respond to the type of action or intervention carried out by the nurse.

Physical Variable

Categories:

Hygiene
Examples of questions in this category:

    Routines
        e.g., Bath, complete Y N   Regular Y N   Frequency _____
    Difficulties or limitations
        e.g., Physical incapacity Y N   Explain _____
    Independence
Nutrition
Rest
Mobility
Female health
Systematic evaluation
Restrictions
Indirect influences

Psychological Variable

Categories:

Behavioral
Examples of questions in this category:

    e.g., Alcoholic intake: Amount _____ Frequency _____

        Circumstances _____ Regularity _____

        Smoking Y N   Amount per day _____
        Uses of leisure time (respondents circle appropriate descriptors)
        Flexibility in daily schedule Y N
        Long- and short-term goals (options provided)
Emotional
Adaptive behavior
Intellectual/academic
Information input
Perceptions
Values and priorities

Figure 11.1. Variables included in the health appraisal of women.

Social Variable

Categories:

Vocational/economic
Examples of questions in this category:

e.g., Attitudes toward responsibility and authority
    e.g., Resentment Y N (client's view)   Y N (nurse's view)
      Respect Y N
    Major concerns about work:
      Health
      Social
      Money
      Job itself
      etc.
    Health hazards and benefits associated with work _____
    Employment history
Communication/interpersonal
Family
Indirect influences

Environmental Variable

Categories:

Physical
Examples of questions in this category:

e.g., Housing
      Type: single-family, apartment, single room, etc.
      Provision: owned, rented
      Cleanliness and general sanitation: adequate, inadequate
      Heat: adequate, inadequate
      Air pollution Y N
      Water pollution Y N
      Excessive noise Y N
      Waste disposal Y N
Social environment
Indirect influences

Figure 11.1. Variables   included in the health appraisal of women. *(Cont.)*

State of Health

How this woman defines health _____

How she describes health _____

Determination that she is _____, is not _____ healthy and the reasons for this

_____

What she does to maintain or improve health _____

When she does comply with recommended health practices and when she does
  not comply _____

Agreed Areas for Nurse and Patient To Work On

Area(s) identified by client _____

Area(s) and/or problem(s) the nurse identifies _____

Possible Approaches

Approach   Criterion/criteria for evaluating approach

_____   _____

_____   _____

_____   _____

_____   _____

_____   _____

Implementation of Nursing Approaches

Dates   List in order of priority

_____   _____

_____   _____

_____   _____

_____   _____

_____   _____

Unpredictable happenings:

_____

_____

_____

_____

_____

Nurse's Evaluation and/or Reformulation of Nursing Process

_____

_____

_____

_____

_____

Figure 11.2. Nurse's conclusions and intervention record after considering assessment data.

STUDY SAMPLE

Subjects selected for this program were derived from women receiving public aid in a selected rural, nonfarm, midwestern area. Their ages ranged from late adolescence to late adulthood. All were judged to be of normal intelligence.

Initially, 20 women were identified for the study, but data are reported on the 13 who remained in the case load for the full four-month period. The subjects' agreement to participate in the project was obtained.

DATA COLLECTION

Student nurses assigned to provide care to the women for four months, as part of a community health field experience, were the data collectors. It was their responsibility to determine at which point in their relationship with the study subjects it seemed appropriate to collect assessment information. Usually this followed a judgment that a trust relationship had been established between them. Some data were gathered over the entire period of time.

DATA ANALYSIS

Analysis of data from this pilot study is qualitative, reflecting an early stage of investigation in a relatively unexplored area. In their explanation of field methodology, Schatzman and Strauss capture the essence of the approach herein employed:

> Field method is more like an umbrella of activity beneath which any technique may be used for gaining the desired information, and for processes of thinking about this information.[20]

> [The] researcher . . . enters and relates himself to a human field in its natural state; that is, in its own time and place, and in its own recurrent and developing process.[21]

> "Method" is seen as an abstraction of the ways the researcher handles, or might handle, the many real situations, problems, and options which present themselves to him as he conducts his inquiry.[22]

FINDINGS

Women in the study sample thought of health predominantly in terms of the presence or absence of physical states usually associated with a disease. "Health" generally meant the absence of disease symptoms or of uncomfortable states, such as flu or colds. On the whole, women in the study evidenced little inclination to incorporate psychological, social, or environmental components into the determination of her own health status.

Physical

General hygiene measures were adequate except for dental care, which rarely met recommended practices. Some women used only mouthwash in their dental regimen, and others reported brushing their teeth two or three times per week. Nearly all said that limited finances affected their hygienic states.

Concern for physical safety in the home varied among the subjects. Some of the women carefully removed dangerous materials from the reach of children, whereas others, for example, let their children live in the midst of furniture bulging with dangerous springs.

The study women were able to assume responsibility for self-care but most needed encouragement or suggestions from the nurse to increase their awareness of hygiene or safety factors important to health.

Generally, the women ate two to three meals per day. For snacks, they preferred breads and cereals. None reported taking nutritional supplements such as vitamins unless the doctor had specifically urged their use. As a group, the women did not self-medicate. Some hoped to lose weight but felt their financial situation limited diet choice.

Rest-sleep data produced little significant information. The only reported dissatisfaction was sleep interruptions from others, usually small children. However, the subjects rarely reported fatigue and did not report that sleep interruptions interfered with their overall sense of sufficient rest.

Most women in the study group were involved in daily household work and child-care activities. Few were sufficiently active to qualify for an activity level above "moderate," and the nurses were inclined to place them, as a group, in the sedentary category.

In the area of female health, the women were questioned about menstrual cycles, use of contraceptives, fertility, and breast self-examination practices. Five of the subject women used no contraceptives, five used oral contraceptives, one had an intrauterine device, and one had been sterilized. All had heard of breast self-examination, but nine never performed it. Two did it irregularly, one did every month, and another did every morning (she had previously had a breast biopsy). None of the women reported irregular menstrual cycles.

Generally, the body-systems evaluation of each woman revealed conditions already known to her and under medical treatment. One woman did have untreated dental problems. The lack of significant findings in this area is in itself interesting. It may be that the findings are consistent with the women's health concepts, since most of them viewed health as the absence of disease and sought treatment only for infections or dysfunctions. Also, the women in the study were primarily young adults, not yet subject to chronic health problems.

One of the subject women could not recall the last time she had seen a doctor, but 12 reported a medical examination within the last two years. Although most sought dental examinations every two years, one had not seen a dentist in eight years, and another had not seen one in four years. None participated in any health screening programs, either because the programs were not offered, the subjects were not aware of the programs, or they were not inclined to participate.

Psychological

Data collected in this health component suggest possible further fruitful explorations.

About half of the study women smoked. Ten were satisfied with the way in which they spent leisure time, usually in the company of family or friends. As a group, the subjects reported few hobbies or other interests not directly related to homemaking.

One women—an 18-year-old mother of a three-year-old child, with no husband in the home—reported boredom. Nine women had daily schedules related to homemaking and child-care activities. Most were financially dependent on another person or on public aid.

Short-term goals of most importance to the women were everyday needs (nine), money (seven), and maintenance (six). Most important long-term goals were money (seven), employment (seven), and everyday needs (six).

Attributes of the subject women that seem to deserve fuller exploration include determination, timidity, and self-concept. Data collectors portrayed the women as "hopeful" if they seemed determined to improve their situations (more positive in self-concept). A description of a woman as "timid" usually corresponded with poor self-concept.

The nurse-interviewers were asked to describe the women's positive and negative adaptive behavior. Six were described as present oriented, four as distrustful of others, seven as accepting of their situation and of the people in that situation, five as trusting, and four as manipulative.

Only one of the subject women reported finishing high school. None received vocational training, but two were now completing their education via the general education degree (GED) program offered through the local school system.

More than half of the subject women made decisions on the basis of impulse, but the same number said they used reason to arrive at decisions. Five viewed their opportunities as limited, whereas two thought that their futures held plentiful opportunity. Nine saw their chances for creative self-expression as low.

A majority of the women (seven) reported that they would be influenced by input or counsel from professionals such as nurses. They would weigh this influence against that of family, friends, and social agencies.

Asked to identify values and priorities, the women placed highest values on family (eleven), health (eight), maintenance (eight), money (nine), and independence (six). Seven women placed no priority on education or learning, whereas eight stressed the importance of recreation. Half listed employment as a priority.

When asked to identify their roles, nine women listed "mother," five chose "individual," another five "homemaker," seven said "single parent," and another seven said "friend." "Student" was listed twice; "wife" once.

Occupation and Work History

Of the thirteen women studied, only one was currently employed. Now a factory worker earning $400 per month, she had passed through many job changes. Most of the women had no paid vacation, no savings, and no retirement plans. Two were supported by their husband's income. The remaining ten were receiving some form of public aid of not more than $400 per month, $300 monthly being a typical figure. Most of the subject women saw their financial situation as inadequate, although some felt it sufficient to sustain them.

Social/Emotional

Ten of the subject women were described as socially isolated in the realm of communication and interpersonal skills. The closest associations reported by this group were with immediate family members. The interviews revealed that three of the women thought their affectional needs were inadequately satisfied. Eight thought their need for achievement was unsatisfied, and four lacked satisfaction of security needs. Five needed greater approval from others, and the same number felt insufficiently recognized by others. Three sensed that they did not belong to a group with a significant identity in the community.

Only six of the women chose to discuss their sex lives. All six were sexually active. The impression gained from study of the data was that most were satisfied with their sexual partners. The women made all the decisions regarding method of contraception, with no discussion or participation by the partners.

Five of the subject women were single, three were married, three were separated, and two were divorced. All shared what the interviewers regarded as a profoundly passive and dependent attitude toward the men in their lives, as demonstrated by decision making in their relationships.

Most of the women, whether married or single, expressed the desire to be successful as parents. Probed on details of child care or perception of children's needs, however, they were often vague. Most appeared unable to understand concepts of mobility, play and environmental needs, and distribution of age-appropriate responsibilities. Their backgrounds limited them in discussions of the physical, psychological, and social needs of young and adolescent children.

Yet the mothers as a group exhibited a remarkable sense of pride in their children and a hopeful attitude toward the children's future development. This pride was evident even though some of the children had created classroom problems sufficient to bring them to the worried attention of school personnel.

Most women in the study reported the family as a source of maintenance, reproduction, and socialization, but not as a source of status within the community. They had given little thought to parenthood beyond the fact that it gave them someone to love and care for.

The subject women had little interest in social issues and little contact with people of other races. They saw themselves as members of a low-income social stratification and acted accordingly. None reported voting, and none belonged to community organizations or took part in community activities. Only one woman was actively involved in a church. The impression of the group was that the churches of their communities were not involved with them.

Environmental

All of the women lived in rented housing facilities. Overall, housing was adequate except for furnishings, general cleanliness, and sufficient privacy for all family members.

SUMMARY

Asked to develop a model description of the women they had interviewed, the nurses agreed on the following:

Generally, the women had been raised in low-income families and were participating in a learned way of life. They considered it normal to have children at an early age. Their relationships with men reflected both a need to be loved and a desire for sexual activity as a form of entertainment. Sexually active women exhibited severe lack of adequate information regarding use of contraceptives.

As a rule, the women had not completed high school and were underdeveloped in job-related skills. Their dim sense of self was manifested in an apparent lack of ability to change their stations in life.

When means could be found to develop skills related to jobs or to home and child care, hopeful attitudes developed among the subject women. As a group, they were oriented to the present time.

The women lacked knowledge about nutrition and about the growth and developmental needs of children.

Television and social activities planned with immediate family members were primary sources of entertainment. The women said very little about close family members in their conversations with outsiders. It was the opinion of the interviewers that the women slept a great deal.

Continued refinement of the health assessment of low-income women may support the hunch that they exhibit masked depression arising from the situation in which they find themselves. It is unlikely that future exploration will uncover genuinely healthy situations among the poor, as long as "health" is tied to notions of productivity, self-sufficiency, and satisfaction with life.

IMPLICATIONS

The nurse's unique function in health state assessment is increasingly recognized as the base for subsequent health maintenance or health promotion actions. The assessment process is itself an interaction that alters the people involved in it. We may anticipate that the person whose health state is assessed will grow in his/her perceptions of what health means and will come to understand what health means to the nurses. The concept of "health" then becomes a heuristic device that can educate both the nurse and the client.

This study aims to initiate an appreciation of the context in which low-income women view themselves and their health states. The description of the women's perceived and reported health status provides data for planning, implementing, and evaluating nursing practice. Nursing actions based on such data more accurately respond to the health needs of women in low-income situations. The ability of such women to obtain health care is partially due to economic restrictions, but it is also related to their ability to differentiate among health states, to find entry into the health care delivery system, and to determine where a paritcular quality or type of care can be obtained.

Nurses have ready access to the socially stigmatized, including low-income women. The extent to which a nurse can function as the advocate of such women in realizing access to good health care depends on how exact and sensitive that nurse is in assessing the woman's health status and practices.

NOTES

1. Constance T. Fischer, "Contextual Approach to Assessment," *Community Mental Health Journal* 9, no. 1 (1973): 38.

2. M.J. Lefcowitz, "Poverty and Health: A Reexamination," in *The Health Gap: Medical Services and the Poor,* ed. R.L. Kane, J.M. Kasteler, and R.M. Gray (New York: Springer, 1976), p. 55.

3. C.S. Chilman, *Growing Up Poor* (Washington, D.C.: U.S. Government Printing Office, 1966), p. 9.

4. National Center for Health Statistics, *Current Listing and Topical Index to the Vital and Health Statistics Series, 1962-1975,* DHEW publication no. (HRA) 78-1301, April 1976.

5. L. Bergner and A.S. Yerby, "Low Income and Barriers to Use of Health Services, in *The Health Gap: Medical Services and the Poor,* ed R.L. Kane, J.M. Kasteler, and R.M. Gray (New York: Springer, 1976), p. 31.

6. Nancy Milio, *9226 Kercheval: The Storefront That Did Not Burn* (Ann Arbor: University of Michigan Press, 1970).

7. M. Bauer, "Health Characteristics of Low-Income Persons," *Vital Health Statistics* 10 (1972): 1-51.

8. Ibid., p. 2.

9. R. Pomeroy, "Comparison of Negro Mothers from Welfare and Low-Income Families," *Poverty and Human Resources* 5, no. 2 (1970): 46.

10. L. Komisar, "Issues: Subsidies and Women," *Poverty and Human Resources Abstracts* 9, no. 1 (1974): 46.

11. B.B. Washington, "Woman in Poverty," *Poverty and Human Resources Abstracts* 1, no. 2 (1966).

12. Stanley Lesse, *Masked Depression* (New York: Jason Aronson), 1974.

13. U.S. Department of Labor, "Manpower Report of the President, Including a Report on Manpower Requirements, Resources, Utilization, and Training," *Poverty and Human Resources Abstracts* 3, no. 4 (1968): 124.

14. J.L. Triplett, "Characteristics and Perceptions of Low-Income Women and Use of Preventive Health Services: An Exploratory Study," *Nursing Research* 19, no. 2 (1970): 140-146.

15. N.A. Polansky, R.D. Borgman, and C. DeSaix, *Roots of Futility* (San Francisco: Jossey-Bass, 1972).

16. D.M. Brinton, "Value Differences Between Nurses and Low-Income Families," *Nursing Research* 21, no. 1 (1972): 46-52.

17. B. LaBelle McElmurry, *The Development of a Nursing Curriculum Design for Health Promotion and Maintenance* (Ann Arbor, Mich.: University Microfilms, No. 73-25, 598, 1973).

18. Ibid., p. 82.

19. Helen Yura and M.B. Walsh *The Nursing Process: Assessing, Planning, Implementing, Evaluating* (New York: Appleton-Century-Crofts, 1973).

20. Leonard Schatzman and A. Strauss, *Field Research: Strategies for a Natural Sociology* (Englewood Cliffs, N.J.: Prentice-Hall, 1973), p. 14.

21. Ibid., p. vi.

22. Ibid.

Part III
Crisis Experiences
and Their Resolutions

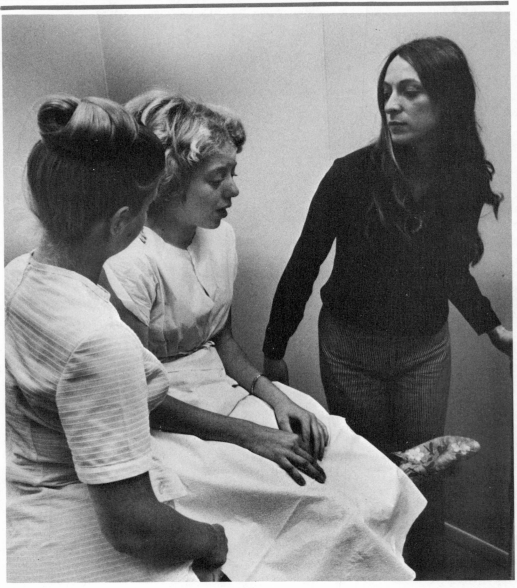

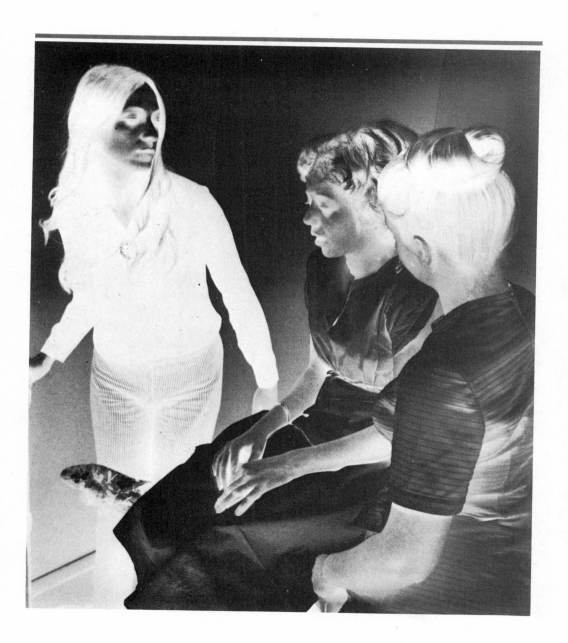

12
Working with the Physically Abused Woman

CAROL VALENTI

Anyone who approaches the area of family violence needs to have an appreciation of the complex nature of the problem. Any form of family violence is obviously a family problem, but it is also a personal, relationship, cultural, social, and legal problem. There are no easy solutions. Professionals working with many aspects of family violence find themselves at times feeling bewildered, frustrated, irritated, and perhaps even hopeless. Professionals must identify and deal with negative reactions to intense situations. Progress is being made in many parts of the country to assist those who find themselves caught in violent situations. The purpose of this chapter is to present material that should be helpful for professionals intervening where family violence, specifically violence against women, occurs.

LABELING THE PROBLEM

One should be aware of the possible danger is using the label "battered woman syndrome." The label "battered woman" has proved to be important in drawing attention to an area that has been ignored and underassessed. It has also been important in gathering statistics and in doing research in this problem area. However, when professionals in a variety of settings attempt intervention, the label has the potential of misleading the professionals and possibly to harming the client. It can mislead professionals into thinking that they are dealing with a very different human problem. Seeing only the label can influence the helping person to ignore the specific dynamics involved in each situation. Physical abuse in one respect demonstrates the existence of a relationship problem. It is a complex problem that shares many variables with other types of relationship problems. If individuals have the expertise to work with relationship problems, they can work with women in physically abusive situations. Professionals far too often believe that they do not have the expertise to work with "battered women" and have the tendency to refer them elsewhere for services. In many situations, making a referral can be a mistake. Individuals involved in helping professions should attempt to work with situations involving family violence in their own setting. Outside assistance should be requested by individuals who have had the courage to try to work with this problem. Information on community resources such as emergency housing, criminal prosecution, and financial assistance can be crucial to a woman caught in a violent relationship. Information should also be sought on factors that help perpetuate violent situations and on the concerns one should have for women who find themselves in violent relationships. Information such as this will serve as an important adjunct to professionals' existing abilities to work with individuals experiencing relationship problems.

Labeling also has the potential of harming the client. An individual with the label "battered woman" may begin to view herself as different or "sicker" than another woman who might be experiencing relationship problems without physical violence. This faulty perception can lead to an increase in the amount of shame and embarrassment that a woman in a physically abusive situation is already experiencing. There has been much damage done in the mental health field by the labeling of mentally ill patients. For many individuals it has been difficult to overcome the stigma involved in the frequent usage of such labels. We certainly have not reached this point with physically abused women, but we must be aware of the possible negative effects of labeling on those involved in violent situations.

FACTORS OR DYNAMICS INVOLVED IN UNHEALTHY RELATIONSHIPS

If professionals expect to be effective in working with relationship problems, they must be aware of factors or dynamics involved in the perpetuation of unhealthy relationships. One factor is one's personal or family background. It is generally believed that a large number of adults who find themselves in physically abusive situations have been exposed to models of family violence as children, the idea being that violence passes from one generation to another. Such individuals either were abused as children or witnessed violence between their parents. In a study done on three generations of abused children, the theme that violence passes through generations was supported. [1] The study concluded that the abused child might cope with abuse by identifying either with the aggressor or with the victim. As an adult, the abused child might become either another violent member of society who abuses others or an adult victim of physical violence. The abused child may have learned that love equals being hurt, and abuse received as an adult reinforces this theme. A study done by Gayford in England on 100 abused women showed that 23 of the women and 51 of the abusing men had been exposed to models of family violence as children. [2] Added to the learned belief that love equals being hurt is the fact that violent situations can become familiar. It should be stressed that physically abusive situations are never acceptable to the victim. However, it is understandably difficult for individuals who have been exposed to violence all their lives to leave a violent situation if they think there is a high likelihood that they will be in a similar situation again.

Another variable at work in helping to perpetuate unhealthy relationships, although it takes a particular turn in physically abusive situations, is the low self-concept of the people involved. There are many situations in which the woman develops an intimate relationship with her self-concept intact. The devastating effects, however, of even one beating, along with the psychological abuse that is usually involved, can be devastating to her self-worth. There are other instances in and out of physically abusive situations in which the individuals come to the relationship with a diminished self-concept. A woman in this instance may have a tendency to choose an inadequate man with the hope of being able to improve him. An inadequate man is defined here as one who is chronically unemployed, chemically dependent, or in trouble with the law. By improving this man, the woman can validate her own worth. The woman's self-concept is then reflected in the accomplishments or failures of her partner. Eventually, the woman realizes the impossibility of the task that she has set for herself but stays with the man because she experiences such a personal sense of failure. In many instances in which physical abuse is occurring, the abusing man admits to the fact that he perceives the woman as being more adequate than himself — occupationally, socially, and educationally. If the man lacks good verbal skills, feels threatened by the woman, and is also violent, he may strike out at the woman. Striking out by the male in these situations can be done in an effort to maintain the superior role that he has been socialized to believe he must maintain in order to qualify as a male. The more inferior and frightened a violent man becomes, the more likely he may be to strike out at his partner. In one of his studies, the sociologist Richard Gelles discovered that family violence was more prevalent when the husband's occupational and educational status was lower than his wife's.[3]

Another factor that helps to perpetuate unhealthy relationships for women is the socialization of women. There is strong emphasis in our culture on the importance of being a good wife and mother. One of the functions of a good wife and mother is taking almost total responsibility for keeping the family together. Women many times feel a tremendous sense of failure if they are unable to keep the family unit together no matter what the cost. The situation becomes even more intense if pressure is put on the woman by her family and friends to stay and "grin and bear it." Particularly when physical violence is present within a family system, having detrimental effects on the children as well as the adults involved, encouraging the woman to stay seems, indeed, unhealthy and foolish.

The financial bind that women often find themselves in can be a strong force which helps to keep them in unhealthy relationships. In our society it has been common for a woman to choose marriage or involvment with a man at an early age. This can mean not only that she is now without a profession, but also that she has never worked outside of the home. If dependent children are involved, a woman at times is at a loss as to how she can independently support herself, let alone the children. Leaving a physically abusive situation often engenders tremendous fear of physical reprisal by the abusing party. It may mean that the woman has to leave everything she knows and owns and accomplish much with dependent children and no money. Where, then, does the physically abused go with her children for safety? The homes of friends and relatives are usually not acceptable, for the abusing party will often look first for the woman at such locations. Women who live in communities that have shelters for them and their children are indeed fortunate, for often shelters are the only safe place to which a woman can escape.

In physically abusive relationships, fear can be an overwhelming factor which makes it difficult for the woman to make the choice of leaving her situation.

Often the woman has been threatened with a knife or a gun and has been told that she will be killed, possibly along with her children, if she attempts to leave. If there is no safe place for the woman to go, she may feel trapped in an impossible situation.

For many individuals, the thought of a relationship ending mainly means that they will be alone. Fear of the loneliness that might result from such a separation can keep both men and women in relationships that they have defined as unhealthy. Both men and women sometimes feel that being in a bad relationship is better than being alone. When the fear of loneliness is so great that it will force someone to stay in an unhealthy relationship, individuals can and perhaps should become more aware of the dynamics involved in their personal fears. Such an awareness can help individuals to see their situation more clearly and to make better choices for themselves in relationships.

Many times people stay in unhealthy relationships because they hope that the unpleasantness will disappear. A relationship is rarely all bad. There are often good times as well as traumatic times, and ambivalence about terminating the relationship can certainly stem from such mixed experiences. In physically abusive situations, a woman is often treated well after a beating. Her partner often does special favors for her or her children or buys them presents. Frequently this is the only time the physically abused woman is treated in such a positive manner. There is the hope that after such a pleasant experience the physical abuse will not happen again.

Another justification given by individuals for remaining in a bad situation is, "But I love him/her." Such a statement made after individuals have defined a relationship as unhealthy for them can be indicative of what they think they deserve in life. The motivation for leaving a bad situation is low if individuals believe they do not deserve or will ever find anything better.

Chemical dependency is often involved in unhealthy relationships. Reliable data are not available on how often chemical dependency is involved in physically abusive situations, but it is generally thought to be high. Chemical usage by the abusing party has generally been regarded as the cause of violence. There is a growing belief, however, that many men may drink as an excuse or justification for becoming violent.[4] After the violent incident, both the assailant and victim can blame the behavior on alcohol. It is often assumed that, if an individual has been drinking, he is not responsible for his behavior. The use of chemicals by the victim in violent situations needs to be examined and can be a factor in making it difficult for a woman to leave an unhealthy relationship.

One must have an appreciation of the tremendous amount of energy it takes a woman to plan and execute a move away from a family situation, particularly if there is violence. Living in a psychologically and/or physically abusive situation erodes a woman's self-concept. Eventually, she begins to believe the cruel, disparaging remarks and may begin to believe that somehow she deserves the physical abuse as well. The more worthless and depressed a woman feels, the less energy she has and the more difficult it becomes to harness that energy to plan and carry out a move. Support and help from outside resources is sometimes the only way a woman is able to make a move away from a violent situation.

INTERVENTION

Effects of Attitude on Behavior

Professionals can and should attempt to intervene in family situations when violence is present. One's attitudes toward violence, and specifically violence toward women, is an important consideration in any discussion of intervention for attitudes have a direct effect on one's behavior.

Dealing with physical abuse evokes certain attitudes and feelings in professionals that might not be apparent when working with other types of problems. Often there is an implicit and at times unrecognized attitude by professionals that, if a woman does not define physical abuse as a problem and/or does not display a readiness to act, she is somehow "sicker" than another woman who might not be ready to get out of an unhealthy, nonviolent relationship. Holding such attitudes can affect professionals' behavior. At times, individuals in the helping profession urge a woman to leave a physically abusive situation before she is ready to do so. By taking such a stance, a professional can lose the woman to her/his services or influence her to leave a situation before she is psychologically ready. In the latter situation, there is a high likelihood that she will either return to the same situation or find herself in similar situation.

There appears to be a personal and perhaps even societal attitude that, at some level, violence against women, particularly if the perpetrator is her husband, is acceptable, understandable, or at least justifiably provoked by the woman. Attitudes such as this have been reflected in a study conducted at Michigan State University. [5] In this study, fights were staged and observed on a city street. In the first three situations, a woman was being attacked by a woman, a man was being attacked by a woman, and a man was being attacked by a man, respectively. In all of these situations, a male bystander came to the rescue of the victim. In the last staged situation, a woman was being attacked by a man. No male bystander came to the rescue of the victim in this situation. The experiment was repeated several times with the same results. Many people can recall the tragic Kitty Genovese murder in New York City, in which not one of the 38 witnesses attempted to intervene. [6] When the witnesses were questioned, many of them said that they did not intervene because they thought the attacker was the victim's husband. Implicit in such a tragic, frightening lack of response may be the attitude in our society that the use of violence against women within the family system is acceptable or understandable.

Another shocking development in our society and that of Europe is the growing commercial trend in which the motif of violence against women is used to advertise and successfully sell clothing and records. A revealing article in *Time* magazine entitled "Really Socking It to Women" describes how prominent fashion photographers and advertising people, as well as record companies, are using violence to sell their products. [7] It also describes how *Vogue* magazine abroad and in America has used situations depicting violence against women to stimulate sales of their products. There have been pictures showing women as killers and victims and one in which a woman's head is being forced into a toilet bowl. American *Vogue*, in a 12-page spread, shows a man intermittently caressing and menacing a female model. The grand finale occurs when the man smashes the woman across the face. On the next page, the female model is pictured affectionately nudging the abusing man. The Jon Anthony jumpsuit that the model wears in this picture spread has sold beautifully. Needless to say, the manufacturer of the jumpsuit thinks the ad was successful. The most distressing question to be asked is, Why can violence and maltreatment of women stimulate sales in a predominantly female market?

This *Time* article also describes a store window in a Boston boutique. Displayed in the window was an apparently dead woman with blood running out of her mouth tumbling out of a garbage can with a pair of men's shoes on her head. The sign in the window read "We'd kill for these." One could certainly offer innumerable cultural, sociologic, or sexist reasons for the use of this form of advertising. One thing that cannot be denied is that trends such as this are promoting and perpetuating the attitude that violence against women is acceptable and, in some cases, even enjoyed by the victim. Promoting such attitudes in any manner will drastically affect society's and one's individual motivation to assess and intervene when violence against women occurs.

Professionals working with family violence must become aware of their personal attitudes toward violence, specifically violence against women, and reflect on how these attitudes affect their behavior. This awareness can be accomplished by providing opportunities for individuals in the helping professions to come together and talk openly about their thoughts and feelings on the subject and to acquire information on and insight into some of the factors involved in the perpetuation of family violence. Only after helping people have reflected on their personal attitudes are they ready to consider some of the specifics involved in intervention.

Helping Process

The helping process is a framework that can be used effectively by professionals to assess and intervene. The author defines the helping process as professional activity with the purpose of assisting individuals, couples, or families with emotional states or practical situations that they have defined as a problem and have a desire to act on. It is the professional's responsibility to help the individual, couple, or family define the problem and to either help them assess their readiness for action or attempt to motivate them toward action for change. It is not the professional's responsibility to decide unilaterally what a problem is to the individual, couple, or family or when and how they should act on the problem. These are rules or concepts that many of us hold to be true in working with people. It is particularly important to stress them in any discussion on violence against women.

When utilizing the helping process, the professional must first discover if physical abuse is occurring in a situation and then ascertain whether the individual, couple, or family is defining such abuse as a problem. When the professional is working specifically with a woman, she may regard other problems in her life, such as chemical dependency of her spouse or of herself or other family problems, to be of more concern to her than physical abuse. It is clearly the professional's role to identify whether violence is occurring and never to lose sight of it when working with a woman or her family but at the same time to respect the woman's position in defining such violence as a problem.

There are many situations in which women do define physical abuse as a problem. The next step in utilizing the helping process is to assess her readiness to act on the situation. Often, even though the woman sees her situation as a problem, she does not demonstrate a readiness to act on it. As previously discussed, there are many factors and dynamics that help to perpetuate unhealthy, physically abusive relationships and that directly affect a woman's readiness to act. The professional should help the woman to discover what dynamics and factors are involved in her resistance to change. It is also appropriate for the helping person to give the woman feedback on the negative effect that the situation may be having on her. The professional must never go beyond this point and force or pressure the woman to leave the situation before she is ready to leave.

Intervention in the Health Care Setting

The health care setting provides many opportunities for assessment and intervention when violence against women is occurring. Health care settings include emergency rooms, physicians' offices, outpatient clinics, and inpatient hospital units. Women are frequent users of health care services. They often go to physicians or other health personnel for birth control, pregnancy, and gynecologic problems; they also take their children to health care facilities for treatment. Whenever a social or family assessment is done in a health care setting, consideration should be given to relationships within the family. If there is any indication of problems in these relationships, it is necessary to sensitively question whether there is any physical abuse. When the woman's symptoms are anxiety, depression, or various somatic complaints, one should thoroughly assess her social and family situations. There have been many situations in the author's experience in which, even though the presenting problem has been anxiety or depression, the real but concealed problem has involved physical abuse. Women also come to a health care setting for treatment of injuries. It is always appropriate for the physician or allied health professional to ask the cause of injury. If there is reason to think that the woman might have been assaulted, it is appropriate to sensitively ask her whether she has been assaulted and by whom.

There is usually a great deal of shame and embarrassment associated with being caught in a violent situation. One should not expect a woman coming to a health care facility for help to offer information about physical abuse without some assistance by a professional. Even after sensitive questioning, the woman seeking help might give an untrue or defensive answer. In addition to shame and embarrassment, there are other factors that might inhibit a woman's response to questioning about physical abuse. Often the woman is fearful of the consequences if she tells someone what has been happening. She also might believe that it is useless to tell anyone because nothing could possibly be done to make the situation any better. The woman might also be reluctant to talk about physical abuse for fear that she will be regarded as "sick" for remaining in the relationship. No matter what the response of the woman, the most important thing is that the question has been asked. Even if the woman is not ready to define abuse as a problem or to act on the situation, by asking the question, the professional has opened the door for her.

If and when the woman is ready to talk about her situation, she knows there is a place for her to go.

Certain considerations in approaching a woman about the possible existence of family violence have been identified by the author in her practice. In view of the previous discussion on the feelings of abused women, it is important to make any questions as nonthreatening as possible. It helps to put a woman at ease if, in questioning about violence, the professional is able to tell the woman that this is a common problem in the health care setting and that the woman is not alone in her experiences. If the woman does admit to physical abuse, consideration must be given to her physical safety. The woman should be asked if a knife or gun has ever been used in a physical attack. The woman should be told about the professional's concern for her safety. She should also be asked if she is afraid of being severely hurt. It takes only a few seconds in a violent situation for the victim to sustain serious bodily harm. If the woman does admit to fear of severe bodily injury, she should always be believed, no matter how extreme or unbelievable her story may seem. A woman who comes to a health care setting for treatment of injuries should be asked if she wants to return home. The woman might be too frightened to return to a situation in which the abusing party can attack her again. At a time such as this it is essential to be aware of community resources that could be of assistance to the abused woman.

There are situations in which both women and their children are being physically abused. A professional must remember this important consideration. It is appropriate and necessary to ask a woman whether the children are being abused. If information is received about child abuse, the professional must fulfill possible legal responsibilities in reporting this to the proper agency. Mandatory reporting of child abuse might force the woman to do something about her situation before she is psychologically ready to do so.

Another important consideration in interviewing a woman who has been physically assaulted is to inform her that she has the right to file criminal charges. The author has interviewed women who did not know that it is a crime for a husband or boyfriend to beat his partner. Knowledge of procedures for criminal prosecution is essential to help the woman if she wishes to press criminal charges. Often the woman is reluctant to initiate criminal proceedings because of the overwhelming fear of reprisal by the abusing party. Informing the woman of her rights and the procedures for prosecution are appropriate activities of the professional. The woman, however, should never be forced or pressured to follow this course.

Group Approach to Intervention

In the author's experience, women's therapy groups have been an effective means of attempting to intervene when relationship problems exist. It is not advisable to put together in a group only women who have been physically abused and then label the group a "battered women's group." As previously discussed, there can be detrimental outcomes to such labeling. Rather, women experiencing a wide range of relationship problems, physical abuse being only one of them, should be considered for this group experience. There are many advantages to having a group with a mixture of problems. It is therapeutic for all group members to see the similarities and differences among themselves regardless of their situations. It helps to reduce the isolation barrier of women in physically abusive situations to see themselves as similar to other women in different situations. Individuals who are experiencing relationship problems or have a diminished self concept generally believe, for a variety of reasons, that they have little self-power and few rights; they do not think that they deserve to have emotional feelings or deserve to express their needs. These factors are often present whether or not physical abuse is occurring. These are issues that can be addressed through a group approach. Group process can be utilized to help individuals who practice and learn new ways of relating to other significant persons in their lives.

In stressing the group experience for women, it is particularly important to state that the women do not have to leave unhealthy relationships in order for personal growth or change to take place. The author has observed in her practice that women can change as a result of a group experience regardless of their personal situations. Through a group experience, women begin to develop their ability to share feelings with others and thus begin to trust and accept the help of other people in and outside of the group in stressful as well as pleasant times. It is generally believed that there are certain pros and cons relating to the ways in which outside relationships affect group process. Considering the extreme isolation of some of these women, it is exciting to see them develop meaningful relationships for perhaps the first time in their lives. The possible negative effects on group process seem minimal in comparison to these growing friendships.

Another area of personal growth for women observed by the author in a group experience, again regardless of the participant's personal situation, is the development of a stronger self-concept and thus the beginnings of healthier behavior. This development is very much connected with the first area discussed, for from the building of trusting relationships also comes a better opinion of oneself. There are declarations that women can make to promote a more positive self-concept. Setting limits within a relationship on the type of behavior that will be tolerated is such a declaration. Women do reach the point where they state that further physical violence will not be allowed. Sometimes this limit setting is accomplished by the real threat of separation or even by the threat of physical reprisal by the woman. Women who make decisions to seek employment or job training or enroll in school also find that they eventually begin to feel better about themselves. Another behavior that helps promote a healthy self-concept is asking for what one wants and needs in a relationship. This behavior can be initiated, practiced, and learned within a group context.

As mentioned at the beginning of this chapter, working in this problem area can become quite frustrating to the professional. It is undoubtedly more frustrating to work in settings where the professional, rather than the woman, is identifying the problem. There is a high likelihood in these situations that the woman might not be ready to do anything about her situation. Questions regarding family violence still need to be asked. Individuals in a helping profession, therefore, must identify and deal with their own frustrations and irritations. It might be helpful if professionals in a variety of settings dealing with family violence formed support groups for themselves. These groups could provide not only a good opportunity for the expression of thoughts and feelings, but also the impetus for discovering new and better approaches for dealing with this complex problem area.

NOTES

1. Larry Silver, Christina Dublin, and Reginold Lourie, "Does Violence Breed Violence? Contributions from a Study of Child Abuse Syndrome," *American Journal of Psychiatry* 126, no. 3 (September 1969): 152-155.

2. J. J. Gayford, "Wife Battering: A Preliminary Survey of 100 Cases," *British Medical Journal* 1 (January 25, 1975): 194-197.

3. Susan Edmiston, "The Wife Beaters," *Women's Day*, March 1976, pp. 61-63.

4. Ibid.

5. G. I. Borofsky, G. E. Stollack, and L. A. Messe, "Sex Differences in Bystander Reactions to Physical Assault," *Journal of Experimental Social Psychology*, 7 (1971):313-318.

6. Edmiston, "Wife Beaters."

7. "Really Socking It to Women," *Time*, February 7, 1977, pp. 58-59.

13

Impact of Rape on Victims and Families

Treatment and Research Considerations

LINDA E. LEDRAY
SANDER H. LUND
THOMAS J. KIRESUK

Rape is a problem of great national, local, and personal concern. A rape has far-reaching effects on a woman's social, psychological, and physical being, often leading to involvement with the police, the court system, medical personnel, and counselors. This chapter deals with some of these issues. It includes the incidence and reporting of rape, the impact of rape on the woman and her family or significant other, the post-rape experience, and some of the recent changes in the medical and legal system that make it more responsive to the needs of the victim.

This chapter also outlines some of the difficulties related to clinical research in the area of sexual assault, suggests some strategies for surmounting these obstacles and developing useful research designs, examines some of the themes that might be important in such research, and describes a research project currently underway at Hennepin County Medical Center in Minneapolis that addresses some of the issues raised in the foregoing discussion.

INCIDENCE AND REPORTING OF RAPE

According to FBI statistics there were over 56,000 forcible rapes in the United States in 1976. This represents one *reported* rape for every 1,000 adult females, an increase of 166 percent in the past 15 years. In the state of Minnesota the increase has been even more dramatic. There has been a 528 percent increase from 1960 to 1976. Whereas all other violent crimes decreased nationally 5 percent in 1976, rape increased 1 percent during the first six months of the year. There also appears to be a shift in the incidence of rape from the major urban areas to the suburbs. In 1976 forcible rape decreased 1 percent in the large cities and increased 3 percent in the suburbs surrounding the large core cities. However, 42 percent of all rapes still occur in cities with a population of 250,000 or more.[1]

Although rape is the most frequently committed violent crime in the United States, the *Uniform Crime Report* states that rape is reported to the police less often than any other *Crime Index* offense.[2] Officials cannot be certain if this increase is due to better reporting, an actual increase in the incidence of rape, or a combination of the two. Even if better reporting is responsible for the higher statistics, officials estimate today that only 1 out of every 10 to 14 rapes is reported.[3] This means that there is an estimate of 1 actual rape for every 50 to 100 adult women. Reporting is lowest in major urban areas with high population density and low income levels.[4,5] It appears that many rapes go unreported because of the pervasive myths regarding rape and rape victims generally held in our society. These myths tend to disparage the victim and to demonstrate sympathy for the assailant.[6-8] It is probable that rapes also go unreported because of the humiliation and depersonalization of the victim by police, medical personnel, and the legal system.[9-11]

COMMUNITY ATTITUDES

Pervasive but unfounded myths about rape have been long accepted as fact and have a profound effect on the way that society views the rapist and rape victim, on the way that the victim sees herself, and on the number of rapes that are reported. The acceptance of these myths appears to be the result of a lack of understanding of the nature of forcible rapes.

One such myth is that rape is usually an impulsive act which occurs because the woman acts or dresses seductively and that rapists are driven mad with sexual desire and cannot help themselves. This view has been discredited by the research of Amir and others, who have shown that rapists plan their rapes, and their intent is often aggressive rather than sexual.[12] Amir's research also questions the commonly held belief that rape is a sex crime and supports the belief that rape is an assault, an act of aggression by one person against another. The findings of Price concur and show that the rape victim is reacting to an aggressive act of violence rather than a sexual act.[13]

A paradoxical twist of this myth has been reported by Jones and Aronson, who find that, the more socially respectable the victim, the more she is seen to be at fault by society. Rape victims are faulted more if they are either a virgin or married than if they are divorced. The authors interpreted these data as evidencing the belief in a "just world," where people get what they deserve. According to this theory, if a victim is perceived as respectable, there is a greater cognitive need to attribute fault to her actions, because fault cannot be attributed to her character.[14] This theory is based on Lerner's just-world hypothesis[15,16] and the cognitive dissonance theory.[17]

Rape myths include beliefs that women enjoy or secretly desire to be raped, that nice girls do not get raped, that rapes occur only in dark alleys, and that a woman cannot be raped unless she is willing ("a woman can run faster with her skirt up than a man with his pants down"). These and many others are discussed and refuted by Amir,[18] Brownmiller,[19] Medea and Thompson,[20] and many reputable scientific investigators. However, these myths continue to be believed by otherwise intelligent, knowledgeable individuals, and, no matter how unfounded, these myths have a profound effect on both the victim's view of herself and the family's or significant other's view of the victim.

IMPACT ON THE VICTIM

Rape is a violent crime with physical, social, and psychological consequences that are often of great magnitude. However, until recently there has been little concern about the impact on the victim. Rape has been considered a crime by one man against the property (wife or daughter) of another man.[21]

The way a woman responds to rape depends to a great extent on her prior adaptive capacity, coping style, and social support.[22] Certainly the 946 women raped in Minneapolis from 1973 to 1976 reacted in a variety of ways and to various degrees. Preliminary research, although limited, provides some insights into the nature of the physical, social, and psychological suffering of the victim regardless of age, race, occupation, or personal history.

Physical Trauma

The physical trauma is perhaps best documented because of records kept by hospitals. The rape victim may have sustained injuries from being beaten and other forms of physical violence, as well as from forceful intercourse leading to vaginal and rectal trauma. From the limited statistics available it appears that the need for hospitalization after a rape is low. Hayman and Lanza reported that only 1 percent of the rape victims seen in a Washington, D. C., hospital needed to be hospitalized, and only 3 percent needed emergency room treatment for severe injuries.[23] Hennepin County Medical Center in Minneapolis found that 32 percent of the rape victims treated in 1976 had been beaten severely enough to require medical treatment. Statistics are not readily available on the number of deaths related to or subsequent to rape, since these are usually reported by the police as homicide. However, fear of death or serious injury is often the greatest concern of the woman at the time of the incident.[24,25]

Statistics show that the risk of pregnancy following a rape is low, about 1 percent, as is the risk of contracting verereal disease, less than 4 percent but increasing. However, these are both of great concern to a woman following a rape. It is difficult to ascertain the actual risk of becoming pregnant or contracting verereal disease after a rape, because the statistics available are based on the small percentage of women who report the incident and receive care after the rape. This care usually includes prophylactic penicillin to prevent venereal disease and prophylactic diethylstilbestrol to prevent pregnancy.[26] The above statistics would undoubtedly be much higher were they to include the many victims, possibly 13 out of 14, who fail to report the rape, receive no prophylaxis, and are therefore much more vulnerable to both venereal disease and pregnancy.

Other, often long-term physical problems may occur. These include changes in eating habits and in sleeping patterns, often due to recurrent nightmares.[27]

Social Impact

The social impact of rape on the victim is not documented in systematized research; however, implications can be drawn from case studies. Rape has been recognized as a time of crisis for the victim. However, it differs from other crises because the victim's usual support system is more likely to be disrupted.[28,29] The victim may be isolated after rejection by the husband, family, friends, and/or lover because of their preconceptions regarding her role in the rape.[30] Peters and Medea and Thompson found that many victims voluntarily withdraw socially and emotionally from all contact with friends and family, while they are at the same time afraid to be alone.[31,32] Brownmiller has shown that rape may often be used by the man as a means of conquering, suppressing, and subjugating the female to his authority or of punishing her.[33]

Case studies document incidents of victims being evicted from their apartments following rape because the landlord was upset when the police arrived and believed it to be a drug bust. Other victims may move to another city, either voluntarily or after being ordered to leave home. For many this move represents a way to escape the social disgrace still associated with rape.[34] If the rape occurred in their home they may fear that the rapist will return and therefore move to ensure their safety.[35] The literature alludes to some long-term effects of the socially disruptive consequences of rape; however, the extent and prevalence have not yet been determined.

Psychological Impact

Although the physical and social impact of rape is great, the psychological trauma is the most devastating.[36] Research studies of the psychological impact of rape are just beginning to appear in the literature and evidence a pattern of response, which Burgess calls the "Rape Trauma Syndrome."[37] This pattern is generally broken down into three phases. Phase 1, the *acute reaction*, is characterized by shock and disbelief, physical symptoms, gross anxiety, emotional breakdown, and disorganization and disruption in the normal pattern of behavior and function. Phase 2, the *outward adjustment*, includes resolution of the acute anxiety, denial and suppression, and return to normal function at work, school, or home. This usually occurs a few days to a week after the incident. Phase 3, that of *integration and resolution*, often goes unnoticed. It is characterized by the onset of depression, the need to talk about the experience, anger at the assailant and at oneself and eventually a realistic appraisal of one's view of oneself.

Case studies have revealed the existence of long-term psychological effects of rape. Some of the long-term traumas noted are recurrent nightmares, depression, phobia to men, fear of being alone, fear of being outside if the rape occurred outside, fear of being inside if the rape occurred inside, sexual fears, fear of crowds, fear of people behind them,[38] and fear of looking provocative.[39] In Operation De Nova, a Hennepin County Juvenile Division program in Minneapolis, it has recently been found that the first sexual experience of 70 percent of the juvenile prostitutes was either rape or an incestuous relationship.[40] This finding raises additional questions about the long-term effects of rape.

Burgess also identified what she calls a compound reaction. This was noted in individuals with current or past physical, social, or psychiatric difficulties and consisted of additional symptoms such as depression, psychosis, and suicidal behavior.[41] Two rape victims seen in the Hennepin County Medical Center emergency room in a six-month period have attempted suicide subsequent to the rape.

IMPACT ON THE FAMILY OR SIGNIFICANT OTHER

Borges,[42] Peters,[43] Medea and Thompson,[44] and Brownmiller[45] all recognize that the attitude about rape and the reaction of the family or significant other to the rape incident are of great significance to the rape victim, but they give no clear indication as to how or the extent to which this is significant. Emergency room nurses at Hennepin County Medical Center have found that often the first question asked by the rape victim is, "Should I tell my husband/parents/boyfriend?" and, if so, "How should I tell them?"

Mental health professionals have accepted for some time that the family is an interacting social system. Whatever affects one member has an effect on another member. The rape victim, as a member of a social system, interacts with family and with friends. However, very few research data are currently available regarding the family's/significant other's reaction to a rape or how their reaction affects the victim.

Many families decide to keep the rape a secret. This practice may "protect" both victim and family immediately, but case studies show that problems may arise in therapy at a later date.[46] From these case studies we have learned that families are often inconsiderate and rejecting, blame the victim, and misplace their anger at the rapist onto the victim instead of providing the support she so desperately needs.[47] Although no statistics are currently available, Brownmiller states that husbands often divorce their wives after a rape, further escalating the trauma and isolating the victim.[48] Burgess concurs that the adverse reaction of the significant other is often part of the further traumatization of the victim after the rape.[49]

One would expect that the traumatization of the victim would end when the rape incident ends. This is not always the case. All too often, the trauma is compounded during what should be treatment.

TREATMENT OF THE VICTIM

The treatment needs of rape victims include medical intervention, psychological intervention, and legal intervention by the police and perhaps the courts.

Medical Intervention

The first need of most rape victims is medical care, yet many hospitals still refuse to treat rape victims. Peters reported that every hospital in Philadelphia, except the General Hospital, has been turning away rape victims for years.[50] Hayman reported a lack of success in encouraging hospitals in the Washington, D. C., area to treat rape victims because the hospital administrations, staff physicians, interns, residents, and private physicians still greatly fear having to testify in court about a sexual assault.[51] Because of this, rape victims are often refused treatment at the first hospital they go to and must find another. This is a rejection they do not need at this time of crisis.

Some hospitals that do treat rape victims have not yet developed adequate protocols to collect the necessary corroborative evidence that will later be needed in court; thus, they do the victim a further disservice. In Hennepin County, the largest county in the state of Minnesota with a population of close to 1 million people, only five of the major hospitals have developed protocols and treat rape victims. Hennepin County Medical Center is the primary rape treatment center and last year saw 239 of the 402 county rape victims.

Once the victim finds a hospital where treatment will be provided, her problems still have not ended. The literature is filled with examples of the degradation, blame, moralizing, and lack of understanding by medical staff members who do not really believe she was raped.[52,53] Male hospital staff members have admitted to feeling guilty, as men, when they have to deal with a rape victim.[54]

Hospital personnel have just recently recognized the problems and are developing better treatment programs. The goals of a good medical treatment include (1) immediate care of injury, (2) prevention of venereal disease, (3) prevention of pregnancy, (4) proper medical-legal examination with documentation for law enforcement agencies, and (5) psychosocial crisis intervention.

In many hospitals the initial examination may cost from $50 to $150, adding an additional burden for the victim and her family. Hennepin County in Minnesota as well as other facilities have recently made provisions to absorb this cost if the victim is willing to report the incident to the police. They do so because this evidence is essential to the presentation of the case in court.

Hospitals are just beginning to pay attention to the emotional component of rape. Knowing that the physical examination can be traumatic to the rape victim, many hospitals try to have a female staff member available to be with the victim, explain all procedures, and provide emotional support.[55]

Psychological Intervention

The counseling needs of rape victims have also just recently been recognized. Burgess identified the counseling needs as a need to talk, confirmation of concern, ventilation, clarification, and advice.[56] McGee cautions mental health professionals to remember that people in crisis, and rape victims are in crisis, are not sick. They are not mentally ill, but they do need immediate, active, and aggressive crisis intervention.[57] Other authors indicate that the counseling needs of the rape victim are mainly support and advocacy.[58] An important implication for the mental health professional, which Bard and Ellison pointed out, is that without effective avenues for talking the experience through, there can be long-term damage to psychological functioning.[59]

Legal Intervention

The other agency with which the victim will most likely have immediate contact is the police department and later perhaps the courts. She must decide if she wishes to press charges and fill out a police report. Her credibility may be questioned. The police, not believing the rape charge, may change the charge to a lesser offense. The police report goes into specific detail regarding the rape incident and asks questions about intimate sexual contact that are difficult to answer, especially to a disbelieving, insensitive male.[60] A strong effort is presently underway to change both the attitudes of the police and police treatment of the victim. Many cities have established special sexual assault squads with well-trained, sensitive policemen and policewomen.[61]

Should the victim decide to prosecute and should the assailant be apprehended, the victim must then undergo the ordeal of the courtroom. In many states her character is literally put on trial. Her credibility, morality, and past sexual conduct are questioned.[62] Not only must she relive the experience in detail but she must do so in a public courtroom where members of the press may be present to report the incident in the media.

Even after she undergoes this ordeal, the chances of obtaining a conviction are very low. Nationally about 40 percent of those taken to court are convicted.[63] The situation is not as bleak in Hennepin County, where for the past two years the Sexual Assault Services have made a concerted effort to change the legal system and protect the rape victim rather than only the rapist. The present conviction rate in Hennepin County is 75 percent, one of the highest in the nation. This has been possible because of a coordinated effort between the police, courts, and medical/counseling personnel.

COORDINATION OF SERVICES

Rape is a law enforcement, legal, and medical problem. The groups of professionals involved cannot work in isolation and expect to solve a problem they do not have all the resources to deal with. To function effectively an interlocking system must be established with mutual support and cooperation among these professionals and the agencies they represent.

In the past each of these groups worked independently. The police brought the victim to the hospital and later completed their report on the incident. The hospital treated any injuries and did routine venereal disease and pregnancy tests. When the woman chose to prosecute the courts later became involved.

The result of this situation in 1970 was that in the entire state of Minnesota, only 23 charges of rape were made and only 12 of these resulted in convictions. The police did not understand rape and in many instances did not believe a rape had actually occurred, as evidenced by their changing the charge to breaking and entering or burglary. When the police did make an arrest for rape, often after expending considerable time and effort to apprehend the suspect, the courts could not prosecute because of the lack of evidence. In many instances there was nothing to go on; it was the woman's word against the suspect's. The physicians and nurses in emergency rooms had no idea what evidence would be useful, how to collect it, or what to do with it if it was found. So the evidence was lost or not admissible in court because it was improperly handled. Victims did not want to prosecute because of revictimization in the courtroom, nor did they choose to call the police or see medical personnel because of the lack of understanding and empathy others had experienced and reported.

When this situation was finally identified and the problem recognized, a concerted effort was made by legal, medical, and law enforcement groups to discuss the issues in interagency meetings. Their goals were not only to improve their own understanding and handling of the rape situation but, even more importantly, to learn from each other and integrate and coordinate their efforts so that they could provide support and assistance to each other and deal more effectively with victims of sexual assault.

The police received training to increase their understanding of the rape situation and the needs of rape victims. The police and the courts worked with hospital personnel to develop an evidentiary examination that would allow physicians and nurses to collect evidence that could later be used in court. The hospitals trained interested physicians and nurses to collect this evidence and provide support to victims of rape. When necessary, they would go to court and testify as expert witnesses. Since these professionals were now providing a very useful service, their frustration was greatly diminished and replaced by a satisfaction with the service they were providing.

Since 1970 the county attorney's office has made dramatic changes that have greatly enhanced the total impact of services to victims of sexual assault. This began with the establishment of the Sexual Assault Program, a division of the county attorney's office. Their efforts have led to changes in the laws relating to criminal sexual conduct, making them much more comprehensive, humanistic, and nondiscriminatory and, most important, making it easier to more appropriately charge and prosecute offenders. In addition, the laws now protect the victim and do not allow her character to be put on trial. The county attorney also issued a directive that offenders would be charged with the sexual crime; they would not be allowed to plead guilty to a lesser crime and the sex charge dropped.

Under the present coordinated services, the following is a typical case:

> A 24-year-old white woman, Mrs. Mary K., was brought to the Hennepin County Medical Center emergency room at 11:30 p.m. by two policemen. She had called the police after an unknown man had broken into her ground-floor apartment and raped her. Her husband was out of town.

> Upon arriving at the emergency room she was tearful and frightened. The policemen were both understanding and sympathetic. While one comforted her, another identified her as a rape victim to the nurse in charge of the emergency room. She was taken immediately to a quiet section at the back of the emergency room specifically set aside to deal with rape victims. The nurse who had been trained to deal with rape victims remained with her throughout the medical-legal examination. While the evidentiary examination was being completed, the rape crisis counselor on-call arrived.

> The emergency room nurse introduced Mary to the rape counselor, who Mary would later learn would be available to meet with her for up to one year. Mary was afraid to go home; so the counselor found her a safe place to spend the night.

The next day the rape counselor called Mary and arranged to pick her up and take her to the police station to complete the police report. Based on Mary's statement and the evidence collected by the emergency room staff, the police were able to apprehend the offender, who later pleaded guilty. The counselor would have accompanied Mary to court had this been necessary. The counselor met with Mary and her husband weekly for the next two months to discuss their feelings about and reactions to the rape. She also met Mary at the hospital on her return visits to see if she had contracted venereal disease or was pregnant. After the first two months they decided the visits could be less frequent, although they continued to meet for the next ten months and terminated the meetings one year after the incident.

Mary and her husband moved to a new location shortly after the incident. Mary was still a little uncomfortable when her husband was out of town; otherwise, their lives had returned to normal.

Once these groups integrated their services, other groups working with victims and offenders became involved in the Sexual Assault Task Force. Representatives from various community agencies met regularly to share information and concerns. The agencies represented included hospitals, rape crisis centers, police, the county attorney, homes for battered women, counseling services for victims and offenders, Department of Corrections, Court Services, and witness assistance programs. By meeting on a regular basis to share interests and concerns, to solve problems, and to continually coordinate their programs, these groups can offer more effective services to offenders, victims, and families or significant others.

Since this coordination has occurred, the number of cases of sexual assault charges has increased from 23 in the entire state of Minnesota in 1970 to 136 in Hennepin County alone in 1976. This compares with a 1 percent increase in a neighboring county, where no changes in the system occurred. While only 50 percent of the cases were convicted in 1970, 83 percent of the cases were convicted in 1976. Only 10 percent of these ever had to go to court. The evidence was so well established that the defendant pleaded guilty, greatly decreasing the trauma to the victim. The Hennepin County police state that at least 70 percent of the case is made by the evidence presently collected by hospital personnel. The coordination of efforts and the integration of programs are recognized by all involved as essential in providing the services that must be available to victims and their families or significant others.

The more closely the sexual assault situation is examined the more we are faced with a dearth of systematic research about the impact of rape and needs of rape victims and their families or significant others, who are also affected by this experience and must deal with their feelings as well as those of the victim.

OBSTACLES TO CLINICAL RESEARCH IN THE AREA OF SEXUAL ASSAULT

Like most human problems, sexual assault is a topic that has little potential for study in the controlled conditions of laboratory research. Neither the event, nor the conditions of the event, nor the characteristics of any of the main actors are subject to the control of the investigator, and as a consequence most research in this area is descriptive, involving ex post facto analysis of rapes. Threats to validity due to poor control of spurious sources of variation are legion, and the inappropriateness of research designs that incorporate experimental safeguards means that many of the conclusions generated from such research must be interpreted with caution.

The efficacy of various approaches to the treatment of victims of sexual assault, however, is a subject that can be addressed with greater methodologic confidence. Once a victim of sexual assault has been identified and has sought services, it is possible to institute appropriate research controls (i.e., random assignment of victims to treatment conditions that embody various kinds of therapy modes of untested effectiveness) to mitigate the effects of contaminating variables.

A major obstacle to effective research in this area accrues from the absence of a body of useful empirical generations from previous research. Not only are there no generally accepted theories and principles to guide research, but the field is often still obfuscated by popular myths, half-truths, and untested convictions, which must be dealt with before formative research can begin. Inquiry must literally start at the most rudimentary level.

Related to this is what might be called the problem of definition. Meaningful research requires a clear specification of the variables under study. In research regarding sexual assault, this is impeded by the absence of previous research to (1) point out the important variables to study and (2) provide a commonly accepted definition for further inquiry.

A severe threat to the validity of research regarding sexual assault comes from the difficulty in drawing unbiased samples for study from the true universe of sexual assault victims. In the first place, not all instances of sexual assault come to public attention. For a variety of reasons, many of those who are victims of such attacks do not report it, which means that it may never be possible to make an unbiased estimation of the essential characteristics of victims of sexual assault. This problem may be mitigated in the future as rape is destigmatized and positive efforts are made to construct means to facilitate the entrance of rape victims into the human services delivery system.

With regard to clinical research in this area, the problem of the nonrepresentativeness of those who seek services as opposed to the whole universe of those who are victims of sexual assault is not so acute. The function of clinical research is to determine the efficacy of a given treatment for those who receive services. However, a related problem is that, because of the nature of sexual assault, many victims refuse or are unavailable to participate in research. Often this means that clinical research generalizations are founded upon work focused on a small and probably nonrepresentative segment of the universe of victims of rape. The various "quasi-experimental" designs catalogued by Campbell and Stanley do not solve the problem but are helpful in highlighting which assumptions are required in various designs for statistical inference to be valid.[64]

Rape research is also greatly hindered by the special circumstances attendant on sexual assault. One special issue, alluded to above, is that rape involves violence, humiliation, and potential stigmatization of the victim. Because of the special vulnerability of the victim and because research may exacerbate the aftereffects of rape (and may also bring attention to the victim that she wishes to avoid), special safeguards are necessary to insure that the research procedures are innocuous regarding the victim's recovery and do not contribute to potential stigmatization.

In addition, because sexual assault is a crime, any research in this area must be managed so that it does not compromise the legal processes. Confidentiality is always a crucial issue, but particularly in this instance it is vital that client records be guarded with absolute security. Also, records, if they are liable to be used in a legal case, must be kept so that they do not inadvertently compromise the prosecution of the perpetrator of the sexual assault.

Measures

One critical consequence of the absence of a cohesive body of past research data in the area of treatment of victims of sexual assault is that there are few measurement devices specific to this area. Investigators may borrow or adapt measures from fields with related emphases (e.g., crisis intervention), but, since there is no guarantee that such measures actually assess variation in appropriate variables reliably, the results may, to one extent or another, be compromised.

Related to the above issue is the fact that the absence of measures means that there are no baseline data on the recovery of rape victims from assault. There has been little empirical validation of the kinds of problems experienced by rape victims, and overall there are no commonly accepted empirical standards for evaluating treatment accorded to victims of sexual assault. Without such information, it is problematic for clinicians, community, and policy makers to assess the impact of rape treatment programs.

A technical difficulty regarding most measurement in the area of treatment of sexual assault is that most of the measures employed thus far have been reactive; that is, the method and content of the measure are apparent to the subject and in consequence may alter her attitudes and behavior regarding the assault and her recovery from it. Even in routine social research, reactive measures have been shown to bias outcomes.[65] In the turbulent setting of rape therapy research, where the victim may be confused and disoriented in the immediate aftereffects of the assault, all reasonable effort must be made to control the effects on results of intrusive research methodology.

RESEARCH STRATEGIES

The existence of these and other related problems means that the conduct of rape treatment research in the coming years will be guided and controlled by a series of issues and needs.

Exploratory—Multivariate Designs

Since systematic empirical inquiry regarding the causes, constituents, and consequences of sexual assault is only now beginning, a major emphasis in the field will be upon establishing the parameters of the field, identifying the most important variables for study, developing common definitions of concepts, devising special research methodology, and constructing empirical models that can be employed in wide subsequent research. In this process there is a need for both wide-ranging exploratory studies and tightly focused field experiments. The exploratory studies help the field develop a clinical focus, common vocabulary, and formative theoretical framework. The field experiments provide small amounts of empirical information that can be woven into the general theoretical formulations. At both the macro and micro levels, it is important that the designs include provision for the study of the effects of multiple variables.

As research gets underway, it is vitally important that an information network be formed among rape researchers and that central offices be established to coordinate activities, evaluate research, identify needs, and facilitate development of theoretical and empirical generalizations. The impetus for research in. this area comes from various sources, and those who will conduct the research represent almost all of the major academic and human service disciplines. Redundant actions and wasted effort (not to mention potential hostility among disciplines) will probably occur unless those involved in studying and preventing sexual assault can link themselves to an entirely new and unencumbered communication system. A helpful sign is that the National Institute of Mental Health has established and funded the National Center for the Study and Control of Rape.

Measurement

The lack of meaningful measures in the area of sexual assault will be alleviated, at least in part, as a natural consequence of the implementation of theoretically meaningful and technically sound research designs, the development of technically sound measurement being an inevitable aspect of the implementation of effective research. At least two strategies are possible with regard to development of meaningful measures to assess the effectiveness of treatment of rape victims.

Standard Measures

The usual procedure in clinical rape treatment research has been either to borrow measures from related fields like crisis intervention or to develop questionnaires and measurement forms specifically for the immediate situation. The difficulty with the former is that instruments developed for other purposes may not be sensitive to the essential processes involved in the treatment of victims of sexual assault. The difficulty with the latter is that program-specific measures tend to be of variable psychometric quality, are not norm-referenced, are difficult to interpret, and are difficult to generalize with other research findings. Examples of standardized measures that may be appropriate to research in sexual assault are the Hopkins Systems Checklist, the Holmes Stress Inventory, the Menninger Health Sickness Rating Scale, and the Self-Rating Symptom Scale.

An essential prerequisite for the development of fixed-content measures of the efficacy of the treatment accorded victims of sexual assault will be the identification and specification of the constructs that are important in the therapy process. Some such constructs will, of course, generalize from other field measures, but some will be specific to recovery from sexual assault. Most needs will be identified through the successive formulation, testing, and reformulation of research hypotheses. Once such constructs are identified, "indicators" (usually scales that are intended to reflect variation in behavior or attitudes) may be selected (or constructed) to signify changes in the quality or quantity of variables under measurement. These scales can then be evaluated to determine their reliability (the degree to which they measure whatever it is they measure consistently) and validity (the degree to which they measure whatever it is they are supposed to measure), and statistical norms may be developed to show how the scopes of the measure vary when generated from populations with various characteristics.

Individualized Goal Attainment Measures

The development and validation of meaningful standard measures will inevitably be a lengthy process. One form of assessment appropriate to determine the effectiveness of the services provided victims of sexual assault is already in existence. This is individualized goal attainment (IGA) measurement. A characteristic of this form of measurement is the determination of treatment outcome according to the attainment of specific, predetermined clinical goals that have been tailored to fit what is known both about the client and about the probable effects of the proposed treatment. With roots in idiographic psychology, psychotherapy research, and management science, IGA measurement currently is constituted by a loosely comparable set of goal-setting methodologies. Perhaps the best known of these is goal attainment scaling,[66] which at last count had been formally implemented by over 300 human service organizations throughout the world. Goal attainment scaling is a flexible, patient-specific technique for quantitatively assessing attainment of specific, predetermined goals. Goal attainment is measured on a grid-shaped form called a goal attainment follow-up guide (Fig. 13.1). Such a form consists of a succession of discrete five-point scales, each of which represents an individual client concern arrayed along a qualitatively ordered series of possible outcomes. The nature of these outcomes ranges from "most unfavorable outcome thought likely," to the "best anticipated success," with the expected level of success at the middle level. The content of each scale is determined prior to treatment and is tailored to the needs, capacities, and expectations of the person receiving services. There are a variety of strategies possible for determining the content of a goal attainment follow-up guide. One strategy is for a clinician, or group of clinicians, to fill in the content without client participation. Another strategy is for a clinician and client to determine the content through negotiation. A third strategy is for the client alone to determine the content.

At a predetermined time following the construction of the goal attainment follow-up guide, the client is contacted and, on the basis of each scale of the follow-up guide, the degree to which the specified goals have been achieved is determined. From this information it is possible to calculate a goal attainment score. A goal attainment score is generated through a formula that transforms the weighted ratings on the individual scales on a follow-up guide into a single overall numerical value. A goal attainment score of 50.00 indicates that, on the average, a client has exactly attained the "expected outcome" level on the goals scaled. A score of more than 50.00 indicates that expectations have been exceeded, and a score of less than 50.00 indicates they have not been met. A distribution of goal attainment scores typically approximates a normal curve, with a mean of about 50.00 and a standard deviation of about 10.00. This makes it possible to use parametric statistical procedures to analyze results.

Level at Intake: 29.4
Goal Attainment Score
(Level at Follow-up): 62.2
Goal Attainment Change Score: +32.8

PROGRAM EVALUATION PROJECT

GOAL ATTAINMENT FOLLOW-UP GUIDE

Level at Intake: ✓
Level at Follow-up: *

Check whether or not the scale has been mutually negotiated between patient and CIC interviewer.

SCALE HEADINGS AND SCALE WEIGHTS

SCALE ATTAINMENT LEVELS	SCALE 1: Education Yes __ No X__ (w_1=20)	SCALE 2: Suicide Yes __ No X__ (w_2=30)	SCALE 3: Manipulation Yes __ No X__ (w_3=25)	SCALE 4: Drug Abuse Yes X__ No __ (w_4=30)	SCALE 5: Dependency on CIC Yes X__ No __ (w_5=10)
a. most unfavorable treatment outcome thought likely (-2)	Patient has made no attempt to enroll in high school. ✓	Patient has committed suicide.	Patient makes rounds of community service agencies demanding medication, and refuses other forms of treatment. ✓	Patient reports addiction to "hard narcotics" (heroin, morphine).	Patient has contacted CIC by telephone or in person at least seven times since his first visit.
b. less than expected success with treatment (-1)	Patient has enrolled in high school, but at time of follow-up has dropped out.	Patient has acted on at least one suicidal impulse since her first contact with the CIC, but has not succeeded. ✓	Patient no longer visits CIC with demands for medication but continues with other community agencies and still refuses other forms of treatment.	Patient has used "hard narcotics," but is not addicted, and/or uses hallucinogens (LSD, Pot) more than four times a month. ✓	Patient has contacted CIC 5-6 times since intake.
c. expected level of treatment success (0)	Patient has enrolled, and is in school at follow-up, but is attending class sporadically (misses an average of more than a third of her classes during a week).	Patient reports she has had at least four suicidal impulses since her first contact with the CIC but has not acted on any of them.	Patient no longer attempts to manipulate for drugs at community service agencies, but will not accept another form of treatment. *	Patient has not used "hard narcotics" during follow-up period, and uses hallucinogens between 1-4 times a month. *	Patient has contacted CIC 3-4 times since intake.
d. more than expected success with treatment (+1)	Patient has enrolled, is in school at follow-up, and is attending classes consistently, but has no vocational goals. *	*	Patient accepts non-medication treatment at some community agency.	Patient uses hallucinogens less than once a month.	
e. best anticipated success with treatment (+2)	Patient has enrolled, is in school at follow-up, is attending classes consistently, and has some vocational goal.	Patient reports she has had no suicidal impulses since her first contact with the CIC.		At time of follow-up, patient is not using any illegal drugs.	Patient has not contacted CIC since intake. *

Figure 13.1. Sample clinical guide: Crisis Intervention Center (CIC).

Systematic investigations regarding the reliability[67,68] and the validity[69,70] of goal attainment scaling have found them to be within accepted psychometric parameters.[71] The special relevance of goal attainment scaling to clinical research regarding sexual assault relates to the current absence of accepted measures of the impact of rape and the corresponding need to determine appropriate problem areas and recovery rates. The goal attainment follow-up guides constructed for clients of rape treatment centers will serve as a depository of information regarding what must be done to alleviate the consequences of rape for a victim and how long it takes to do it.

Attrition

As in most field studies, the utility of data collected in clinical rape research will depend largely upon success in recruiting appropriate subjects and following them up in an appropriate and timely fashion. If a significant portion of the sample leaves treatment or declines follow-up, the research will have to contend not only with asymmetric cells and a computationally difficult method of analysis, but also with logical limitations on the inferences that can be drawn regarding treatment effects. The topic under investigation is very sensitive; most research methods are somewhat intrusive; and the length and intensity of commitment by victims to a study are sometimes demanding. These factors, together with the manifest need to avoid even the subtlest pressure on subjects to participate in a research project, mean that attrition of the sample may become a serious threat to the integrity of a study. Fortunately, there is some evidence that victims of sexual assault who seek, or are brought to, medical services are typically willing, even enthusiastic, to help find more effective means to assist other rape victims. For example, during a survey of rape victims who were receiving services at Hennepin County Medical Center, 25 out of 25 approached said they would participate in a study that involved multiple follow-ups, randomized assignment to different kinds of treatment, and potential family involvement in therapy. Although this finding is a hopeful sign for the future conduct of research in this area, it seems self-evident that our future success will vary according to our ability to devise and implement special means to mitigate the effects of sample attrition. A straightforward means to reduce attrition is to insure both that the research has a realistic potential to add to what is known about treatment of rape victims and that the purpose and methods of the study are clearly communicated to the potential participant. People seem more likely to participate in a project when they are convinced that it is worthwhile and they understand how it works. Victims will also be more likely to participate if their prior commitment is elicited through the use of a consent form and if the research procedures are either intrinsically rewarding to the subject or are linked to events that are rewarding. Particularly in longitudinal studies, follow-up success can often be increased if the application of the research measures are linked to some form of treatment intervention. Minimizing paperwork, insuring that staff members are sensitive and efficient, and assuring clients of absolute confidentiality will also help increase participation.

Of course, no field study will ever prevent all attrition of research subjects. One means to mitigate the bias occasioned by the differential loss to the study of subjects is to implement a very aggressive follow-up policy for a small, randomly selected subset of the sample. Although often too costly to adhere to on a large scale, making every effort to follow-up a limited number of subjects provides a means to estimate the characteristics of those who reject or are unavailable for follow-up. Such findings can be used during data analysis to correct for the effect on results of differences between subjects who do and do not receive follow-up.

Sensitivity

Few crimes are as physically and psychologically deleterious to a victim as is sexual assault. The pain, horror, and confusion occasioned by rape greatly increase the vulnerability of a subject to further injury and require that special safeguards be implemented to see to it that her recovery is in no way hindered by the research. To insure, for example, that victims are able to make a truly "informed consent" regarding participation in a given piece of research, presentation of the consent form and subsequent initiation of research procedures should be delayed until the immediate turmoil surrounding the attack has subsided and the victim has a chance to examine the research critically. As an additional safeguard, the content of the consent form can be reviewed at every follow-up so that the victim will have ample opportunity to withdraw from the study.

It is vitally important that follow-up contacts be absolutely confidential and as unobtrusive as possible. No one should be contacted regarding the victim's participation in the study without her explicit approval. Follow-up workers should be matched with victims on racial and ethnic variables and should dress in a style that blends with the victim's neighborhood and life style. If the victim does not wish the follow-up to take place in her home, arrangements should be made for an interview at another site and free transportation provided. Concern that follow-ups will interfere with the victim's full recovery is mitigated by the findings of a study by Halley and Baxter.[72] In this research, clients of Hennepin County Mental Health Service who had previously been followed-up to determine treatment outcome were surveyed again to assess reaction to the previous follow-up. Over three-quarters reported being pleased with the previous follow-up and many had shown a marked clinical improvement subsequent to follow-up (suggesting that research follow-ups are not contraindicated clinically and may even have salutory side effects).

A source of great concern for those who participate as subjects in research regarding rape treatment is that their records remain strictly confidential. To protect each subject's right to privacy, all records must be treated as privileged communications. Storing research data in locked files in locked rooms (or, if the data are stored in an automated information system, seeing to it that appropriate security measures are adhered to) is a good beginning, but in addition steps should be taken to insure that the research workers who have access to the data are unable to determine the identity of the subject. One means to do this is to store records according to a randomly selected identification number, with all identifying information (e.g., name, address, telephone number) deleted. A master list identifying each subject can be maintained by the coordinator of the research, but after a subject's active involvement in the research is over (and it is no longer important to be able to identify a subject as an individual) the link between the identification number and the subject's name is destroyed. This makes it impossible to identify the subject at any future time, either inadvertently or by design.

THEMES IMPORTANT IN CLINICAL RESEARCH REGARDING SEXUAL ASSAULT

Overall, relatively little seems to be known about how people recover from the trauma of sexual assault.

Treatment

The most obvious and pressing research topic in this area relates to determining the relative effectiveness of various methods of helping rape victims recover from their attack. Often rape victims receive little more than perfunctory medical care following the assault, but sometimes they also receive intense, long-term, crisis-oriented counseling. The relative (comparative) effects of these two forms of treatment are not known and clearly require investigation.

Once base rates have been established regarding effectiveness, it·will be important to inquire as to how the treatment process is influenced by the characteristics of those who render treatment. As Strupp[73] observed regarding psychotherapy, it is no longer legitimate to treat therapy as a "blackbox" that will have the same effect on all clients. Complex problems require complex solutions, and, just as each client is individual in terms of needs and capacities, each service provider is individual in terms of therapeutic philosophy and skill level. The central task in clinical research regarding sexual assault will be to find the optimal means to match different kinds of treatment and different kinds of treatment providers with specific client problems. Questions must be answered in a variety of areas:

1. *The assault*: How is the victim's recovery affected by the characteristics of the assault and the assailant (e.g., the degree of violence of the attack, the number of attacks, the relationship of the attacker to the victim, the physical location of the attack)?

2. *The victim*: How is the victim's recovery affected by the characteristics of the victim herself (e.g., her age and background, her attitude toward rape, her previous sexual experiences, her previous level of "mental health")?

3. *The treatment*: How is the victim's recovery affected by the characteristics of the treatment she receives (e.g., long term or short term, medical alone or medical plus counseling, immediate or delayed)?

4. *The therapist*: How is the victim's recovery affected by the characteristics of the person who provides treatment (e.g., professional or paraprofessional; level of skill and training style, therapeutic opinions and attitudes; degree to which therapist is similar to victim in terms of personal characteristics)?

5. *Other circumstances*: How is the victim's recovery affected by the immediate circumstances of the assault and its aftermath (e.g., the victim's financial/vocational situation, the sort of treatment received from police and medical personnel, the existence of a support group or family or friends)?

The overall course of clinical research regarding rape will be guided by past research, by experiential observations of those already in the field, and by evolving theoretical formulations. Initially, most research will be summative in nature, dedicated to determining whether particular forms of clinical intervention are worth continuing. As effective treatment modalities are identified, research will become increasingly formative, aimed at refining and improving clinical practices and determining situations in which they are most likely to have maximum impact.

Family Involvement

Although the act of rape is usually a solitary event for the victim, recovery often takes place in the midst of a complex social network composed of family, friends, and casual acquaintances. Little is currently known about how this support system can influence a victim's recovery from sexual assault. Common sense would suggest that an open, loving, and supportive family that allows expression of anger and rage would provide the backup needed by a rape victim at a time when she would feel most vulnerable and unloved. Yet some families would clearly have a potential for being destructive in the aftermath of an assault (e.g., might blame the victim for the attack), and others might need therapeutic guidance to know how best to assist the victim.

Many questions must be answered. Should families be involved in planning and providing treatment for a rape victim? If so, how soon after the attack should they be brought in? What kind of families should not be involved? What should be done with victims who have no immediate support system? (Can artificial support systems be created?) If the victim has an enduring outside relationship with a male (husband/lover/boyfriend), how, if at all, should this person be involved in treatment? Clearly, different victims in different situations have different needs and different potential for benefiting from services. Research into the complex interaction of the various factors described above is needed to develop guidelines for rape treatment definitions.

Goal Setting

One specific, practical, and easily implemented means to maximize the impact of treatment of victims of sexual assault may simply be to involve them in clinical goal setting. There is substantial evidence that client goal setting has a facilitative effect on mental health therapy.[74-76] It will be important to determine if such an effect is also operative with regard to therapy for victims of sexual assault. The clinical functions of client goal setting are varied, depending on the needs of the client and the therapeutic style of the counselor. Often client goals stimulate treatment motivation; sometimes they are a means to keep treatment focused on particular issues; other times they are a catalyst for communication; and yet other times they facilitate mutual examination of expectations. Severe and intransient discrepancies between counselor and client goals have been a rarity in the experience of the authors; to the extent that disagreements occur, they typically serve as a basis for further discussion and negotiation. Davis[77] describes the basic process at work as "target tropism": the inherent tendency for a person to try to move toward any goal held up for her/him. Whatever the underlying mechanism, the success of goal setting as a treatment facilitator in mental health opens a clear line of research in the rape treatment field.

CONCLUSION

Although an ageless social problem, rape has recently become a topic of grave public concern with the recent resurgence of the feminist movement and the subsequent legislation enacted by Congress (P.L. 94-93, Title III, Part D) establishing the National Center for the Prevention and Control of Rape. However, although rape crisis centers have been established in various cities, sexual assault remains a topic about which there is little formal research. Knowledge that exists comes largely from descriptive studies, agitation by women's advocates, and political debate.

The substance of the available information deals with such topics as the effects of immediate intervention and crisis support, prevention of sexual assault, and changes needed within the legal system. Little attention has been paid to determining the hopes and aspirations of rape victims, to trying to anticipate their patterns of recovery, or to developing counseling guidelines. Nor has sufficient attention been paid to the way a family reacts to sexual assault, to the nature of a family's aspirations and intentions, or to changes in the family structure over time. Recently, there have been serious efforts to study and alter attitudes toward rape, but no link has been established between attitude formation and its effects on the behavior of the rape victim and her family.

NOTES

1. U.S. Department of Justice, *Uniform Crime Report for the United States* (Washington, D.C.: U.S. Government Printing Office, 1976).

2. "The Victim in a Forcible Rape Case: A Feminist View," *The American Criminal Law Review, A Symposium: Women and the Criminal Law*, American Bar Association, Section of Criminal Law, no. 2 (Winter 1973): 347.

3. Gary Flakne, ed., *Sexual Assault: The Target is You* (Minneapolis: Hennepin County Attorney's Office, 1976), p. 13.

4. Menachem Amir, *Patterns in Forcible Rape* (Chicago: University of Chicago Press, 1971), pp. 27-39.

5. John M. MacDonald, *Rape: Offenders and Their Victims* (Springfield, Ill., Charles C. Thomas, 1971).

6. Susan Brownmiller, *Against Our Will: Men, Women and Rape* (New York: Simon and Schuster, 1975), pp. 283-308.

7. Amir, *Forcible Rape*, pp. 17-29.

8. Andra Medea and Kathleen Thompson, *Against Rape: A Survival Manual for Women* (New York: Farrar, Straus, and Giroux, 1974), pp. 1-28.

9. Charles Hayman, "What To Do for Victims of Rape," *Medical Times* 101, no. 6 (June 1973): p. 49.

10. Joseph J. Peters, "Social, Legal, and Psychological Effects of Rape on the Victim," *Pennsylvania Medicine*, February 1975, pp. 34-36.

11. Lorraine Judson Carbary, "Treating Terrified Victims," *Journal of Practical Nursing*, February 1974, pp. 20-22.

12. Amir, *Forcible Rape,* pp. 129-194.

13. Vern Price, "Rape Victims: The Invisible Patients," *Canadian Nurse,* April 1975, p. 30.

14. C. Jones and E. Aronson, "Attribution of Fault to a Rape Victim as a Function of Respectability of the Victim," *Journal of Personality and Social Psychology* 26, no. 3 (June 1973), pp. 415-419.

15. M.J. Lerner, "The Desire for Justice and Reactions to Victims," in *Altruism and Helping Behavior,* ed. J. Macaulay and L. Berkowitz (New York: Academic Press, 1970), pp. 205-229.

16. M.J. Lerner and C.H. Simmons, "Observers' Reactions to the Innocent Victim," *Journal of Personality and Social Psychology* 4 (1977):203-210.

17. D.J. Bern and H.C. McConnell, "Testing the Self-Perception Explanation of Dissonance Phenomena: On the Salience of Pre-Manipulation Attitudes," *Journal of Personality and Social Psychology* 14 (1977):203-210.

18. Amir, *Forcible Rape.*

19. Brownmiller, *Against Our Will.*

20. Medea and Thompson, *Against Rape.*

21. Brownmiller, *Against Our Will,* p. 18.

22. Elaine Hilberman, *The Rape Victim* (Washington, D.C.: American Psychiatric Association Committee on Women, 1976), pp. 33-39.

23. C.R. Hayman and D. Lanza, "Sexual Assault on Women and Girls," *American Journal of Obstetrics and Gynecology* 109 (February 1, 1971): 50.

24. Joseph W. Hanss, "Another Look at the Care of the Rape Victim," *Arizona Medicine* 32, no. 8 (August 1975): 634.

25. Price, "Rape Victims."

26. Hayman and Lanza, "Sexual Assault."

27. Peters, "Effects of Rape," p. 36.

28. Hilberman, *Rape Victim,* p. ix.

29. Ann Wolbert Burgess, "Crisis and Counseling Requests of Rape Victims," *Nursing Research* 23, no. 3 (May-June 1974): 196-202.

30. Hilberman, *Rape Victim.*

31. Peters, "Effects of Rape."

32. Medea and Thompson, *Against Rape,* pp. 101-110.

33. Brownmiller, *Against Our Will,* pp. 49, 283-308.

34. Hanss, "Care of the Rape Victim."

35. Ann Wolbert Burgess and Lynda L. Holmstrom, "Rape Trauma Syndrome," *American Journal of Psychiatry,* September 1974, p. 983.

36. Hayman and Lanza, "Sexual Assault," p. 48.

37. Burgess, "Crisis and Counseling Requests," pp. 981-985.

38. Ibid.

39. Price, "Rape Victims," p. 30.

40. Interview with Debbie Anderson, Director, Sexual Assault Services, Hennepin County, Attorney's Office, Minneapolis, June 1976.

41. Burgess, "Crisis and Counseling Requests," p. 985.

42. Sandra S. Borges and Kurt Weiss, "Victimology and Rape," *Issues In Criminology* 8, no. 2 (1973): 71-115.

43. Peters, "Effects of Rape."

44. Medea and Thompson, *Against Rape.*

45. Brownmiller, *Against Our Will.*

46. Peters, "Effects of Rape."

47. Price, "Rape Victims."

48. Brownmiller, *Against Our Will,* p. 124.

49. Broges and Weiss, "Victomology and Rape," p. 99.

50. Peters, "Effects of Rape," p. 34.

51. Hayman and Lanza, "Sexual Assault," p. 49.

52. Cindy Cook Williams and Reg A. Williams, "Rape: A Plea for Help in the Hospital Emergency Room," *Nursing Forum* 12, no. 4 (1973): 392.

53. Medea and Thompson, *Against Rape.*

54. Hayman and Lanza, "Sexual Assault," p. 48.

55. Williams and Williams, "A Plea for Help," pp. 393-394.

56. Burgess, "Crisis and Counseling Requests," pp. 200-202.

57. Richard K. McGee, *Crisis Intervention in the Community* (Baltimore: University Park Press, 1974), p. 182.

58. Price, "Rape Victims."

59. Morton Bard and Katherine Ellison, "Crisis Intervention and Investigations of Forcible Rape," *Police Chief*, May 1974, pp. 68-74.

60. Peters, "Effects of Rape," pp. 34-36.

61. Flakne, *Sexual Assault.*

62. Peters, "Effects of Rape."

63. Price, "Rape Vicitms," p. 29.

64. Donald T. Campbell and Julian C. Stanley, *Experimental and Quasi-Experimental Designs for Research* (Chicago: Rand McNally, 1966).

65. Ibid.

66. Thomas J. Kiresuk and Robert E. Sherman, "Goal Attainment Scaling: A General Method for Evaluating Comprehensive Community Mental Health Programs," *Community Mental Health Journal* 4 (1968): 443-453.

67. Robert E. Sherman, James W. Baxter, and Donna M. Audette, "An Examination of the Reliability of the Kiresuk-Sherman Goal Attainment Score by Means of Components of Variance" (unpublished report, Program Evaluation Resource Center, Minneapolis, Minnesota, 1974).

68. Geoffrey Garwick, "An Introduction to Reliability and the Goal Attainment Score" (unpublished report, Program Evaluation Resource Center, 1972).

69. Robert E. Sherman, "Content Validity Argument for Goal Attainment Scaling" (unpublished report, Program Evaluation Resource Center, 1972).

70. Geoffrey Garwick, "A Construct Validity Overview of Goal Attainment Scaling" (unpublished report, Program Evaluation Resource Center, 1972).

71. Howard R. Davis, "Four Ways to Goal Attainment: An Overview," *Evaluation* 1 (1973).

72. Coleen Halley and James Baxter, "Client Perception of Evaluation at Hennepin County Mental Health Service" (unpublished report, Program Evaluation Resource Center, 1971).

73. Hans H. Strupp, "The Outcome Problem in Psychotherapy Revisited," *Psychotherapy: Theory, Research and Practice* 1 (1964): 1-13.

74. Susan Jones and Geoffrey Garwick, "Guide to Goals Study: Goal Attainment Scaling as Therapy Adjunct?" *Program Evaluation Report Newsletter* 4, no. 6 (July-August 1973): 1-3.

75. Lorraine LaFerriere and Robert Calsyn, "Goal Attainment Scaling: An Effective Treatment Technique in Short Term Therapy" (Ph.D. diss., Michigan State University, 1975).

76. David L. Smith, "Goal Attainment Scaling as an Adjunct to Counseling," *Journal of Counseling Psychology* 23, no. 1 (1976):22-27.

77. Howard R. Davis, "Change and Innovation," in *Administration in Mental Health Services*, ed. Saul Feldman (Springfield, Ill.: Charles C. Thomas, 1973).

14
Child Abuse

LA VOHN JOSTEN

Stress is one of the factors that has been shown repeatedly to be associated with child abuse. Nurses have contact with families when many of these stressful events occur. Numerous other factors including history of poor parenting, inadequate self-esteem, and inadequate support system have also been associated with child abuse. Nurses also have contact with families who are at risk for or are actually experiencing child abuse because of the presence of one or more of these factors. Thus, nurses are a key professional group in the process of identifying, treating, and preventing child abuse. If the nurse is knowledgeable about her role, she can successfully intervene in some family situations in which actual or potential child abuse is present.

In order for a nurse to provide nursing care effectively in these situations, she must have knowledge of the dynamics of child abuse as they are influenced by stress. She must understand the usual patterns that persons exhibit when coping with stress as well as the factors that enhance coping. With that knowledge, she can use the nursing process to develop and implement nursing care plans aimed both at facilitating the family's attempts to cope with stress and at dealing with the other factors so that child abuse is less likely to occur.

The first step in understanding the dynamics of child abuse is to have a clear definition of child abuse. Common to all cases of abuse is a child who has suffered or is at risk of suffering some type of injury. The injury can result from a purposeful action or from the absence of any action when purposeful action is necessary for the child's well-being. The injury can be physical, emotional, intellectual, sexual, or social. The degree of damage may be so minute that it is impossible to detect or so severe that the child dies. Examples of various forms of child abuse include those that lead to readily definable injury: a 4-year-old who is hit repeatedly in the abdomen until his spleen ruptures; a toddler whose legs are twisted until the bones break; an infant who is shaken so severely that his brain begins to bleed; an infant who is not adequately fed, stimulated, or loved so that his body or mind does not grow. Other forms of abuse result in injuries that are more difficult to detect: an adolescent girl whose father fondles her genitals; a toddler who is left alone in the parents' apartment for a period of time; a 7-year-old who is not allowed to go to school because her mother does not like to be alone. Common to all of these examples is an act or absence of an act which results in a child receiving either physical, emotional, sexual, or intellectual injury. Throughout this chapter the term "child abuse" refers to all forms unless otherwise indicated.

The number of children who are abused each year in the United States is not known. Some data are available on cases that have been reported for investigation by the legally mandated reporting agency in each state. In most states this is the Department of Welfare. Twenty-nine states and territories participated in the National Study of Child Neglect and Abuse reporting for 1975,[1] in which 289,837 reports of neglect and abuse were made. Of the cases that were investigated, 59.6 percent were judged to be actual cases of abuse or neglect. Since many cases are not reported and not all states participate in this study, a fair conclusion would be that the validated cases do not reflect the total number of abused children. However, it has been estimated that in the United States there are 2,000,000 cases of abuse yearly, 500 to 1,000 of which result in death.[2]

Who are these parents that have injured so many children? Characteristics of abusive parents suggest that they have many things in common with all parents. Past studies have shown the majority of abusing parents to be married and living together at the time of abuse and to have an average age of 26 and 30 for the abusive mother and father, respectively.[3] Galub states that in three-fourths of child abuse cases natural parents were involved with the mistreatment of the child and that mothers were more often responsible for abuse than fathers, probably because they spend more time with the children.[4] The abusive parents are a part of all educational levels, social strata, and ethnic groups.[5] Education ranges from partial grade school to advanced postgraduate degrees, and IQs range from the 70s to the 130s.[6]

A number of specific factors have been repeatedly reported to be present in the life of an abusive parent. A specific crisis or stressful event has been reported to be associated with child abuse.[7] One study suggests that the actual incidence of abuse is highest among families in which the stress of low income and high unemployment is present.[8] Other studies report the following stressful events. Very often the father is absent from the home or unemployed;[9] when he is employed, his occupational status is lower than his level of skill.[10] When the father is present, there is quarreling with the wife and often heavy drinking by the father.[11] Various studies suggest that the child herself/himself is a stressful presence. There is a higher incidence of child abuse among children born premaritally, extramaritally, or from unplanned pregnancies.[12]

The factor of abusive parents not having supportive relationships in their lives has also been reported. In a study comparing 50 mothers of abused children with a group of nonabusive mothers, Elmer[13] found that the abusive mothers rarely belonged to church, PTA, or other social groups and had almost no close friends. They also stated that they had no adults in the family on whom they could count for help, being isolated from their extended families.[14] Other studies of parents have found similar patterns of a lack of supportive relationships.[15] Some parents see their children as competitors for their mate,[16] and other parents show resentment and hostility at having to meet another person's needs. This implies that they see their children as competitors for resources and attention.[17]

Some researchers have proposed that abusing parents share misconceptions about child rearing. These parents often expect more of their children than the children are able to give physically, intellectually, or emotionally. On a questionnaire given to a group of parents receiving public health nursing services, 7 percent of whom were known to have abused or neglected their children, 25 percent of the parents indicated that they expected their child to be toilet trained by a year, and 50 percent expected their child to know right from wrong at 1 year or sooner.[18] When a child is not able to satisfy the needs of her/his parents, punishment and even abuse often occur.[19]

The concept of role reversal, i.e., the parent expecting the child to parent or take care of the parent, has also been set forth as a factor in abuse by parents. This theory[20,21] proposes that parents perceive their children from birth as having adult powers for deliberately displeasing or judging them. Aggression is often used by parents for dealing with these seemingly disapproving infants.[22] Other studies[23] add that abusing parents are unable to empathize with their children.

It has also been reported that abusive parents frequently possess feelings about self that could be categorized as reflective of a poor self-concept.[24] Clinical observation of abusive parents reveals that parental inadequate self-esteem is a common problem. Numerous studies of abusing parents[25,26] indicate that they were themselves victims of some form of abuse as children. When one combines childhood experiences of receiving negative messages about oneself while currently experiencing life stresses, many of which contain negative messages such as loss of employment, with an inability to form positive relationships, the presence of low self-esteem in abusive parents is readily understood.

Since child abuse is a problem of family function, knowledge about the other member of the family, the abused child, is also helpful. The average age of the abused child is under 4 years, with the majority being under 3 years.[27-29] The child between 1 month and 6 months seems especially vulnerable, for it is estimated that a child of this age experiences one-third of the child abuse, and child abuse is the second-ranking cause of death for this age group.[30] Usually there is no sex differentiation with respect to the abused child, and the average period of time during which abuse occurs prior to detection is from one to three years.

Independent of demographic conditions and parental factors, other factors must be considered in order to determine why one child is abused and another is not. According to Leonard et al., neglected children may show extremes of temperament.[31] They are either vigorous, active, and irritable or quiet, placid, slow moving, and undemanding. In Terr's sample, many children were mentally retarded or hyperactive.[32] The parents characterized their abused children as different from their siblings, e.g., sickly, spoiled, and problem children. Studies have not shown whether the characteristics were present in the child from birth or resulted from interactions with the parents. Kempe discovered that the adopted child, the premature baby, and the precocious child are high risk for abuse.[33] Helfer adds that the infant of a cesarean delivery and the child separated from his mother before age 11 years are more vulnerable to abuse.[34]

The pregnancy itself is also a stressful factor. Many of the high-risk infants, i.e., premature or adopted, have birth experiences that are more stressful to the infants and their mothers. For many of them, there is a longer period of time between contact with the mother in utero and contact with the mother after birth. Separation of the newborn from his mother appears to have long-term effects on the mother-child relationship, placing those infants at higher risk of abuse. Kennell reports on a study in which one group of mothers was given contact with their infants shortly after birth and an increased amount of contact in the first three days of the infant's life.[35] At infant age of 1 month and 1 year, the mothers receiving the increased contact remained closer to their infants, comforted them more, and had more visual and tactual contact with them. Helfer reports on a study in which mothers of premature infants had more contact with their infants;[36] those infants at 42 months of age had higher IQs than premature infants with less contact. Increased contact with the infant gives the mother a greater opportunity to get to know her infant. Barnard reports on giving a modification of Brazelton's "Neonatal Behavioral Assessment Scale" to a group of parents.[37] This scale evaluates the neonate's ability to respond to a variety of stimulants including the human face. When the infants were 1 month of age, the study parents expressed feelings that were significantly more positive toward their infants.

Rather than looking at the individual characteristics or factors of the parents and child, several authors have attempted to clarify the occurrence of child abuse by examining the interrelating dynamics of the family situation when abuse occurs or when a family is at increased risk of it occurring.

Helfer proposed that three components are necessary in order for child abuse to occur:[38] (1) the potential for abuse, (2) a special kind of child, and (3) a crisis or series of crises. The potential for abuse includes (1) poor parenting received by the parents, (2) poor support systems, (3) poor marital relationship between parents, and (4) lack of knowledge regarding normal child growth and development. After the potential is present, there must be a particular child and, finally, a crisis or series of crises.

Justice and Justice proposed a psychosocial system model of child abuse, which facilitates understanding of the complex interrelationships of factors present in abusive families (Fig. 14.1).[39] This model includes the characteristics previously ascribed to the child and the parents, expectations and definitions of parenting present in any cultural group, and factors from the family's environment that impede or support its ability to function. The latter includes the stresses that this family unit has experienced.

The significance of stress as a factor contributing to child abuse within this model has been substantiated. Justice and Duncan (1976) administered the Social Readjustment Rating Scale to 35 abusing parents and to 35 controls.[40] In assessing the degree of stress experienced by the study group, Justice and Duncan gave the questionnaire to the abuser and his/her spouse because of their belief that if both parents are involved in the family both are involved in the abuse. They found that the abusive families in the year preceding the abusive incident had suffered more stressful events than nonabusive and those events were more severe. The overwhelming frequency and intensity of stressful events adversely affected the parents' ability to constructively deal with even minor stress and made them vulnerable to responding in a destructive manner.[41] The abusive parents were also more likely to feel a sense of rivalry with the other members of the family, including the child, as to which member was going to get her/his needs for nurturance met within the family system.[42] Obviously, if the child is not meeting the parents' needs, she/he is a readily available object for the parents to vent their frustrations on when overwhelmed by stress.

Although this psychosocial system model does not include an explanation of the relationship between child neglect and stress,[43] the description of neglectful mothers as "the apathetic-futile, the impulse-ridden, the mentally retarded, the mother in a reactive depression, and the psychotic" suggests a relationship. Does the neglectful

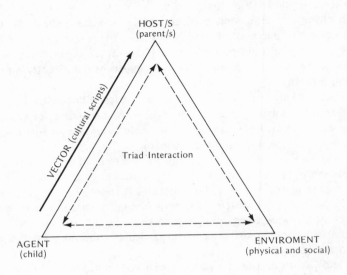

HOST/S
(parent/s)

VECTOR (cultural scripts)

Triad Interaction

AGENT
(child)

ENVIROMENT
(physical and social)

Figure 14-1. Psychosocial system model of child abuse.

parent respond to stress by coping mechanisms such as withdrawal, denial, passivity, escape, which in effect make her/him unavailable either physically and/or emotionally to care for the child? It is this writer's clinical impression that neglectful parents frequently do use those coping mechanisms when overwhelmed with their life situation. Gelles clarifies the relationship between stress and various kinds of abuse including neglect by suggesting that a person learns how to deal with stress within his family of origin and tends to use the modes of adaption to stress utilized by his parental models.[44] As previously noted many abusive parents themselves were victims of child abuse, suggesting that they may have learned nonconstructive coping methods.

Authors of theories of response to stress give further insight into the relationship between stress and child abuse. Understanding the family characteristics that facilitate positive crisis adjustment is essential if the nurse is to help families in crisis. Hill suggests that these characteristics include "family adaptability, family integration, affectional relations among family members, good marital adjustment of husband and wife, companionable parent-child relationships, family council type of control in decision making, social participation of wife and previous successful experience with crisis."[45] It is apparent that many of these characteristics are in opposition to the characteristics ascribed to abusive families. LeMasters adds that certain features of the crisis affect the family's success in mastery of the event, including, "(1) the nature of the crisis event; (2) the state of organization or disorganization of the family at the point of impact; (3) the resources of the family; and (4) its previous experience with crises."[46] Rapoport identified steps in the process of aiding the family to cope with a stressor.[47] They include the family's need to understand the event, ventilation and clarification of the feelings the individuals have concerning the event, as well as bringing into play the potential aids the family has either within itself or its environment to support constructive coping. Thus, it is apparent that, after experiencing repeated stress including unmet needs for nurturance, many adults have a greatly diminished capacity to adequately parent a child.

Nurses can help families to deal more constructively with stressful events if they are cognizant of the significance of the stress and know how to effectively enhance the families' coping abilities, thus decreasing the likelihood of abuse. Nurses at the Minneapolis Health Department are helping families with many of the problems abusive families experience. Records of 12 families receiving public health nursing services from the Minneapolis Health Department were audited for the presence and improvement of the following parental problems: history of abuse toward a child, inadequate parenting received by parents, inadequate emotional support, inadequate cognitive functioning ability, abuse of one parent by the other, mental health including inadequate self-concept, personal immaturity, poor emotional control, chemical dependency, lack of knowledge of normal growth and development, major stress or stresses in the past year, rejection of child, and inappropriate utilization of services. The average number of problems present per family was 7.9, and the range of problems was from 4 to 11 per family. The audit suggested that nurses can intervene positively in many cases. Of the 12 families in this group, 10 showed improvement in their parenting abilities after receiving public health nursing services.

During or after many of the life events or stresses listed on the Social Readjustment Rating Scale,[48] the family would also have contact with a nurse. The most obvious include death of a spouse, death of a close family member, personal injury or illness, change in health of a family member, pregnancy, sex difficulties, and death of a close friend. One mode of coping with stress may be to develop illness symptoms. The nurse having contact with a parent who is seeking medical care and is diagnosed with psychosomatic illness should also be concerned. Mogulnicki et al.[49] reported on three cases in which functional symptoms were used by the parents as a mode of coping with impending child abuse.

The family in which child abuse has occurred or is highly likely to occur also has contact with a nurse for a variety of reasons. Some examples include the following. A child is brought to the emergency room and/or hospitalized because of a physical injury, or an infant is examined and/or hospitalized because she/he is failing to grow and develop appropriately. A child is brought to the doctor's office or public clinic for a routine examination or immunizations. A family is visited by a public health nurse for routine health promotion or a specific family health problem. A child is brought to the school nurse's attention because of numerous absences, behavior problems, or a physical injury.

To clarify the role of the nurse in helping the family under stress that is vulnerable to or actually experiencing child abuse, an outline for the nursing process is presented below followed by two case situations using that process outline. In both cases more than one nurse had contact with the family, so the activities of each nurse involved in the cases are presented. In actual work settings, which nurse performs which activity may vary depending on the unique features of the work setting and the community.

NURSING PROCESS OUTLINE:
STRESSFUL EVENT*

1. Data to be collected.
   a. Meaning of current stressful event to this family.
   b. Other stressful events that this family has experienced in the past year.
   c. Level of family functioning at the time of the most recent stressful event.
   d. Family style in coping with stressful events.
   e. Strengths family has that will aid them in coping constructively with the stressful event.
   f. Resources available and acceptable in the family's environment that will support their efforts to cope.
   g. Level of family functioning in the weeks and months following the stressful event.

2. Sample data collection questions.
   a. Have you ever lost anyone close to you?
   b. Have you yourself or anyone close to you been ill or hospitalized in the past few years?
   c. At the time (specific stressful event) occurred, what was going on with your family?
   d. What kinds of things did you enjoy doing together?
   e. When something upsetting happens to your family what do you usually do?
   f. Who is the person most helpful to you when you are upset?
   g. How has your life changed since (specific stressful event) occurred?

3. Sample nursing diagnosis.
   a. Family denies impact of stressful event.
   b. Family is unable to meet basic needs for food, rest, or shelter since occurrence of stressful event.
   c. Family members blame each other for causing stressful event.
   d. Family refuses to accept assistance in coping with stressful event.
   e. Family has made a constructive plan to cope with stressful event.

4. Sample objectives for nursing care plan.
   a. Family will resolve their feelings about the stressful event.
   b. Family will cope with the stressful event.
   c. Family will be able to reestablish homeostasis within the family unit.

5. Sample nursing care plan.
   a. The nurse will give the family members an opportunity to express their feelings about the stressful event including its effect on them as a group as well as individuals.
   b. The nurse will help the family members identify strengths and resources among themselves that will aid them in coping with this stressful event.

---

*Minneapolis Health Department: Parenting Assessment and Intervention Tool.

   c. The nurse will help the family members identify methods of coping that they have used effectively in previous stressful events and that would be appropriate in this situation.

   d. The nurse will help the family identify and use constructive methods of coping to replace previously used nonconstructive methods.

   e. The nurse will refer the family to resources that can facilitate constructive coping with the stressful event.

6. Sample expected outcome criteria.

   a. Family is able to meet their basic needs for food, rest, and shelter.

   b. Each adult family member makes supportive statements to other family members.

   c. Family is able to manage activities necessitated by the stressful event.

CASE SITUATION 1

Frank Smith, a 46-year-old fireman, was severely burned in a factory fire. He was hospitalized but died 36 hours after admission to the hospital. His wife Martha is 38, a full-time homemaker, and mother of four children: Bill, 21, married with two children; Harvey, 17, a senior in high school; Jim, 14, a sophomore in high school; and Frank, Jr., 9, in the third grade. A month after the father's death, the school nurse brought Frank, Jr., to the hospital emergency room with a broken arm, which he had when he arrived at school that morning. Upon examination, Frank, Jr., was found to have numerous welts on his back and chest. A diagnosis of suspected child abuse was made.

What could either the hospital or the school nurse do to help this family better cope with the father's death and decrease the likelihood of abuse occurring? The first step was to determine the meaning of this stressful event to the family. A sympathetic interviewer used open-ended questions to ascertain the role played by the father in the family and subsequently the roles of the other family members. Most persons seek reasons or explanations for the cause of an event which go beyond the facts of the event itself. Many persons believe that it is God's will; others think that they have always had bad luck and that this is simply another example of it. Some families are very vocal about their beliefs. Some beliefs are comforting; some are upsetting. If a family's beliefs are the former, it may add to their ability to cope with the event.

One of the things the nurse assessed was who made the decisions in the family, which helped to clarify the dependency needs of the family. If Mr. Smith made all the decisions and none were made by each or mutually, Mrs. Smith will feel more stressed by the decisions she will now be facing. Also, if Mr. Smith made all the decisions, Mrs. Smith may have played a dependent role in the family system and perhaps is less confident in her decision-making ability. In addition, to the father's role in family decision making, the affectional ties of all family members including the father relationship with the children are significant. Obviously, the children needed help in dealing with their father's death. If they were perceived by the mother to have been closer to their father, she may resent them if they now turn to her for comfort.

Persons who have resources available to help in a crisis will more likely use positive methods of coping. By asking about persons perceived to be helpful to the family, one hopes to determine the availability of persons who are willing and able to support the family through the crisis as well as the family's willingness to accept that help. As previously noted, abusive families tend to be isolated families.

The nurse also assessed whether the family's coping abilities had been decreased by previous stressful events. As stated earlier, many families who have experienced numerous stressful events may experience more child abuse. If stressful events have occurred, it is helpful to determine the family's method of coping with those crises as a clue to how they may cope with this crisis. One wants to determine if the family is able to reach out for help if their methods of coping are ineffective. Knowledge of the acceptability and the mode of expressing negative feeling within the family system is also helpful. Is crying accepted? When upset, does anyone go out and get drunk? The nurse had data about how the family responded during Mr. Smith's hospitalization, and the especially significant data included initial family response to the accident, including their ability to manage the necessities of life for themselves, i.e., food, rest, transportation, and arrangements necessitated by the accident such as insurance papers and notification of other family members.

The nurse also had data on their ability to emotionally support each other. If extended family members and/or friends were present, did they increase or decrease the family's ability to function? Was Mrs. Smith able to be at all supportive to her children, or did she expect them to take care of her during this stressful event. The nurse also had data on the family's concept of their ability to cope. Healthy families recognize that they can cope with some crises but, if the crises are too severe, they seek help. Families who are overconfident may be denying the significance of the stress, which may lead to later difficulties, or may be afraid to accept help because of problems with trusting helping persons. Other families may convey the belief that they are incapable of managing the crisis and expect others to take care of them completely. Either situation puts the child at risk for neglect or abuse.

The school nurse had additional data on the Smith family which aided in her assessment of the impact of Mr. Smith's death on the family. She had information on previous stressful events that this family had experienced. The school records contained such data on the family as moves, absences by Frank, Jr. because of illness, and problems Frank, Jr. had had. Abused children often have problems getting along with their classmates or teachers because they are either overly aggressive or withdrawn. The school nurse knew whether the family had shown appropriate interest in Frank's performance in school. The unrealistic expectations that many abusive parents have of their children may be reflected in excessive concern about the child's grades.

Nursing Diagnosis

Whether a hospital nurse, school nurse, or public health nurse has assessed the previously described data, she will be able to make a nursing diagnosis about the impact of Mr. Smith's death on the family's ability to function. Several possible diagnoses include the following. (1) Mrs. Smith is unable to express her feelings about Mr. Smith's death. (2) Mrs. Smith has unrealistic expectations of Frank, Jr.; she looks to him for comfort. (3) The family is unable to make decisions, e.g., those necessitated by Mr. Smith's death.

Nursing Care Plan

Specific activities the nurse might wish to include in her nursing care plan aimed at the overall objective of helping this family cope constructively with Mr. Smith's death include helping the family with the necessary decisions by referring them to someone such as the hospital chaplin, family minister, social worker, or other person acceptable to the family or, if the time is available, helping them herself. The person helping the family with decision making should help them clarify which decisions need to be made immediately and which can be delayed. She should help them to identify the various alternative decisions. She should help each family member feel comfortable in expressing her/his opinions on the possible alternatives and establish for the family that all opinions are to be respected. She should help them reach a consensus regarding a decision. Throughout the process, she should identify the positive behaviors exhibited by each family member including their willingness to participate in the decision-making process. The latter is especially important since it shows the persons involved that another person recognizes the difficult situation they are experiencing, and it may decrease their feelings of isolation.

Specific activities by the nurse aimed at helping Mrs. Smith express her feelings about her husband's death call for a great deal of sensitivity. She must recognize Mrs. Smith's right to not express them or to select someone else with whom to share them. Mrs. Smith may have acquired cultural problems that might dictate how to behave in this situation; i.e., her cultural group is stoic rather than expressive at the time of a death. However, the nurse has the responsibility of making Mrs. Smith aware that she can express her feelings to the nurse. In order to give Mrs. Smith this message, the nurse must do more than ask Mrs. Smith how she feels about her husband's death. She must be ready to accept those feelings, which might range from "I'm glad; he was a terrible person," to overwhelming grief. She must also provide a private place where both she and Mrs. Smith can sit without interruption. At times, the nurse is the best person to do this, especially if the nurse has had previous supportive contact with the family. At other times, it may be better for the family minister or a friend or relative to serve this role, but the nurse has the responsibility of seeing that someone is available to help Mrs. Smith.

Having someone available immediately and over the next year to help Mrs. Smith express her feelings may help with the problem caused by the unrealistic expectation that her young son will be able to comfort her. This problem as well as the fact that Mrs. Smith was very dependent on Mr. Smith place Frank, Jr. in a precarious position. He is too young to replace his father, and his mother could respond to his inability to take his father's place by abusing him. The activities of all the nurses and other professional personnel involved in helping the Smith family must be coordinated. In many cases, the public health nurse coordinates the family's care. Other activities of the public health nurse include the following: ongoing assessment of the family's ability to cope with Mr. Smith's death, sympathetic listening to help the family through the grief process, and intervention as needed if other stressful events occur. All the activities mentioned, because they are aimed at helping the Smith family to use constructive coping mechanisms, may help in preventing the stressful event of the abuse of Frank, Jr.

When a child is seen in the emergency room because she/he has been abused, there are things the nurse can do to decrease the negative impact of this event on the family. Some of these include the following. Since Mrs. Smith was not present when Frank, Jr. was brought to the hospital, the first step would be to notify her. Abusive parents need the same caring concern that the relatives of any person admitted to the emergency room need. They are concerned about how serious the injuries are and feel very guilty because their anger resulted in their child's injury. The nurse should recognize and positively reward Mrs. Smith for being concerned about Frank, Jr. Most abusive parents have feelings of low self-worth. The feeling common to many abusive parents is "I must be a terrible parent to do this to my child," which adds to their low self-esteem. Treating the parents with respect, involving them in the child's care, as well as recognizing and rewarding them for the positive behaviors observed by the nurse are important activities the nurse in the emergency room can perform in the treatment of a family in which abuse is suspected.

Cases of suspected physical abuse are required to be reported to the legally mandated reporting agency in all states, which is usually the child protection unit of the local welfare department. The nurse or the physician must tell the parents that a report is being made. Most abusive parents, because of their experience of being abused themselves, find it difficult to trust people. Basic to the establishment of a trusting relationship is honesty; thus, it is essential that the parents be told that a report is being made.

Being reported for child abuse is frightening. The nurse should recognize that the parents will be very concerned about what will happen to them and their child as a result of the report; thus, the consequence of the report should be made clear. For example, the nurse might say, "Tomorrow a social worker will be calling you to arrange a time to come and talk with you. She knows you do not want Frank, Jr. to be hurt again. She and we are going to try to help you so it doesn't happen again."

If Frank, Jr. were hospitalized because of his injury, the hospital nurse would also have an important role in helping this injured family. Neill and Kauffman have identified eight goals for the hospital nursing care of abused children and their families.[50]

1. Setting a tone of treatment rather than one of punishment
2. Promoting a sense of parental adequacy
3. Supporting strengths of the parent-child relationship
4. Decreasing the trauma of hospitalization for child and parent
5. Identifying needs of parents and child and sharing these with the team
6. Promoting the child's return to wellness
7. Implementing principles of crisis intervention
8. Modeling for parents and the child alternate ways of handling behavior, feelings, and interactions with others

Because parents who have abused their children have experienced frequent rejection and criticism, e.g., have been abused themselves as children or have had negative life experiences, they are extremely sensitive to behaviors that indicate the professional staffs disapproval. Nursing care plans that are aimed at the goals identified by Neill and Kauffman should decrease the likelihood of the parents having experiences with the professional staff that will lower their feelings of adequacy as parents. At times, professional staff members, because of their competence and efficiency, believe that they are, and actually are, giving better physical and/or emotional care to the child than the parents are able to give. The professional responsibility of teaching child care to the parent can also add to the parental sense of inadequacy. When one is being taught one frequently gets the message that the person teaching is better or more adequate than oneself. Persons with low self-esteem sometimes cannot tolerate that additional blow to their self-esteem. Some persons respond verbally with a statement such as, "What do you know? He's not your kid." Others withdraw from further contact with persons they think are being critical of them. This is one of the reasons some abusive families do not visit their abused child in the hospital. It is too painful for them emotionally.

The hospital nurse needs to acknowledge to the abusive parents their parental expertise—for example, the parents' knowledge of their child's likes and dislikes. The nurse should first explain to the parents what she must do for the child. Then by asking the parents to help her plan the approach to this nursing activity, she is recognizing their importance and value in this situation. By involving the parents in many of the care activities, the nurse can set up a situation in which the nurse and parents are equals, each of whom brings something special to the situation. The nurse should also be comfortable sharing with the parents some of her mistakes or frustrations if they occur while she is interacting with the child. By sharing her mistake and how she would handle it next time, she is role-modeling an area with which many abusive parents have difficulty, i.e., learning from one's mistakes.

The majority, if not all, parents who have abused or neglected their children can benefit from the services of a public health nurse. The hospital nurse should refer the family to the public health nurse shortly after the child is admitted to the hospital. This will give the public health nurse time to begin the establishment of a long-term supportive relationship with the family before the child goes home. She can also assess the impact of the current stressful situation, i.e., the hospitalization of the child as well as the stress of the investigation on the total family. Of special importance is the effect of this stressful event on the parents' ability to care for their other children. The role of the public health nurse is described in some detail in the next case situation.

CASE SITUATION 2

Jerry Jones, a 3-year-old boy, was brought to the doctor's office for his yearly examination. As the nurse was reviewing the record in preparation for updating the child's medical history, she observed a child run down the hall followed by a very disheveled-looking mother, who grabbed him and yanked him back to the waiting area, saying, "Why do you always have to be so bad?'' According to the records of the previous examination, Jerry was essentially a well child. The social notes included reference to the fact that neither set of grandparents was available to assist with child care; the paternal grandparents lived out of state, and the maternal pair were alcoholics.

As the nurse called the patient and his mother, she noted that Jerry was the child who she had previously observed running down the hall. After introducing herself, she asked Mrs. Jones if she had any special concerns regarding Jerry.

MRS. JONES: "Yes, I want the doctor to give him something; I think he's hyperactive."

NURSE: "What makes you think that?"

MRS. JONES: "He's always getting into something. He never sits still. In fact, he knows how to get to his mother. He's always doing things to upset me."

NURSE: "What sort of things does he do to upset you?"

MRS. JONES: "Oh, like this morning all he would do was play with his cereal. The nursery school also had trouble getting him to eat."

NURSE: "Has his teacher at nursery school said he's hyperactive?"

MRS. JONES: "No, but it doesn't matter; he doesn't go anymore. My husband and I separated about a month ago, and I can't afford to send him. I had to quit my job so I could take care of him and go on welfare."

NURSE: "You sure have been having a rough time. Had you and your husband been having trouble getting along?"

MRS. JONES: "At times. See, he kept messing around with other women, and the times before I let him come back, but this time I'd had it."

NURSE: "I can see why you feel you've had it. Have the two of you considered going in for counseling?"

MRS. JONES: "No, he wouldn't go. Besides, I don't want him back; he can just drop dead."

NURSE: "You have reason to be very upset; do you have anyone you can talk to?"

MRS. JONES: "Well, I've got a sister in town, but she's got a couple of kids who give her trouble. I've got a couple of girlfriends, but I don't have money for a phone, so I can't call them."

NURSE: "So at the moment it's not easy for you to reach anyone to talk to."

MRS. JONES: "No, but I'm hoping to go down to welfare next week to get my worker to help me get a phone. I worry about what I would do if I or Jerry suddenly got sick."

NURSE: "Yes, I can believe that would be frightening. I'm glad you're going to ask your worker for a phone, but I'm concerned about how you'll manage even if you get a phone. I think it's very hard for a mother to be cooped up all day with a three-year-old child and no one to talk to. Do you have anyone you can leave him with so you can have some fun in your life—we all deserve some fun."

MRS. JONES: "Yes, but I can't afford to use her very often."

NURSE: "Are there any fun things you and Jerry do?"

MRS. JONES: "Sure, he likes it when we color together, or he likes to sit on my lap and name my nose, eyes, and so forth."

NURSE: "He's lucky to have a mother who will play with him."

MRS. JONES: "Yes, I like to play with him except when he gets so hyperactive."

NURSE: "Does that happen a lot?"

MRS. JONES: "Yes, and he's getting worse."

NURSE: "Did it start before you and your husband started having problems?"

MRS. JONES: "Yes, he's always been that way."

NURSE: "It would be very normal for him to react to the separation by being upset, and I sure can understand why with all you're going through it would be harder to manage alone. Has it been harder to take now that you have all the responsibility and very little time to yourself?"

MRS. JONES: "Yes, I think it's been harder for me to take. I just haven't been myself."

NURSE: "How haven't you been yourself?"

MRS. JONES: "Oh, I've been upset alot."

NURSE: "In the past when upsetting things happened to you, what seemed to help?"

MRS. JONES: "Oh, nothing really. I've always had to get by on my own, but nothing like this has ever happened before."

NURSE: "Did anything like this ever happen to your parents?"

MRS. JONES: "Oh, they were always having trouble, but they'd always get drunk, and I'm not doing that."

NURSE: "So you can't count on them for any help."

MRS. JONES: "No."

As the nurse interacts with Mrs. Jones, she notices that Mrs. Jones's face is very drawn, her hands and feet are frequently moving, and she is chain smoking. These observations in conjunction with the data collected in the interview and from the record lead the nurse to wonder if Mrs. Jones had inadequate models as a child on how to handle stress, since her parents were alcoholics. She has recently experienced a number of stressful events: her husband's infidelity and their subsequent separation, termination of her job, and a change in child-care responsibility. This combination of events and Mrs. Jones's feeling that Jerry is hyperactive contain many of the dynamics that Helfer[51] and Justice and Justice[52] have described in their models of the dynamics of child abuse. The nurse has no data to suggest that abuse has occurred, but she recognizes her responsibility to intervene and try to reduce the likelihood of abuse.

Nursing Diagnosis

Several possible diagnoses exist, including the following: (1) Mrs. Jones is overwhelmed by stress. (2) Mrs. Jones has inadequate supportive relationships. (3) Mrs. Jones perceives Jerry to be hyperactive. (4) Mrs. Jones is at high risk of abusing Jerry. There are some additional potential nursing diagnoses for which additional data are needed: (5) Mrs. Jones has received inadequate parenting. (6) Mrs. Jones has unrealistic expectations of Jerry. (7) Either Jerry is hyperactive or his level of activity is normal for his age.

Objectives for the nursing care plan for Jerry and his mother include the following. (1) Mrs. Jones will be able to cope with the current stress. (2) Mrs. Jones will have at least one supportive relationship. (3) After the cause of Jerry's hyperactivity is determined, Mrs. Jones will be able to manage his behavior in a way that fosters their mutual growth and development.

Expected outcome criteria include the following. (1) Mrs. Jones will be able to identify two ways in which her management of their situation has improved. (2) Mrs. Jones will be able to identify someone who she feels is emotionally supportive to her and available to her either on the telephone or in person.

Nursing Care Plan

1. Help Mrs. Jones identify ways to improve her management of the situation until other activities are underway.
   a. Help Mrs. Jones decide specifically what she will do if Jerry's behavior makes her so upset that she wants to beat him, such as put Jerry in his room and shut the door while she takes a warm bath or take herself and Jerry to a crisis center.
   b. Help Mrs. Jones identify the positive actions she is taking to make the situation more manageable such as her plans to see the social worker next week and her ability to discuss her problems with the nurse.

2. Refer Mrs. Jones to a mothers' support group at a local social services agency that also provides baby-sitting services.

3. Collaborate with the physician in evaluating Jerry's hyperactivity.
   a. Administer Denver developmental screening tool.
   b. Check Jerry's vision and hearing.
   c. Observe Jerry's behavior in office playroom.
   d. Request that a public health nurse observe Jerry's behavior in the home.

4. Refer Mrs. Jones to a social worker to help her get Jerry back into nursery school and to assess if she needs further assistance such as legal aid, emergency financial assistance, and employment.

5. Public health nurse should visit in the next few days to work on the following:
   a. Help Mrs. Jones learn to constructively deal with feelings of frustration with Jerry.
   b. Demonstrate methods of managing Jerry's inappropriate behavior.
   c. Teach age-appropriate normal growth and development.
   d. Provide empathetic listening regarding Mrs. Jones's anger at her husband. Reassess her desire for further counseling regarding marital and other problems.
   e. Identify practical means whereby Jerry and his mother can get pleasure from life individually and together such as going to the park and story hour at the library.
   f. Further assess Mrs. Jones's own childhood, health needs, personal goals, etc.

6. Offer Mrs. Jones the opportunity to call the office nurse each day for the next few days so that she will not feel so alone.

After the nurse made the care plan with Mrs. Jones, she made plans for Jerry and Mrs. Jones to have an appointment with the nurse the following week to reassess how they were doing and how the plan was working. She also made plans to discuss with the other professional workers the possible need to have a joint case conference after the completion of their initial assessments.

Two days after Jerry's appointment, the public health nurse made her first home visit. During the visit, Mrs. Jones told the nurse that her parents beat her with a leather strap when she was bad or when they were drunk. Her son Jerry reminds her of her older brother, John, who was her parents' favorite child. Her parents made her feel like they drank only because she was such a bad person. Throughout the visit Mrs. Jones made negative statements about Jerry and herself. Also, Mr. Jones had been quite critical of Mrs. Jones in justifying his infidelity. He said it was due to her frigidity. Mrs. Jones's life experiences with criticism and rejection make the fact that she has a negative self-image understandable. The nurse plans to verbally reward Mrs. Jones for all positive behavior she observes.

As the nurse observed Jerry, she saw a very active 3-year-old who was busy exploring his world. She noted that the only time Mrs. Jones acknowledged him was when he did something she did not like, at which time she would yell at him to stop.

Based on the data, the public health nurse provided the care for that visit as follows. She knew that before Mrs. Jones could change her parenting from the parenting she received, she must reject her parental models and have available acceptable positive models. This process has been described by Josten.[53] The nurse was able to get Mrs. Jones to identify that she wants Jerry to feel love for her rather than the anger she feels toward her parents. The nurse then offered to help her to identify specific things that she could do with Jerry that were more likely to lead to a positive feeling between Jerry and herself.

Acknowledging Mrs. Jones's concern about Jerry's level of activity, the nurse asked the mother if she had had any experiences with Jerry when his level of activity was acceptable. Mrs. Jones acknowledged that her husband used to "rough-house" with Jerry and he enjoyed that, but she didn't like to do that. The nurse then helped her identify other acceptable ways in which Jerry could be active.

The nurse was concerned about Mrs. Jones's negative perception of Jerry and her apparent failure to give him attention for his positive behaviors. She encouraged her to talk freely about her frustration in caring for him, her resentment at her husband at having left her with all the responsibilities, and the anger she felt when Jerry reminded her of her older brother. The nurse helped her to identify ways in which Jerry was different from her brother and then asked her to identify something he'd done in the last 24 hours that she'd liked. She could not identify anything. The nurse said it would be helpful for her to know both the things Jerry did that she liked and the things that she disliked. She then asked Mrs. Jones, for the next week, to write down both the liked and disliked behaviors. They would talk about them during the nurse's visit the following week. The nurse plans to use that list as the first step in making Mrs. Jones's perception of Jerry less negative. The next step will be to ask her to say one positive statement to Jerry a day and then two, etc. After the successful accomplishment of each of those tasks, the nurse plans to positively reward Mrs. Jones, which may help her self-esteem. She also plans to assess and discuss with Mrs. Jones the list of Jerry's activities to teach Mrs. Jones which of Jerry's behaviors are normal for his age.

The public health nurse plays an important role in coordinating the services the family is receiving as well as in assessing the impact of those services on the stress the family is feeling. The nurse, although recognizing many needs in this family, realizes that, in view of all the stress, change can occur only over time. So her immediate concern is to redirect Mrs. Jones's anger and frustration from Jerry while laying the groundwork for helping this family unit learn to function in a manner that will facilitate healthy development for each of them.

Common to both these case situations is stress of such a nature that the family ceased to function adequately and a child became the obvious victim or potential victim of that dysfunction. However, the cases also illustrate that all the family members were victims of the stressful situation.

Stressful events can cause any family to have problems in adequately meeting their needs. Families in which the parents, because of inadequate role models, have learned ineffective modes of coping with stress, whose life experiences have made them feel inadequate, and whose environment does not include supportive persons to aid in successful coping are vulnerable to losing control. If there is a child, especially a child who is perceived by the parent to be unable to meet parental demands, child abuse is a real possibility. The nurse, in her role as a helping person, has contact with many persons involved in stressful life events. If she has knowledge of the interrelationships between stress and abuse she can deliver nursing care aimed at helping the parents increase both their parenting abilities and their coping abilities and thus decrease the likelihood that a child will be abused.

NOTES

1. Vincent DeFrancis, "American Humane Association Published Highlights of National Study of Child Neglect and Abuse Reporting for 1975," *Child Abuse and Neglect Reports*, DHEW Publication No. (OHD) 77-30086 (Washington, D.C.: National Center on Child Abuse and Neglect, February 1977).

2. David Gil, as reported by Randy Furst in "Child Abuse," *Minneapolis Star*, Section B, (May 20, 1974): 1.

3. Theo Solomon, "History and Demography of Child Abuse," *Pediatrics Supplement* 51, part 2 (April 1973): 773-776.

4. Sharon Galub, "The Battered Child: What the Nurse Can Do," *RN*, (December 1968): 43-45, 66-68.

5. Brandt F. Steele, "Parental Abuse of Infants and Small Children," in *Parenthood: Its Psychology and Psychopathy*, ed. E. James Anthony and Theresa Benedik (Boston: Little, Brown & Co., 1970).

6. E. Elmer and C.D. Gregg, "Developmental Characteristics of Abused Children," *Pediatrics*, 40 (1969): 596-602.

7. J.M. Giovannonii and A. Bullingsley, "Child Neglect Among the Poor: A Study of Parental Adequacy in Families of Three Ethnic Groups," *Child Welfare* 49 (1970): 196-204.

8. D.B. Satten and J.K. Miller, "The Ecology of Child Abuse within a Military Community," *American Journal of Orthopsychiatry* 41 (1971): 675-678.

9. D.G. Gil, "Physical Abuse of Children: Findings and Implications of a National Survey" *Pediatrics* 44 (1969): 857-864.

10. L. Terr, "A Family Study of Child Abuse," *American Journal of Psychiatry* 127 (1970): 665-671.

11. Elizabeth Elmer, "Child Abuse: A Sympton of Family Crisis" (paper read at American Psychiatric Association, Washington, D.C. (November 17, 1967).

12. S.R. Zalba, "The Abused Child: A Survey of the Problem," *Social Work* 2 (1966:3-16).

13. E. Elmer, "Child Abuse: The Family's Cry for Help," *Journal of Psychiatric Nursing* 5 (1967): 332.

14. Elmer and Gregg, "Characteristics of Abused Children."

15. Barton D. Schmidt and C. Henry Kempe, "The Pediatrician's Role in Child Abuse and Neglect," *Current Problems in Pediatrics* 5 (March 1975): 3-47.

16. Terr, "Family Study."

17. Zalba, "Survey of the Problem."

18. *Parenting Assessment and Intervention Tool* (Minneapolis Health Department, 1977).

19. B.F. Steele and C.B. Pollack, "A Psychiatric Study of Parents Who Abuse Infants and Small Children," in *The Battered Child*, ed. R. Helfer and C.H. Kempe (Chicago: University of Chicago Press, 1968).

20. Steele, "Parental Abuse."

21. Beatrice Kalisch, "Nursing Actions in Behalf of the Battered Child," *Nursing Forum* 4 (1973): 365-377.

22. M. Morris and R. Gauld, "Role Reversal: A Necessary Concept in Dealing with the Battered Child Syndrome," *American Journal of Orthopsychiatry* 33 (1963): 298-299.

23. B. Melmick and J. Hurley, "Distinctive Personality Attributes of Child Abusing Mothers," *Journal of Counseling and Clinical Psychology* 33 (1969): 746-749.

24. Steele, "Parental Abuse."

25. Galub, "The Battered Child."

26. Ray M. Helfer, "The Etiology of Child Abuse," *Pediatrics Supplement* 51, part 2 (1973): 777-779.

27. Terr, "Family Study."

28. R. Galdston, "Observations on Children Who Have Been Physically Abused and Their Parents," *American Journal of Psychiatry* 122 (1965): 440-443.

29. Elmer and Greg, "Characteristics of Abused Children."

30. Schmidt and Kempe, "The Pediatrician's Role."

31. M.F. Leonard, J.P. Rymes, and A.J. Solnit, "Failure to Thrive in Infants," *American Journal of Disease in Children* 3 (1966): 600-612.

32. Terr, "Family Study."

33. C.H. Kempe, "Pediatric Implications of the Battered Baby Syndrome," *Archives of Disease in Children* 46 (1971): 28-37.

34. Ray Helfer, "The Relationship between Lack of Bonding and Child Abuse and Neglect," in *Maternal Attachment and Mothering Disorders*, ed. Marshall H. Klaus, Treville Leger, and Mary Anne Trause (Sausalito, Calif., Johnson & Johnson Baby Products Co., 1975).

35. John Kennell, "Evidence for a Sensitive Period in the Human Mother," in *Maternal Attachment and Mothering Disorders*, ed. Marshall H. Klaus, Treville Leger, and Mary Anne Trause (Sausalito, Calif., Johnson & Johnson Baby Products Co., 1975).

36. Helfer, "Etiology of Child Abuse."

37. Kathryn Barnard, "The Acquaintance Process," in *Maternal Attachment and Mothering Disorders*, ed. Marshall H. Klaus, Treville Leger, and Mary Anne Trause (Sausalito, Calif., Johnson & Johnson Baby Products Co., 1975).

38. Helfer, "Etiology of Child Abuse."

39. Blair Justice and Rita Justice, *The Abusing Family* (New York: Human Sciences Press, 1976).

40. Blair Justice and David F. Duncan, "Life Crisis as a Precursor to Child Abuse," *Public Health Reports* 19, no. 2 (March-April 1976): 110-115.

41. Justice and Justice, *Abusing Family*.

42. Justice and Duncan, "Precursor to Child Abuse."

43. Abraham Levine, "Child Neglect: Reaching the Parent," *Social and Rehabilitation Record* 1, no. 7 (July-August 1974): 26.

44. Richard J. Gelles, "Child Abuse as Psychopathology: A Sociological Critique and Reformation," *American Journal of Orthopsychiatry* 43, no. 4, (July 1973): 611-621.

45. Reuben Hill, "Generic Features of Families Under Stress," in *Crisis Intervention: Selected Readings*, ed. Howard J. Parad (New York: Family Services Association of America, 1965).

46. E.E. LeMasters, "Parenthood as Crisis," in *Crisis Intervention: Selected Readings*, ed. Howard J. Parad (New York: Family Services Association of America, 1965).

47. Lydia Rapoport, "The State of Crisis: Some Theoretical Considerations," in *Crisis Intervention: Selected Readings*, ed. Howard J. Parad (New York: Family Services Association of America, 1965).

48. T.H. Holmes and R.H. Rahe, "The Social Readjustment Rating Scale," *Journal of Psychosomatic Research* 11 (1967): 213-218; *Public Health Reports* 91, no. 2 (March-April 1976): 110-115.

49. Peter Mogulnicki et al., "Impending Child Abuse: Psychosomatic Symptoms in Adults as a Clue," *Journal of the American Medical Association*, 237, no. 11 (March 14, 1977): 1109-1111.

50. Kathleen Neill and Carole Kauffman, "Care of the Hospitalized Abused Child and His Family: Nursing Implications," *American Journal of Maternal Child Nursing* 1, no. 2 (March-April 1976).

51. Helfer, "Lack of Bonding and Child Abuse."

52. Justice and Justice, *Abusing Family*.

53. LaVohn Josten, "The Treatment of an Abused Family," *Maternal and Child Nursing Journal* 4, no. 1 (Spring 1975): 23-34.

15
Women in Pain

HOLLY BRANCH

Pain is exciting. That's correct, exciting. Pain is perhaps the most crucial challenge to the nurse; the common denominator of our professional role identity is to provide for the relief of human suffering. The provision of that relief and the actualization of our professional self-image, then, should be approached with great excitement. However, many nurses practicing with persons in pain have quite the opposite feeling. In fact, expressions of inadequacy, anger, and guilt can be heard from nurses who seem to be almost universally frustrated in their attempts to care for those in pain. Perhaps the reason for this frustration is the nature of pain itself. Its subjectivity prevents nurses from achieving true empathy; its lack of physical substance lends a barrier to its eradication; and its complications leave a formidable responsibility for rehabilitation.

Much has been written on nursing management of women in acute pain, such as the pain of childbirth, and on terminal pain, as with cancer. Relatively little attention has been paid to the nursing care of women with chronic, intractable pain. It seems almost as if these persons are given up as hopeless and told that they must learn to cope with their situation. Unfortunately, many nurses have no idea how to create a plan of care and implement it to assist in coping with chronic pain. One obvious reason for this lack of understanding is the absence of or a misconstrued conceptual framework for chronic pain, for it can be a disease, whereas acute and terminal pain are symptoms. The second reason is that many nurses find it difficult to achieve a satisfactory nurse-patient relationship with those in chronic pain because of their feelings about chronicity, chemical dependency, and psychological dysfunction. These three factors are threatening to a nurse and she/he may think that she/he lacks the necessary psychosocial skills needed to deal with them.

To provide effective and appropriate nursing care one needs mastery of two areas, which can be described as theory base and interaction technique. Theory base is the collection and organization of one's academic knowledge into a conceptual framework that is applicable to clinical experience. Interaction technique refers to one's ability to integrate the professional and personal self and present a caring human being to the nurse-patient relationship. Both theory base and interaction technique are integral to the meeting of the pain challenge and are both given due attention in this chapter.

THEORY BASE

What does one need to know about pain? Isn't it enough to know that pain is indicative of human destruction and suffering and that it is the responsibility of nurses to provide for the cessation of the agony by whatever means are delegated to them by physicians, requested of them by the suffering, or seem appropriate on the basis of their professional nursing assessment? No, that is not enough, and that statement is not even necessarily correct. What one does need to know is a conceptual framework for chronic pain that can account for the many phenomena of that disease and from which appropriate interventions will follow.

To understand phenomena it is usually logical to begin with a definition. Throughout the literature several authors have defined pain in several ways. Typically, the various disciplines of medicine, psychiatry, ministry, sociology, surgery, psychology, and often nursing have attempted to define pain according to their experiences with pain through their own theory base and social institution constructs. Such definitions demonstrate a rigid and myopic comprehension of pain and its resultant diagnosis and management. This author asserts that pain simply cannot be defined. No social institution can define a naturally occurring phenomenon such as pain. Pain is subjective and for that reason is not subject to definition. Because of nursing's tradition of viewing the human person as a whole being, it is appropriate at this point to cite nursing's most well-known author in the field of pain, Margo McCaffery. She states that pain is "whatever the experiencing person says it is and exists whenever he says it does."[1] To define pain in that way, as a completely subjective phenomenon, is the only viable alternative for those who deal with persons in pain.

It is necessary to differentiate between pain as a sensory experience and the resultant behaviors that are exhibited as a response to this stimulus. Pain behaviors are indeed open to definition and, to insure proper assessment and treatment, must be defined accurately and objectively. Pain behaviors consist of any action that can be objectively denoted. These may include verbal manifestations varying from a simple "ouch" to a tirade of complaints and expletives; physiologic manifestations ranging from changes in autonomic functions such as pulse, blood pressure, and diaphoresis to gross behaviors such as limping, limited range of motion, and use of assistive devices such as crutches or braces; and psychosocial pain behaviors such as withdrawal, hostility, agitation, dependency, and social, recreational, and vocational dysfunction. This division between pain the experience and pain the behavior must be kept in mind and will be of great significance for the learning of both the interaction technique and the theory base.

It is appropriate to backstep a bit to provide a historical perspective on the development of theories on pain transmission. Among the first people to talk about pain and pain relief were the ancient Chinese. They believed that the human ear simulated an upside-down fetus and that every part of the human body corresponded to a part of the ear. At that time, when a person complained of pain the physician would locate the part of the ear that corresponded to the part of the body in pain and attempt to relieve the pain by inserting a metal staple or needle into that part of the ear. It is interesting that it was taboo for a physician to look at or touch any part of a woman's body except for her ear.

In early Western medicine, Aristotle made the assertion that pain was an emotion which was the absense of pleasure. Today we know that pain is not an emotion but rather a bodily sensation. This is not to say, however, that the experience of pain cannot elicit emotional reactions or that emotional states cannot affect the intensity of the pain experience, for surely this is the case.

In the 1600s Descartes' assertions were the forerunners to the theories of pain belonging to this century. Descartes supposed that there were connections or strings connecting every part of the body with the brain. He termed these strings "tendons." When a person stepped on a tack or injured herself/himself, it caused a tugging on the tendon, which traveled up to the brain. Descartes conjectured that the sensation of pain was a result of this tugging on the brain.

Early this century the specificity theory was developed. The theory stated that there are specialized pain receptors all over the body that are designed to react to noxious stimuli and send pain impulses along specialized nerve fibers to a specific pain center in the brain. Hence, the specificity theory claimed that there is a direct connection between the part of the body that hurts and the pain center in the brain, so that when a person steps on a tack the pain receptors in the foot send messages of pain along the pain nerve pathways directly to the brain, which then allows for the sensation of pain. This concept of pain transmission is most common among the lay patient population and is surprisingly prevalent in the thinking of health professionals.

There are, however, two pieces of evidence that confound the viability of the theory. The first comes from the research of Beecher[2] into the amount of pain perceived by wounded soldiers. According to classic specificity theory, there should be a direct correlation between the amount of nerve damage and pain perceived, but Beecher found quite the opposite. In fact, he found many soldiers with extensive injuries who were actually unaware of pain. The second piece of evidence comes from clinical exposure to amputees. Phantom limb pain, which is actually sensed in the missing part itself, is initiated by gentle or non-noxious stimuli and can often be agonizing. It is apparent that there cannot be a direct connection between the pain receptors in the hurting part and the pain center in the brain because the part that hurts is not there. That along with the fact that the pain receptors in this case are not specific to noxious stimuli lends to the inadequacy of the specificity theory.

There subsequently followed a group of pain theories known as pattern theories, which stressed the concepts of stimulus intensity, central summation, or input control system. The idea behind stimulus intensity was that all nerve endings are alike, so that pain is a result of the intensity of stimulation as opposed to specificity. Central summation refers to the concept of reverberating circuits of pain in the spinal column that may be triggered by noxious or non-noxious stimuli and are interpreted centrally (in the brain) as pain. This is opposed to the previous opinion that excessive peripheral stimulation was the mechanism for pain and afforded an explanation for phantom limb pain. The input control system proposed that the rapid velocity of certain nonpain nerve fibers inhibited the transmission of impulses in the slower-firing pain fibers. Although each of these theories offered individually valuable concepts, they were too narrowly constructed to account for the overall nature of pain transmission.

In 1965 Melzack and Wall[3] hypothesized the gate control theory, which appears to be the most widely accepted in current practice. The gate control theory utilizes certain concepts from both the specificity and pattern theories in addition to some innovations to provide a theory that is generally applicable to clinical findings. Before exploring the intricacies of this theory it is necessary to diverge and cover some basic neuroanatomy and physiology.

Pain transmission commences with cell destruction, which results in the release of certain proteolytic enzymes. These act on gamma globins to produce a series of polypeptides, which dilate blood vessels and trigger afferent nerve fibers. The pain pathway continues from these afferent fibers to the spinal cord via the dorsal root, up through the reticular brainstem and on to the thalamus, where pain is perceived, and finally to the cortex, where the cognitive, affective, and motor responses are determined.

There are three types of afferent nerve fibers, each responsible for different sensations. Beta fibers are large in diameter, have the fastest conduction velocity and lowest firing threshold, and are responsible for nonpainful or touch sensations. The gamma-delta, or A, fibers have a moderate diameter, conduction velocity, and firing threshold and are responsible for pinprick or knife-like pain, which is often characteristic of acute pain. The C fibers are of small diameter, slow velocity, and high threshold and are responsible for burning and aching, which is usually the nature of prolonged pain.

The gate control theory recognizes the idea of fiber specificity but qualifies it with stimulus intensity. In other words, there are specific fibers for transmission of pain as mentioned above, but smaller fibers are also capable of being triggered by non-noxious stimuli so that one additional factor in determining if pain will be sensed is the intensity of the stimuli. The main assertion of the gate control theory is the existence of a gate in the spinal cord which, when open, allows the transmission of pain to the brain for perception and reaction. When the gate is closed, pain messages are not allowed to reach the brain. The gate operates by degree; there are degrees of being open and being closed, as opposed to an either/or situation. As persons dedicated to assisting in the relief of suffering it is of vital importance that nurses know what opens and closes the gate, because that is how they will control pain.

The gate is not any visible structure but rather a complex biochemical reaction. It consists of cells of substantia gelatinosa in the dorsal column of the spinal cord and operates as part of the input control system by collecting and modulating incoming impulses before sending them on to the T cells, whose function is to fire them up to the brain. The gate can be opened or closed in response to afferent activity from the body or efferent activity from the brain. One special characteristic of the gate is its relationship to the impulses of the beta, or touch, fibers. When these impulses reach the gate they are able to influence it to close to incoming messages from the A and C, or pain, fibers. The gate is also influenced by the central control trigger of the brain, whose efferent messages about the psychological status of the individual affect the afferent conduction. The exact mechanism of the central control trigger is not known. To gain a more comprehensive understanding of pain in a clinical sense, the concepts of pain threshold and the pain loop will be introduced.

The pain threshold can actually be divided into two areas: the pain perception threshold and the pain reaction threshold. The pain perception threshold is that level or intensity of pain that reaches one's awareness, or perception. Pain perception thresholds are presumably the same for all persons regardless of demographic variables. The pain reaction threshold is the level pain reaches when it produces an observable behavioral response or reaction. This threshold does indeed vary according to age, sex, race, religion, childhood experiences, and many other variables. Hypothetically, then, if one could apply the same pain to a group of individuals they would all perceive the pain at the same time, but their reactions to it would vary widely in terms of both degree and time.

To best explain the psychosocial aspects of pain, the concept of the pain loop will be utilized. An arbitrary value of 50 points will be assigned to the pain perception threshold, and a value of 75 points will designate the pain reaction threshold. Remember that it is at the level of the gate in the spinal column that these thresholds exist and that messages received by the gate may either come up from the body or down from the brain. The "points" will denote the quantity and quality of the messages coming to the gate. So at 50 points the combined messages from the brain and the body reach the pain perception threshold of the gate, and the gate opens to the degree that pain is perceived. Similarly, if the combined messages from the brain and the body accumulate to 75 points, the gate opens to the degree that the person will react to the sensation of pain.

With these things in mind, some examples of various pain situations will be explored. The first three examples will focus on the healthy person, and the latter three examples will describe chronic pain states. The first example concerns the situation of a healthy woman on an average day (Fig. 15.1). The messages reaching the gate from the brain emanate from the problems and attentions of daily living, such as getting to work on time or sending the children off to school, and perhaps total 25 points. On an average day in this healthy woman's life she steps on a tack, and the messages from that injury bring 35 points to the gate. Thirty-five points

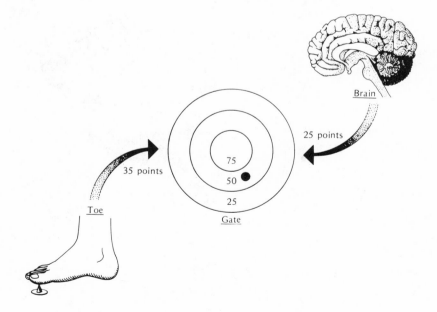

Figure 15.1. Pain in the life of a healthy woman: Example 1.

from the body and 25 points from the brain total 60 points at the gate. Sixty points surpasses the pain perception threshold, and the gate opens to the degree that the woman will perceive the pain associated with her injury. However, after this perception she goes about her daily activities without reacting to her perceptions.

The second example makes reference to the same healthy woman in the first example but under different circumstances (Fig. 15.2). On this particular day she is very relaxed and calm, well rested, and generally satisfied with her life situation. For these reasons the messages from the brain total only 10 points. Stepping on the same tack and receiving the same injury, she again accumulates 35 points from her foot. Ten points from the brain and 35 points from the foot total 45 points at the gate. Forty-five points is under the pain perception threshold so that the gate remains closed, and the woman is not aware of the pain from her injury. Certainly, many of us have received bruises and minor cuts and have been unable to explain their origin; the above dynamics were probably in operation during those injuries.

In the third example the same healthy woman is utilized but in a third set of circumstances (Fig. 15.3). This time the woman is experiencing a day that is not going particularly well; perhaps the car won't start, or there is a family argument, or performance at work was not satisfactory. The tensions and worries of a day such as this send messages worth 45 points down to the gate. Stepping on that same tack yields the same 35 points from the foot. Forty-five points from the brain and 35 points from the foot total 80 points at the gate, which constitutes the pain reaction threshold. This woman will not only perceive the pain in her foot but will react to it with observable behavior that may range from a slight wrinkling of the brow to a loud scream or an exaggerated limp.

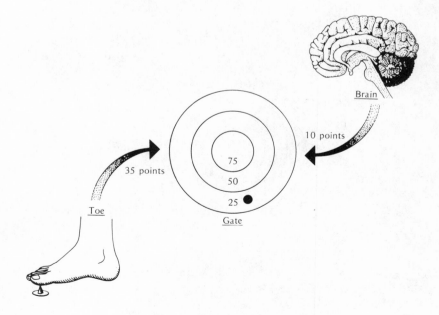

Figure 15.2. Pain in the life of a healthy woman: Example 2.

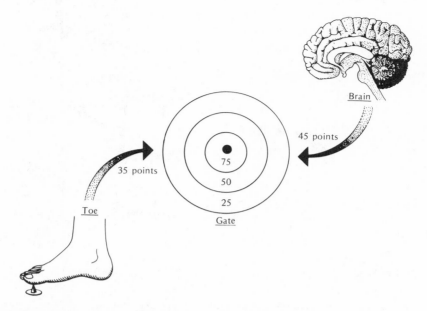

Figure 15.3. Pain in the life of a healthy woman: Example 3.

Before beinning the last three examples, which deal with chronic pain states, there are some vital issues to clarify. The first of these concerns the amount of organic damage present in the hurting part of the woman with chronic pain. Regardless of medical diagnosis or results from diagnostic testing, there is always a certain amount of damage in the painful part. Because persons in pain either underuse or misuse the affected part, there generally exists some organic damage from atrophied muscle at the very least. As an arbitrary figure, 35 points' worth of damage will be assigned to the hurt part of the woman in chronic pain.

In the fourth example the woman is suffering from chronic pain of the foot, and this is an average day in her life (Fig. 15.4). On such a day she is receiving 25 points' worth of average daily tensions at the gate from her brain. Thirty-five points from the chronic foot damage and 25 points from her brain total 60 points. Sixty points surpasses the pain perception threshold, so that on an average day in the life of a woman with chronic pain she is aware of the pain but able to cope with the activities of daily living without reacting to the pain.

In the fifth example, the same woman with the same chronic foot condition is having a relatively good, relaxed day (Fig. 15.5). The same 35 points' worth of disability reach the gate from the foot, and because she is relaxed and calm there are only 10 points coming down from the brain. This combined total of 45 points at the gate is not enough to open the gate, so that on this day the woman is not aware of her pain. Although the time period used in this example is one day, it varies from person to person. But generally there are seconds, hours, or even weeks or longer in the life of a woman with chronic pain when the pain does not break into awareness.

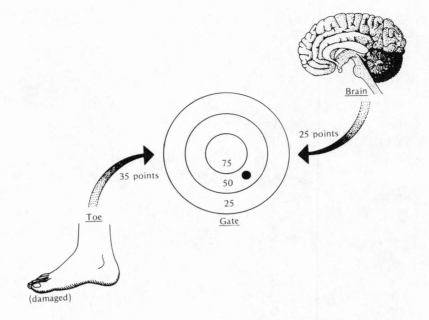

Figure 15.4. Pain in the life of a woman with a chronic foot condition: Example 4.

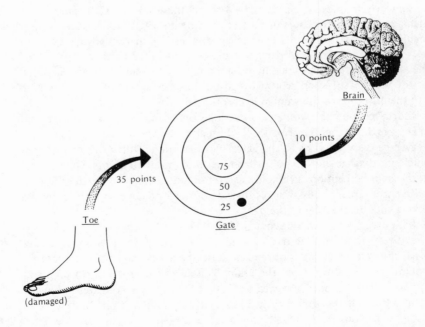

Figure 15.5. Pain in the life of a woman with a chronic foot condition: Example 5.

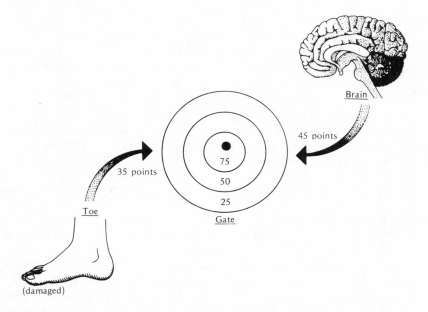

Figure 15.6. Pain in the life of a woman with a chronic foot condition: Example 6.

In the last example the woman with chronic foot pain is receiving the same 35 points at the gate in her spinal column (Fig. 15.6). But because she lives with this chronic disability several changes occur that create an accumulation of points from the brain. If this woman is used to working she may find that she is no longer able to work. If she has been a housewife she is no longer able to care for the house and children. Social and recreational activities become a thing of the past. Even sexual activities are a source of pain. She loses her ability to plan ahead or structure her time because her entire time reference becomes oriented around the pain. When she is in pain she waits for it to stop, and when she is not in pain she fearfully waits for it to appear. Movies, parties, weddings, high school graduations, shopping, picnics, dancing, church services, gardening, and golf have become symbols of hurt. If she starts using narcotics for control of pain she soon notices that they are decreasing in their effect. She fixates on the pills, watching the clock for four hours to tick by. She is preoccupied with refilling prescriptions and perhaps reaches the point where she can't remember when she took the last pill or how many she took last time, but she needs them and becomes indiscriminate in their use with this rationalization. Soon there is no evidence in her life that she is productive or worthwhile in any sense that she was used to. Her existence is without meaning or gratification. Depression, anger, anxiety, and fear set in. All of these events, whether they occur on a small scale in one day or accumulate over time cause 45 points to reach the gate from the brain. Thirty-five points from the chronic foot damage and 45 points from a worried and desperate brain results in 80 points at the gate. These 80 points exceed the pain perception threshold and the pain reaction threshold, and this woman not only is aware of her pain but reacts to it.

Persons with chronic pain typically react to it in two ways, either by underdoing or by overdoing. Those who underdo withdraw, give up, and virtually stop all premorbid activities. They become dependent, passive, and inadequate in their daily responsibilities. Those who overdo tend to dramatically increase their activity level, especially during those periods below the pain perception threshold. All this is an effort to ignore or deny the pain, which usually crops up periodically to an incapacitating degree. Both these reactions are manifestations of an inability to cope with chronic pain, which is also known as the chronic pain syndrome. This is indeed an example of a vicious circle, for the more this woman reacts to her pain, the greater her tension, depression, and worry become, which operates to allow her to feel the pain even more acutely, leading to an even more exaggerated reaction, and so on.

It is important to note that the value of the points used in the above examples is arbitrarily chosen, but not without consideration. Points coming from either the body or the brain are always greater than zero and less than 50, the pain perception threshold. These points are greater than zero because there is no such thing as an absolute state of health in either the mind or the body. These ideals do not exist in reality. The upper spectrum of the points from the body or the mind does not exceed the pain perception threshold because pain is a sensory experience composed of input from both the mind and the body. Absolute organic and psychogenic pain are also pure types that do not exist in reality. But between these limits the possible combinations of points from both body and mind are endless and dependent on the individuality of human beings and their environments.

The major point to be made here is that premorbid psychological dysfunction can never be assumed to be the motive for the acquisition of prolonged pain. This is commonly assumed to be the case, particularly in the case of the woman whose diagnostic testing fails to show organic damage or enough damage to justify her subjective complaints in the diagnostician's opinion. To begin with, there are very few objective data available on the premorbid personality of women in pain, and living with chronic illness, especially pain which has a strong affective component, is generally facilitative of, or concomitant with, personality change. In conclusion, by the time a woman with pain reaches the point of chronicity (medically defined as six months' duration), it is a certainty that she will manifest emotional difficulties. It is simply not important to know whether the psychological difficulties were a part of the etiology of the pain state or exist as a secondary complication. In fact, making the assumption that psychological illness is the sole cause of the pain state is a tragic error for any diagnostician to make and certainly leads to mismanagement of a case. Such labeling only tends to alienate the patient, create an atmosphere of distrust, and close off any possibility of a therapeutic relationship. In addition, whole areas of treatment options are closed off to the patient as she is ignored while awaiting referral to a psychiatrist. The same mistake can be made by the nurse who fails to see the patient as a person whose existence is painful and is concerned only with the traction set up for the low back in room 233. Nursing care is ineffectual if it focuses only on physical or psychosocial needs. Whole people be-

come ill and require whole nursing care, which brings us to a consideration of interaction technique.

INTERACTION TECHNIQUE

Interaction technique, as mentioned earlier, is the ability to integrate the professional and personal self to present a caring human being to the nurse-patient relationship. Learning the interaction technique is a delicate matter and deserves lengthy
consideration. In many ways it is comparable to learning to ride a bicycle. One can
read books and receive verbal guidance from others, which will be helpful, but the
integral learning comes from interaction with the bicycle itself. Riding a bicycle is a
function of both the person and the machinery, and it is a skill that is learned, not
a natural talent or ability. The situation is similar when one is working with women
in pain. One can read what is written here, which will be helpful, but one must
ultimately learn to develop her/his own skills and style in clinical practice. One may
fall down and scrape her/his knees a few times, but the actual learning must come
from repeated interpersonal interaction. It is not easy, but it can be learned. The
following is a statement made by a woman in pain which, it is hoped, will stimulate
an appreciation of the importance of learning from patients themselves.

> Four years ago I was working on a television documentary, and normally
> I have alot of energy; I like to work, keep busy, and am very social. I began
> not to feel well and as I planned to go away for the winter I decided to have
> my check up and pap smear before leaving. I got a letter back saying that my
> pap test had come back positive, cancer. I was sent to the hospital for a
> culdoscopy, which was a totally devastating experience. Needless to say, I
> was terrified of what was going to go on, but the doctor refused to answer
> my questions when I asked him to please explain what he was going to do so
> that I could relax. He told me I wouldn't understand it because it was all in
> medical terms. After he got me into the stirrups set up for the culdoscopy,
> he brought in a class of interns without even asking my permission. They all
> took their turns looking. Obviously it really put me on edge. Then the doctor
> began to do biopsies without giving me an anesthetic or telling me what he
> was doing. He took 12 slices out of my cervix and then walked out of the
> room, leaving me bleeding and in a great deal of pain. I then had a long con-
> versation with a doctor, who explained my options: that I had cancer very
> badly and that if I didn't have something done he didn't know how long I
> would have to live. He told me I could have surgery right away and possibly
> live a long time, or I could travel as I had planned and not come back. Of
> course, I was scared; I really did not know what to do. At that moment I
> became a very passive person and started to let things happen to me. I let
> myself get talked into a hysterectomy, which may or may not have been
> necessary—I still don't know.
>   I entered the hospital and was taken up to a ten-bed obstetrics-gynecology
> ward, which I thought was incredible: putting in the same room with mothers
> someone who was going to have a hysterectomy, though I had already de-
> cided I didn't want to have any children. However, when the choice is taken
> away from you at 28 years of age, it is still kind of devastating, and I hadn't

gotten it all straight in my mind. It was hard to be in there with all those mothers; I was pretty anxious.

They took me up to the preoperative room and got me ready. I was talking a mile a minute just because I wanted someone to tell me what was going on. I was scared. The operating room nurse seemed upset by the fact that I wasn't more drugged, so she gave me another preop hypo. I don't remember much after that, but I found out later I was hemorrhaging and almost died because no one had come to check on me or paid any attention when my mother told them something was wrong. It was a hard time for me because it was very painful. I had IV needles in me everywhere, and yet they came and took blood out every hour to check my hemoglobin. I couldn't figure out why they were taking it out in one place and putting it in another. I tried to be as cooperative as I could, but about the fourth day I broke down and cried because I couldn't deal with the situation. I was discharged early because they told me they needed by bed, but I had no where to go except a nursing home.

Finally it was arranged that my parents would drive 500 miles to pick me up and take me back to their home. I was in so much pain that I had to stop at several hospitals along the way for hypos. I was at my parents' house for two days, and I ended up in the hospital there. The doctor was our old family doctor, and he was very upset that I had had the operation. He felt it was unnecessary and had been bungled. He didn't even examine me. All this time I kept trying to tell someone that something was wrong because I still had alot of pain in my side. Finally, I decided to leave. I just needed to be alone to deal with all of it. It was hard staying with my parents because they expect a great deal of people and have a hard time dealing with illness in their children.

For the next five months I was in an incredible amount of pain but continued to work and be very active, hoping it would go away. Then I began to grow hair on my face, developed severe headaches, and gained 30 pounds, and the pain went on without end. I went back to the hospital, but I couldn't get anyone to listen to me about what was wrong. I knew I was going through menopause. This went on for five days; I went back every day for a pelvic exam and a pap smear. By the fifth day I was furious because I had seen a different doctor every day, had to go through the same story every time, and none of the doctors could imagine why I was going through this, because I was "too young." So the fifth day I got hysterical, screamed and hollered, hit the desk, and things like that. I was at the end of my rope. By this time I was in a severe depression, which frightened me because I've never been depressed. I seriously thought about killing myself, and I just sat for hours alone trying to cope. So the day I had hysterics in the hospital they called in someone from the mental health unit to take me away so that I would not disturb the other patients, which only made me more furious. Finally an endocrinologist came in and told me I was in menopause. He suggested that I seek counseling, as all the doctors seemed to think that my uterus was connected to my personality, even though I could not find that on any anatomy charts. They thought my problem was that I had not accepted the hysterectomy, but to me that was beside the point by that time. I just didn't want to feel so awful. I went to the mental health unit. I took their tests, and I talked with their counselors. The consensus of doctors who saw me was that I was in better shape mentally than most of the people who worked there.

After that I was referred to another hospital for the regulation of my menopause. The doctor there looked at all women as inferior and neurotic, but I was still in my passive state and went along with everything he said. He gave some hormones, a tranquilizer, and some pain pills, as the pain was still there. I finally stopped taking the pain pills because I didn't want to get addicted, and I was determined to lick it on my own. But, again, I had totally cut myself off from all my friends, I wasn't seeing anyone, I was in a bad mood all the time, and I refused to talk to anyone. I was in a great deal of pain all the time, and pains were starting in other parts of my body, which really frightened me. When I tried to tell the doctor about the new pains in my chest and arm, he told me it was all in my head.

One day the pain was so bad that I couldn't breathe so I went to the emergency room, and they told me I have costalchondritis and that the tranquilizer I was on was making it worse. When I told my doctor about this I found that he had not looked at my chest x-ray at the time he prescribed the tranquilizer, and the x-ray already showed evidence of the disease at that time. So I went back to the first hospital and was assigned another doctor, who I thought would be the answer to my prayers—someone who would understand what I was going through, that I did not function solely in a six-by-nine office, that I functioned in the world, and that I was having a hard time dealing with the pain continually and still trying to straighten out things that were the aftermath of my operation.

By last spring I was once again in a desperate situation. I was ready to kill myself, just to end the suffering. I wasn't trying to get even with anyone; I was just tired of hurting. My brother referred me to a nurse-psychotherapist, and I can't say enough about what a help it has been to deal with someone who understands what is going on. I now understand that pain is not all in my head. It comes from my body as well and, when the two meet, a person's tolerance levels change. I'm back to functioning as a normal person, my creativity has come back, I have alot of energy, I'm becoming more social, and I'm not in pain nearly as much as I was before. I hardly ever have a bad day now. The weather still affects me somewhat, but there are some things you learn to accept, and that's part of it—acceptance. Therapy has done me wonders.

I think it's really good that women are pioneering in this field because I think we know more about pain than anyone. We deal with it more in our lives than men do; we are more willing to acknowledge it, perhaps. The doctor who was seeing me refused to have anything to do with me when I decided to seek counseling. He felt it was a quackery program, particularly because it was run by women and nurses. He also made the comment that he wasn't there to listen to patients; he was there to look at their hearts and lungs. He told me he wasn't a psychiatrist, that he was just concerned about organs. That seems to be a prevailing attitude, particularly in the case of women because the implication is that everything is tied to your reproductive organs. You are treated as if you have no identity other than that. I think it is important that people in health care begin to work together for the good of the patient and help the patient realize what is going on in her/his life. Doctors and nurses are only human like anyone else. The knowledge you have is the knowledge you have, and how you put it to use is up to you.

Therapy is helping me deal with the stresses in my life, pain being the biggest stress, though it is now somewhat eliminated. Also, my resentment toward how I felt and how I was treated is being worked through. I think it is important to have this kind of counseling available because it is essential to vent resentful feelings; otherwise you magnify them all out of proportion and you make yourself sicker. Men and women are the cause of their own disease in the first place, which is a pretty hard thing to realize. We would like to blame it on some almighty power, but we've done it to ourselves. The hardest thing to realize is that you are in charge; that is very frightening. But then you realize you are also in charge of making things better, and that is good because you are only as strong as you want to be. If you want to be strong you can fix it. And I want to be, and I am fixing it.

This woman has indeed lived painfully. She has experienced the acute and chronic pain of physical illness; she has suffered the psychological pain of depression, anger, and fear; she has encountered that spiritual pain involved with accountability; and she has coped with the cultural or sociologic pain that plagues women seeking assistance in a male-dominated health care system.

How have health professionals compounded the pain in the lives of persons such as this woman? This can best be understood by looking at the development of the pain career and the role that health professionals play in that development. As mentioned earlier, it is inherent in the role identity of health care professionals that they are dedicated to providing relief for human pain and suffering. Their first contact with the woman in pain is obviously after the onset of the initial pain symptoms, the acute phase. Following their role script, they make every effort to alleviate both the pain and what appears to be the source of that pain. Seemingly, the most appropriate approach during this acute phase is to directly treat the pain with rest and medication. The problems arise somewhere between the acute and chronic phases of pain, which is a rather nebulous span since, according to medical definition, pain does not achieve chronicity until it is of six months' duration. Utilization of the treatment approaches for acute pain generally produces iatrogenic complications after prolonged application. Specifically, three such iatrogenic situations will be discussed.

Persons in pain who are advised to rest or to exercise or work until they feel pain can learn more pain—and pain can be learned. This is called a work to tolerance prescription and operates according to the following diagram:

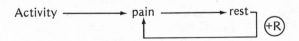

The person is active until she experiences pain, and then she is allowed to rest. Rest (R), then, assumes the characteristics of a positive reinforcer that increases the likelihood of pain occurring again because it is rewarded by rest. In addition to reinforcing pain, prolonged periods of rest reduce self-worth by eliminating sources of worth such as the performance of daily responsibilities and social interaction. Such situations are breeding grounds for depression, fear, anxiety, and dependency.

Similarly, medications used for acute pain are frequently extended beyond the acute phase and into the chronic. The use of pain medications, particularly narcotics, operates like rest as a positive reinforcement to the reappearance of pain:

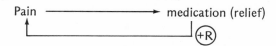

Iatrogenic chemical dependence and its ramifications are often a part of chronic pain states.

There is a third aspect of this acute care approach that is confounding when used beyond the acute stage, and that is the concept of direct intervention to the hurting part. During the acute phase efforts are geared toward diagnosis and treatment of the affected part. After this point diagnosis is no longer engaged in, for it generally shows no organic damage, a healed injury, or intractable damage for which there is no appropriate direct intervention. The patient is then told that she must learn to live with her condition, without any clue as to how to go about doing it. In addition, another factor begins to operate. By this time the patient is a threat to health professionals because she is failing to be relieved of her pain, which indicates that they are failing to fulfill their professional role identity. When faced with such a threat, health professionals may resort to many tactics to alleviate or reduce the threat. Among the most common is labeling the patient as a crock who has imaginary pain solely to resolve neurotic conflict, obtain narcotics to maintain an addiction, or secure financial secondary gain through litigation or compensation. Although such factors may be influential, they are rarely a conscious motivation, and such attitudes and behaviors on the part of health care professionals promote distrust and resentment on the part of the patient and lay the foundation for a nonproductive relationship.

So what can be done in a positive sense? The most important factor in the rehabilitation of the woman with chronic pain is the establishment of a therapeutic nurse-patient relationship. The most important component of a therapeutic nurse-patient relationship is trust. Such trust emanates from understanding of and belief in each other. That kind of trust, understanding, and belief are impossible to achieve if the nurse is preoccupied with determining whether the patient's pain is real or imaginary and, if it is imaginary, what the payoff is. This kind of preoccupation is nonproductive. Unless the nurse can come to accept the ideology that all pain is a real sensory experience with both psychological and physical components, the nursing care will be ineffective. It is fairly common to hear nurses say that they know psychogenic pain feels real to the patient, but even this type of thinking is not functional for it still propagates the concept of dualism. All pain is real, or all pain is imaginary, whichever way is easiest to conceptualize, but pain simply is. Unless this frame of reference is adopted the nurse's energies will be misdirected toward direct intervention of the pain itself, which is inappropriate in a chronic situation. When the existence of pain is accepted as a given, the nurse then becomes more free to direct healing energy toward a more appropriate focus—the patient as a person. The patient as a person has suffered physical, emotional, spiritual, vocational, recreational, social, and familial dysfunction as a result of living in pain. In chronic pain states it is these dysfunctions that demand the attention of the nurse. Even though the patient is usually aware of the dysfunctional life style, it is a pattern that she has grown used to and is generally resistant to change. She operates on the misconception that the pain must be eradicated before she can return to a state of health. It is only with the support of the therapeutic nurse-patient relationship that the patient can begin to risk changing despite the pain.

The nursing plan of care must be designed to reduce the incoming points from both the body and the mind, to provide whole nursing care for an entirely ill individual. The expected outcome of such a plan is to assist the patient to achieve control over her situation so that she is able to maintain herself below the pain reaction threshold. A section will be devoted to nursing guidelines for intervention in each of these two areas.

In the physical realm is the concern of chemical dependency, although this also contributes points from the brain. Many nurses are blatantly angry about having to give narcotics to addicted patients, yet many also feel hesitant to bring these concerns to the physicians who are responsible for that delegation. It is indeed the nurse's professional responsibility to bring her opinions about possible addiction to the attention of the physician, for the nurse is in a position to have more information on patient status because more time is spent in patient contact. If the physician chooses not to withdraw the patient from narcotics, the nurse still has the right to refuse to pass that medication if she/he believes it is detrimental to the patient. It may be an inconvenience on a busy medical/surgical floor to get another nurse to pass medications for that patient, but it is imperative to be assertive with professional convictions. For the nurse who is willing to give narcotic medications there is always the problem of the patient requesting medication before it can be given. This can be frustrating to a busy nurse and create irritation toward the patient. One way to alleviate this situation, as well as foster independence and responsibility in the patient, is to provide her with a pen, a blank medication record, and a clock. A contract is then arranged between the nurse and the patient. The patient is to keep track of her medication intake for her own record and not request medication until it can be given, and the nurse will follow through with prompt and unquestioning administration of the drug. This kind of contract can avoid the power struggles that often exist between the nurse and the patient over the administration of pain medication. Such a record can also be a way of making the patient more aware of her chemical intake and possible dependency.

If the doctor is agreeable to a withdrawal from narcotics, this record can be used by the patient to assist in setting up the withdrawal schedule, for surely the patient should be consulted so as to provide her with a sense of control and motivation. The first step in setting up a withdrawal schedule is to establish a fixed rather than PRN routine of medication intake. A fixed intake refers to setting up regular times for giving the medication, regardless of whether the patient requests it. This avoids the learning situation described earlier in which taking pain medication in response to pain positively reinforces the pain. The next step is to eliminate one time of administration per day so that, if a patient is taking a certain pain medication ten times per day, she will be withdrawn in ten days. The use of major tranquilizers and anti-depressants as an adjunct to withdrawal is often appropriate to assist with relaxation. At no time should placebos be used, for they are dishonest and rob the patient of integrity and independence. Remember that chemical dependency is a disease of delusion, and intervention is highly frustrating, for both the patient and the health care professional. But until the patient is able to function with a mind and body free of narcotics she will be unable to take the remaining steps toward overcoming the disability of her pain.

Another aspect of the physical component of the disability is the deteriorated condition of the muscles in the affected part, as well as overall lowered resistance. Depending, of course, on the privileges of the patient, the nurse should encourage the patient to be as active as possible. Activity should be prescribed according to a work to quota program as opposed to the work to tolerance program mentioned earlier. In a work to quota program the baseline activity level of the patient is assessed, and daily goals of improvement in all areas are set up. The patient then is expected to achieve these daily goals regardless of her pain level. In this way, rest is a positive reinforcer to activity, and pain is not a meaningful variable. In addition to strengthening atrophied muscles and improving general stamina, a program of progressive muscle relaxation and deep breathing can be taught to the patient. Exercising tight, spastic muscles can be destructive, and such a relaxation program can potentiate the effects of increased activity. Also, this relaxation helps to reduce the points of tension coming down from the brain.

The therapeutic use of touch, heat, and cold should also be considered in this category of intervention. Stimulation of the beta, or touch, fibers will affect the gate's reception of the pain impulses and possibly reduce the points from the body, so that the gate will close below the pain reaction threshold. Frequent touching of the patient and use of cold packs, ice applications, heating pads, and warm showers and baths are possible alternatives.

At the other end of the spectrum is the challenge of reducing points reaching the gate from the mind. One needn't be a certified psychoanalyst to intervene here; as mentioned earlier, the most important prerequisite is a trusting therapeutic relationship with the patient. One common roadblock to the establishment of this relationship is frequent complaining of pain by the patient. To many nurses this behavior is irritating and lends to their feeling of inadequacy. Patients usually operate on the assumption that nurses need to know every aspect of their pain, and they have grown used to communication with others through their pain. One way to alleviate this confusion is again by the use of a contract. The nurse should explain that because the situation is chronic there is no reason for the patient to continually refer to the pain and that the nurse is aware of and believes in its presence but is unable to do anything directly to make it go away. The nurse should indicate an interest in knowing more about the patient as a person. This is likely to be a new and threatening idea to the patient; so she is likely to continue with the pattern she is used to—relating through pain. When this happens the nurse should state that she/he will leave the room because the patient is talking about pain but that she/he will return in 15 minutes or whatever time period is convenient. It is important that the nurse be warm but firm in this respect so that the patient knows that she is not being personally rejected but that this pain behavior is unacceptable. It is also important to return to the patient after the time period stated. Remaining consistent with this approach will lead the patient to believe that she is of value as a person, not just as a pain patient, and will add considerably to her self-worth. In time, with consistency and support, the pain-legitimating behavior of complaining should cease.

One topic of great concern to nursing is assessment, and this is valid, for without assessment, formulation of a plan of care becomes an impossibility. But without the open honesty and trust of a therapeutic nurse-patient relationship the assessment will most likely be incomplete and heavily focused on physical detail, which is the safest and most familiar material for the patient to reveal. Once the relationship is begun the nurse should also explore the areas of social and recreational activities, family functioning, vocation, finances, emotional status, spirituality, self-image, plans for the future, and sexuality. One framework for this type of assessment is to ask the patient what has changed in each of these areas in her life from premorbid status to present. This outlining of change will give the nurse a clue as to the areas needing special focus so that an individualized plan of care can be created. The importance of utilizing the other members of the health care team cannot be understated. Occupational therapy, recreational therapy, physical therapy, social work, psychology, chaplaincy, vocational rehabilitation, and chemical dependency consultation should be readily available.

Finally, we approach the most crucial aspect of the nursing plan of care: facilitation of coping and acceptance. The structure most adaptable to this task is the grief process outlined by Kübler-Ross.[4] Indeed, with chronic pain, the patient undergoes a multitude of changes in all areas of her life. Concomitant with change is loss. The patient with chronic pain must deal with the grief of her many losses if she is to learn to accept and cope with the pain. But, alas, unlike the patient with terminal illness, there is no resolution, no death. Meaning must be defined for life, not death. The patient with chronic pain is faced with new losses every day, loss of opportunity, loss of chance, and loss of freedom of becoming. Because of this, the chronic pain patient never reaches an ultimate and final acceptance. The stages of denial, depression, anger, bargaining, and acceptance resurface continually throughout this person's life. It is the task of nurses to educate persons in pain with everything they know about the disease. Cognitive clarity is one positive step toward resolution of any dilemma. Nurses must inform these patients of the signs and symptoms of depression, anger, fear, anxiety, dependency, and denial so that they can learn to recognize these feelings and behaviors in themselves. Beyond this, nurses must teach patients how to resolve these states, how to deal with them, and how to move ever forward to acceptance. There is no one correct way to do this, but reference to psychiatric nursing texts can offer specific guidelines for specific behavioral patterns. As the patient gains skill in this area, the stages of acceptance can become longer in duration and be achieved more quickly.

When a patient reaches acceptance, she knows the reality of her situation. This does not mean she has given up. On the contrary, acceptance requires hard work for its maintenance. Acceptance implies a meaningful, productive life style within the reality of the patient's context. Acceptance does not necessarily show itself through undaunted joy but rather through a sense of security in knowing one's past and present and having faith in one's ability to deal with the future. Disability is ultimately only a state of mind.

Nursing care can be the most effective treatment modality for the woman suffering from chronic pain if the focus remains on the woman as a person.

NOTES

1. Margo McGaffery, *Nursing Management of the Patient with Pain* (Philadelphia: J.B. Lippincott Co., 1972), p. 8.

2. H. Beecher, "The Subjective Response and Reaction to Sensation," *Amer J Med* 20 (1956): 107; "The Psychological and Cultural Influences on the Reaction to Pain," *Nursing Forum* 7 (1968): 262.

3. R. Melzack and P. Wall, "Pain Mechanisms: A New Theory," *Science* 150 (1965): 971.

4. Elisabeth Kübler-Ross, *On Death and Dying* (New York: Macmillan, 1972).

REFERENCE BIBLIOGRAPHY

J. Blaylock, "The Psychological and Cultural Influences on the Reaction to Pain," *Nursing Forum* 7 (1968): 262.

K. Casey, "The Neurophysiological Basis of Pain," *Postgrad Med* 53 (6) (May 1965): 58.

R. Sternbach, *Pain: A Psychophysiological Analysis* (New York: Academic, 1968).

_____, *Pain Patients: Traits and Treatment* (New York: Academic, 1968).

M. Zborowski, *People in Pain* (San Francisco: Jossey-Baas, Inc., 1969).

Part IV
The Stress of Loss

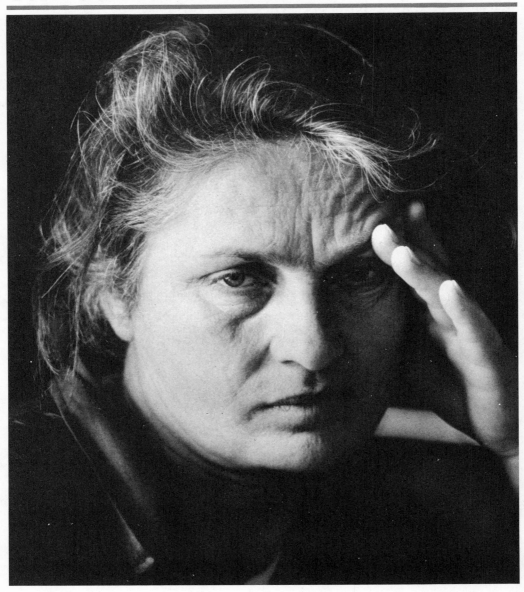

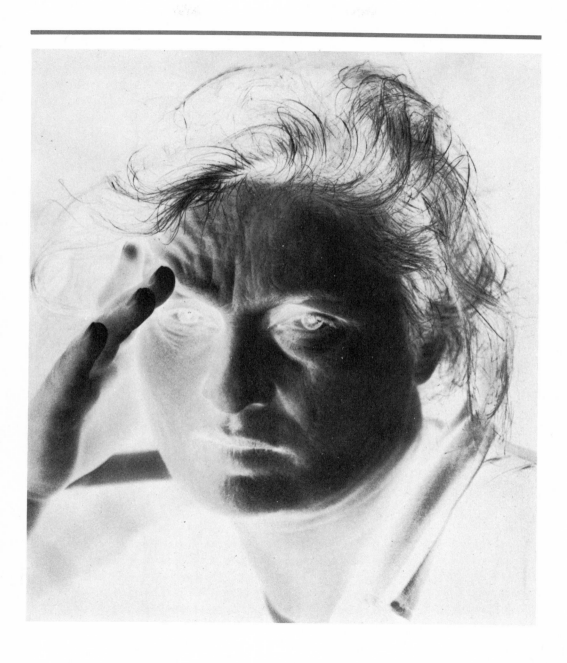

16
Women and Divorce

Implications for Nursing Care

VERONA C. GORDON

"Divorce is one of the most traumatic crises a family faces . . . and nursing is long overdue in taking its share of responsibility in recognizing the powerful impact of change that occurs within divorced families."[1] The eminent psychiatrist Elisabeth Kübler-Ross described divorce as a grief process which nurses still do not recognize as an area of stress that they should become involved in.[2] The purpose of this chapter is to reveal to nurses more information about divorce in our society and its significant effect on the client involved. Nursing implications are still unclear; however, questions needing answers are more apparent.

In 1977, the United States was the leading country in the world for divorce, with one out of three marriages ending in divorce. In Western society it appears that divorce has become a common occurrence. There has been such a growing number of divorce decrees over the past ten years that "divorce is increasing at a faster rate than either the number of marriages or the general growth of the population."[3]

REVIEW OF THE LITERATURE

This author's search of the literature for nursing studies on the effect of divorce on clients with implications for nursing care was discouraging. The paucity of nursing research on divorced mothers and their children was evident. That nurses are slow to write and publish their reactions, experiences, or ideas on intervention with the divorced woman and her children is not astonishing when we read the statement of the prominent therapist Kaplan, "Family-therapy strategies for the child of divorce and his family have yet to be described."[4]

Knowledge about the actual experiences of families approaching, going through, and following divorce is surprisingly limited; literature generally stresses the destructive aspects of divorce, offering little information about the nature of divorces that serves constructive aims.[5]

According to Hertherington et al.: "The latest census data indicate that more than 40 percent of new marriages will end in divorce. Such separation affects all members of a family, yet few studies of divorce have included the father."[6] These authors have also found studies and research lacking in additional areas, i.e., age groups, various minorities (black, native American), professionals and the extremely wealthy or extremely poor classes of people. The problem of chemical dependency among people in the crisis of divorce was not mentioned. A great number of articles have been written which have hypothesized about the causes of divorce and its effects on individuals and family members. These articles have been written mainly by sociologists and psychologists. Family therapists have reported numerous case studies of children of divorce.

That stress and crisis occur with divorce is not questioned. The question is, Are nurses aware that the "divorce factor" is an area of importance that they must assess, be willing to intervene in, and learn and teach about? The lack of nursing literature regarding the concept of divorce indicates that nurses tend to ignore it.

ATTITUDES AND REACTIONS TO DIVORCE

Herman wrote: "Many people withdraw from discussing divorce (or refuse to be open to talk about such topics with family members or friends) because despite the increasing divorce rate, we live in a family oriented culture. The United States values the traditional idea of family life so highly it treats unmarried adults as undeveloped, immature and incomplete, or worse, as failures who cannot or will not take up or maintain a respectable and responsible family role . . . the prejudice against the single adult is evident when she or he attempts to establish credit in the business world, to buy insurance, to find housing, to fill out application blanks, and in the prevailing social attitudes toward single parents raising children."[7]

Psychologists admit that to be moralistically unbiased in America is difficult. "One of the values that blur the objectivity of the clinician's attitude toward divorce is that the survival of human social systems depends upon an enduring, stable family unit. In the Western World, this means that a long marriage with an intact nuclear family is 'good' and that disruption of the family is 'bad,' not only for society, but for the individuals concerned."[8]

It has been pointed out in an interesting article that women tend to be the "scapegoats" or victims of divorce in American society. Brandwein et al. state: "Related to the scarcity of studies on clients with stress of divorce is the assumption throughout the literature that the female-headed single parent family is deviant and pathological. Such families are called 'broken,' 'disorganized,' or 'disintegrated,' rather than recognized as widespread, viable alternative family forms. . . . This is stigmatization. . . . Stigma is ascribed to divorced and separated women for their presumed inability to keep their men. The Societal Myth of the "gay divorcee" out to seduce other women's husbands leads to social ostracism of the divorced woman and her family."[9]

An unusual viewpoint was presented by O'Neil when he wrote that "Christian morality is no longer considered the basis by which to measure the effect of divorce."[10] This may be true; however, in England and the United States, the churches' pressure on people to live up to the marriage vow of "those whom God hath joined together, let no man put asunder" still produces deep guilt feelings.[11] Aguilera and Messick believe that there are some attitudinal changes: "Today there is a greater acceptance of the possibility of divorce; because of this acceptance, divorced persons have lost some of the feelings of failure and guilt that were formerly associated with it. The higher divorce rate may reflect new values placed on marriage. Marriage is no longer accepted as an 'endurance race' that is doggedly maintained 'for the sake of the children.' "[12]

An optimistic view of divorce is reflected in an article by Hetherington et al.: "Divorce can be a positive solution when a conflict-ridden marriage destroys family harmony and harms family members. A stable home situation in which parents are divorced can be better for family members than a troubled intact family."[13]

DIVORCE AND THE MOTHER

Kaseman states: "Like every other segment of our society, the family is in a state of transition. Institutional marriage over the last two decades has undergone radical changes—more and more families are headed by one parent and this single parent family is typically headed by females."[14] Most of the clients seen by Kaseman were women of different cultural backgrounds and moderate to low socio-economic backgrounds with an eleventh- to twelfth-grade educational level. They ranged in age between 19 and 35 years, and the number of children they had varied. As might be expected, most of these women had financial resources for baby-sitting or daycare. Kaseman found that many of these women found a need to be "super-mothers" or "superwomen." They were particularly concerned with proving that they could "take care of everything." They felt guilty about depriving the children of their father, and wondered if divorce had been a good decision. Frequently, they were so caught up with plans for the children and their feelings that their own feelings were given low priority, as were their roles as women. A frequent problem was that of sexual desire. Many women said that they felt guilty about their need for male companionship and sexual relationships. Some admitted feeling helpless and missing the identity associated with their husband's status. There was some ambivalence toward relationships with men. Casual sex brought on feelings of anger, depression, and low self-esteem. Many of the women gained weight and tended to be unkempt. By gaining weight and neglecting their appearance, they could avoid the issue of a male-female relationship. The anger they experienced often prevented or covered up their feelings of loss, which arose later. Most women needed additional support to work through their loss before they were able to discuss the implications of the divorce with the children. Many were unclear as to why the divorce took place, wondering if they could have prevented it, which led to self-blame. They felt isolated and lonely and stated that their greatest need was for companionship. They felt left out of society, not being single or married, but in transition. For many, the children were viewed as the remnants of the marriage, either positively or negatively, depending on the woman's view of the marriage.

DIVORCE AND THE FATHER

In a study by Hetherington et al., it was found that divorced fathers had "day-to-day" living problems that were especially difficult during the first year following divorce.[15] Men whose wives had not worked had a particularly trying time maintaining a household routine, and they fumbled along in what one father called "a chaotic lifestyle." There were three types of problems.

1. *Practical matters.* Divorced men were less likely to eat; they picked up meals at irregular times. They slept less and had trouble managing the basics of shopping, cooking, laundering, and cleaning.

2. *Emotional stress and changes in self-concept.* Fathers complained of not knowing who they were, of feeling "rootless," and of having no structure or home in their lives. The separation induced profound feelings of loss, previously unrecognized dependency needs, guilt, anxiety, and depression. The fathers felt they had failed as parents and spouses and doubted their ability to adjust well in any future marriage. Some of the men were pleased to have the opportunity to date a variety of women and have diverse sexual experiences. They occupied themselves the first year after divorce with dating and casual social encounters at bars, clubs, and parties, but at the end of the year they wanted longer-lasting, more meaningful relationships. Perhaps to alleviate the loss of self-esteem men became more socially active: "I'll do *anything* to avoid going home, to avoid the solitude."

3. *Children.* Most men found that they were lonely for their children, and yet as time passed they saw less of their former wife and children. Some men admitted they could not endure the pain of seeing their children only occasionally and continued to experience a great sense of loss and depression.

Stafford related a different father's reaction: "The real truth is that women are granted custody of children because the male really doesn't want to assume the responsibility of child care."[16] He thinks that fathers do not want custody of their children because it is simply too inconvenient for them, and only when the male has learned to balance the joys of sharing his children's lives against the thrill of his business successes will he pressure for change in laws that will give him equal chances at custody. Stafford reminds us that divorce laws are now written by legislatures dominated by males, the lawyers who handle divorces are mostly males, and the judges who hand down the decisions are mostly males.

DIVORCE AND CHILDREN

The facts indicate that divorce is a family rather than simply a marital phenomenon, because 60 percent of all divorces affect young children, and that most separations occur five years after marriage. Kaplan reports that, with the rising frequency of divorce, the number of children of divorced parents referred to child mental health specialists has increased.[17] His study reveals problems of family configurations as follows:

1. *Mother, child, and maternal grandparents.* Kaplan found that the divorced mother frequently turns to her family of origin for financial and psychological support. This tendency might have been encouraged by the mother's parents, who objected to the marriage initially and supported their daughter's efforts to divorce her husband. An area of dispute between the mother and maternal grandparents is

the child's behavior and the mother's child-rearing capabilities. The children hear and learn things from grandparents and after visits return with different perceptions than those that the mother appreciates.

2. *Overprotective mother and child.* Here Kaplan found that, in the absence of the father, the overprotective child clings more tenaciously to the mother, and the mother tends to focus even more concern on the child than before the divorce.

3. *The helpless and mildly neglectful mother.* This type of mother often finds her child's behavior intolerable. She sees the child as an increasing nuisance and is almost constantly angry with her/him. The child reacts with temper tantrums and hyperaggressive behavior.

4. *The father.* Kaplan felt that in all his cases of children of divorce the father and children remained critically important to each other. Loyalty conflicts arose for the child between choice of parents. In many cases of remarriage a difficult process of beginning a new family occurs. To maintain his relationship with his children, the father must have the support of his new wife. At times the father is forced to either abandon his own children from his previous marriage or attempt to integrate them into his new family. This process of divorce involves a number of disruptions in family organization that takes place over long periods of time.

The psychologist Zigler is concerned with the unmet needs of America's children: "Increased mobility, new housing patterns, life styles have deprived the family life . . . the extended family is now rare in contemporary society, and with its demise the new parent has lost the wisdom and daily support of the older, more experienced family members. Furthermore, many parents today are not well-equipped for the parenthood before them, since over the years most children have been given less responsibility in helping care for younger siblings. There is evidence that child abuse is found more frequently in a single (female) parent home in which the mother is working."[18] Furthermore, the abusing mother in such homes experiences considerable stress, which is exacerbated by her sense of isolation and separation from any effective social support system. The unavailability of quality daycare can only make this situation more stressful. Often children are left unattended or are cared for by older siblings, who are themselves in need of an adult's supervision. Increased efforts in the area of family planning, implementation of widespread education for parenthood programs, an increase in the availability of homemaker and child-care services, and a reexamination of our commitment to doing whatever is in the best interest of every child in America were proposed by Zigler.

CONCEPTUAL FRAMEWORK

The mental health approach to grief and grieving provides conceptual framework within which nurses can guide persons and families experiencing divorce. The grief process as described in the literature by Kübler-Ross and others outlines the five stages people experience in resolving interpersonal separation when caused by death; it can also be applied to the loss experienced in physical separation and divorce. Herman describes these stages:[19]

1. *Denial.* "This can't be happening to me." This stage is necessary to help one collect oneself and, with time, to mobilize other, less radical defenses.

2. *Anger and hostility.* Much of this, which is projected to the former spouse, occurs when the fact that the couple cannot live together is faced. Often a woman experiences the realitites of divorce (lack of money, social isolation) and has valid reasons for anger. The responsibility for the care of children, a need to go to work and to move, and alienation from parents and friends add to the unhappiness, confusion, hurt feelings, fears, and loneliness. The man may experience losing an important job, being with his children, helping make decisions about their growing up, as well as being financially responsible for his wife. Society's norm to be married is additional cultural pressure that may add to the anger, confusion, and hurt feelings one has about being on his or her own. Old friends sometimes become more distant after separation since they do not know how they should act or react to the divorced couple. They, themselves, may be afraid of divorce and consequently do not visit as much and, when they do, talk in superficialities. Even parents often do not know what to do when their children separate or divorce and therefore avoid talking about it to them or anyone.

3. *Bargaining.* "Maybe if I change some behaviors, my former spouse and I can make it together," or "Maybe she'll come back if I can keep feeling good about myself." Bargaining goes on within the person; meanwhile, new friends are made, and new responsibilities become less frightening.

4. *Depression.* In this stage a person's denial, anger, and rage are replaced with a sense of great loss. Depression is a difficult, painful, but necessary stage for divorced people to go through. It is facing the reality that the emotional investment they made in a marriage is lost. The marriage is over, and what it meant to them has ended.

5. *Acceptance.* Now it is possible to tell others that one is divorced without going into details. One realizes that marriage had both good and bad points and finds some direction in her/his life when acceptance occurs.

It is this author's contention that, although being aware that these stages or reactions do occur, health proponents need to recognize that there may be a variety of times and ways that these stages may occur. As a nurse and as a teacher of pediatrics and psychiatric nursing, this author has observed all of these stages occurring simultaneously. I have seen clients using denial and bargaining in anger and depression, even while accepting to some degree their problems. Nurses must try to find "where the client is at" but should not be surprised if she/he is confused, vacillating between stages, or describing feelings arising from a variety of the five stages simultaneously.

IMPLICATIONS FOR NURSING: QUESTIONS NURSES ASK

As people concerned with helping people in stress and crisis, nurses should be more aware of the growing number of hospital admissions and people in their communities who are suffering because with their present physical problems they are additionally experiencing the effects of divorce. To grow in awareness of these added burdens, nurses might consider the following questions:

1.   As individuals, what are nurses' feelings about divorce, the divorced parent, or the child involved?

2.   How do nurses learn that a client (newly hospitalized or in a community setting) is contemplating divorce or is in a stage of divorce?

3.   How do nurses identify and approach the client about her/his feelings and her/his perceptions of the divorce?

4.   What do nurses need to know about the children of a single parent when she/he is hospitalized? How old are the children before they are affected by their parents' separation or divorce? What are they worried about regarding the absent parent?

5.   What are the children of divorce feeling or thinking about when their parent is hospitalized?

6.   Who is caring for these children at home? What is their interpretation of the parent's illness? Is the public health nurse alert to their needs? If not, why not?

7.   What is the single parent feeling when she/he brings a seriously ill child into the hospital alone? How does this parent react to death of the child? How does the absent parent react?

8.   What does it mean to the newly divorced young woman to be admitted to the hospital for serious surgery involving her sexual organs (mastectomy, hysterectomy)? Is she "different" from the single woman in fears and anxieties: What will it mean regarding the possibility of remarriage? Is she concerned about her ability to have children?

9.   How does the older woman (aged 55 to 65 years) feel who faces a divorce? What are her fears and anxieties? How can she be helped to adjust to a new life style (with less financial help)?

10.   Who gives emotional support to the divorced woman or man who has been hospitalized? Are there any special needs to think of in assigning hospital beds to divorced people?

11.   How does the single parent, especially a woman, handle illness or possible surgery when faced with holding her job and caring for her children? Can she afford to take time off to fully recuperate? What alternatives does she have? Is she able to get to doctor's appointments? Does her boss understand when her children phone and ask her to come home? How does she handle this stress? Who can help her with homemaking tasks while the children are small? Is child abuse going on in this home?

12.   How does the divorced single parent help her/his child cope in crisis without the support of her/his spouse?

13. Who might serve as "substitute fathers" in hospitals? Who might visit the sons of single parents during a long hospital stay while the father is absent? Who might be more affected by the father being gone, a son or a daughter? How should nurses approach and help the child?

14. Do the problems of illness or possible surgery seem greater to the divorced woman/man than to individuals who have not married?

15. Are divorced people more dependent clients in the hospital than those who are single or married? If so, why? What might it mean for nursing intervention?

16. Are the sexual needs of the divorced woman greater than those of the single, unmarried woman? How are they satisfied? Is it a concern of nurses? How do we initiate and talk about this need?

17. Are the fears and worries over finances (less income, losing time from a job) greater with the divorced woman than with the single or married woman? Do parents of the divorced couple react differently when their children or grandchildren are hospitalized than if they do not have this additional stress?

18. What times of the day or night does the hospitalized divorced person usually feel most lonely?

19. Can nurses identify the clients, with problems of divorce, who are heavy users of alcohol or other mood-altering chemicals? What help can nurses give the divorced parent whose child is dependent on chemicals?

APPLYING CONCEPTS OF NURSING CARE

Divorce is a difficult and complex crisis, and it denotes loss. Loss and separation are painful. It is crucial that nurses be aware of the feelings of patients experiencing divorce and lend interpersonal support to help them adjust and move through stages of trauma to a more secure, fulfilling life style. To this end, nurses must be informed and understand the stress of divorce. They need to care enough to get involved and to risk using a more direct approach to learn "where the patient is at." Nurses might well expect the divorced woman (who has felt rejection from husband or relatives or friends) to have a hesitant, guarded, mistrusting attitude toward them. She will wait for clues from the nurse indicating a sincere interest in her and a willingness to listen.

That the woman in the hospital is in a divorce crisis might be detected in the initial interview. Examples of verbal clues are "No, my husband won't be visiting," and "My husband isn't with me; we feel we both need time to think about our marriage." Sarcastic remarks about males are easier to pick up, and clarifying them might give information. A woman who does not speak of her husband or mention him phoning her, whose husband does not visit her or send gifts or flowers, and who appears depressed, is seen crying, isolates herself, and eats poorly is giving nonverbal clues about her situation.

Perhaps the best opportunity to become aware of the deep loneliness the divorced woman feels would be open to the night nurse. Nights are long and lonely for most patients; however, this time is acknowledged by the divorced woman (especially newly divorced) to be utterly desolate. She misses her husband to talk to and to touch; she misses knowing someone is in the room who can comfort her and hold her. This is the time for the nurse to stop by her bed, to sit down, and to listen—to use touch for reassurance. The nurse should know and accept that perhaps words will not come but should reinforce that she cared enough to be with the patient.

That the stages the divorced patient goes through are similar to those most people go through in any crisis may be easy to acknowledge. To identify at which stage the patient is requires more perceptiveness. A direct approach is most helpful. (Often we wait for clues to appear and we don't see or hear them. We also wait for the "perfect time," when the patient will talk about her feelings and that time just doesn't come.) Nurses often get vague answers to "How are you feeling today?", "How are things going for you?"—for example, "Oh, pretty good" or "Well, about the same." One might try, instead, "On a scale of zero to ten, with ten as high, where would you rate how you are feeling today?" The patient may reply, "Well, I guess about a two or she/he may say, "Maybe eight." This rating scale gives patients some guidelines to help the nurse understand how they are feeling. It also gives the nurse a clue about their perception of how they actually feel and gives the nurse an opportunity to elaborate clarifying with, "You said you would give yourself a two; that sounds as if you are feeling pretty low today. Do you feel angry or upset about something? Could you tell me about it?"

It is essential for the nurse to *really* listen, to give total attention to the patient by good eye contact, sitting near the patient, and conveying the attitude, "No one is more important right now to me than you and your problems." The nurse must think deeply about what the woman is telling her by observing her nonverbal communication. The patient needs to know that she can weep, shout with anger, or tremble with anxiety. She needs to know that these discharges will release the tension and inner stored-up feelings and that by doing this she will be able to think clearly again, evaluate her situation with the nurse's support, and take better charge of herself.

People in the denial stage are frightened; they need to talk about their insecurity. The nurse must help the patient by listening and presenting reality with perceptiveness. For example, the nurse may ask the patient who, with father absent, would be a good role model for her sons. This is bringing the issue out in the open. Although she may deny that her husband is not coming back, she will be aware of that possibility and that meanwhile her sons need men to communicate with. The nurse needs to accurately interpret the patient's needs by again attempting to clarify what she is saying, without irritating her. The anger stage can be uncomfortable for both client and nurse. It is important that the nurse listen understandingly however the anger is expressed. The feelings of disappointment, the concrete and frightening aspects (finances, housing, automobile), as well as abstract issues (relatives, neighbors, friends, and social outlets) that this woman is facing alone need to be talked about. The thought of helping her children readjust to life without a father can be overwhelming to the mother who is undergoing additional physical problems. Cline believes that the nurse must and can help the

the mother become aware that bitterness and anger of the parents toward each other affect the children far more negatively than any other factor.[20] The mother needs to know that it is normal for a child to try to manipulate his divorced parents. Children usually have a secret wish for their parents to unite, and often they will do all they can to manipulate the situation so the parents will talk to each other. Parents need to talk about how they also tend to manipulate their children by sending messages through them and gaining affection from them unfairly. Cline adds that "children almost always feel guilty and partially responsible for the divorce."[21] Nurses also need to help children express such feelings. Kaseman believes strongly that both parents need to know the understanding that each child has about the absence of one of the parents and what the total picture is.[22]

Marriage counselors have written some "don'ts" for resource people while communicating to a woman/man who is suffering from the effects of divorce: (1) Don't give advice. (2) Don't tell your own stories of distress. (3) Don't make small talk. (4) Don't give comfort and false reassurance: "Everything will be fine. It will all work out for the best; don't worry." (5) Don't give her/him sedatives and tranquilizers. (6) Don't try to get her/his mind off the pain with "Let's go down and play some bridge."

NURSES RELATING TO WOMEN

Most nurses are women. However, sometimes nurses. tend to find it harder to communicate with women clients or tend to expect more from women in coping with problems than men. Do nurses treat the divorced woman "differently" than the single or married client? Nurses tend to forget that women are more alike than unlike. It is helpful to remember we are all "sisters under the skin," that we are women first and single, married, or divorced people second. Basically, as women we have all felt loss, all been lonely, all felt anger and grief. We have found that we can show our emotions, that to do so brings relief, and that there can be an end to unhappiness and pain. As women, nurses must accept that perhaps this woman's marriage might have been a long, horrible nightmare, that by ending the marriage she has brought herself and her children respect and freedom.

The following is a case study that encompasses a woman's dilemma with divorce and nursing intervention. The family involved includes the wife, age 35, a housewife, overwhelmed with grief and anxiety; the husband, age 36, "retired" after a massive stroke six years ago; and the daughter, age 15, who died from brain damage after a car accident three months ago.

S, a short, heavy, tired-looking woman was admitted to the psychiatric unit because of severe depression and anxiety. This was manifested by insommia, lack of appetite, confusion, inability to concentrate, frequent headaches, and crying spells. She was a well-dressed, tense attractive female who used direct eye contact and rapid, articulate speech. She was a chain smoker, had a quick, easy laugh, was noticeably pacing, restless, sighing, tapping fingers, and using rather dramatic gestures with hands. The physical examination was negative. Psychological tests revealed that she was a highly intelligent, hypomanic, psychosomatic, extremely depressed woman.

S's symptoms began three months ago, after hearing that her daughter M had sustained a serious head injury in a car accident on a freeway near Seattle. S, who brought her husband from their home 200 miles away, found M still alive and on a respirator in a hospital's intensive care unit. M suffered from multiple skull fractures and a broken arm. B, the father, a victim of aphasia, was aware of his daughter's injury but was unable to understand S's feelings or needs at this time. He was content to watch television while S made the difficult decision of removing M from the respirator. A former friend of the family, a minister, helped her with counsel. S's grief at the loss of their only child was intensified by B's apparent inability to react to M's death or to give her any support. (At this time S also felt renewed anger at B, who had decided by fiat that S and B would not have additional children.) Other resources such as hospital staff, relatives, and clergy were necessary to sustain S in this situation.

Early Childhood

S was the youngest child and only daughter of deeply religious German parents. She had three older brothers, each passive and introverted like their mother. At 9 years of age, S, a precocious child and a "daddy's girl," had mastoiditis (before the days of penicillin) requiring dangerous surgery, which was complicated by rheumatic fever. There was a great deal of pain experienced by S as well as possible heart damage. Extensive bed rest was required. The parents reacted with overprotectiveness. S became a demanding child with frequent complaints of headaches and neck pains, which increased as she grew older to migraine headaches and dizziness. She visited countless physicians for head pains and allergy problems. S had many temper tantrums, completely controlling the family with her outbursts. She was quite creative in arts and crafts (e.g., painting, sewing, and knitting). After graduation from high school she held a responsible job as an office manager, where she fluctuated from being a highly organized, efficient worker to spending days at home in bed with "splitting" headaches. Again, she spent a great deal of time in physicians' offices and took an excessive number of pills, many of which were tranquilizers. S quickly learned medical and neurologic terminology and seemed to enjoy "keeping the physicians on their toes." Her quick wit and depth of knowledge surprised the physicians, but her mercurial temperment also tended to make people uneasy. Her flash verbal reactions startled the most sophisticated person.

Marriage and Family

S married B, an easygoing and conscientious junior police officer in their city. B was a popular man at work, in the neighborhood, and with relatives. He was a patient, helpful husband for his "nervous," demanding wife, neatly doing the housework when S was in bed with headaches and allergy complaints. M was born to the union and grew to be a kind and energetic, and fun-loving child. Her mother would be exasperated with her antics, such as skipping school, yet enjoyed her humor and her many friends. When M was 10 years old the entire family structure changed: B at age 30 suffered an anuerysm one evening requiring brain surgery. B recovered slowly with aphasia and was retired from his job. His left arm and leg were paralyzed; however, because he was physically very strong and had endless tenacity, he learned to walk with a cane and leg brace. B's halting speech was poor; he could not recall correct words and was frustrated at this loss of memory. He was unable to read and lacked interest and judgment in family affairs. He enjoyed watching cartoons on television or children playing. S took over managing all financial affairs. Financial assistance came from the police retirement benefits and armed service insurance. After his hospitalization B lived at home, where there was a complete role reversal in the family. S rallied to become the staunchest advocate of rehabilitating B. She demanded the top specialists in speech pathology, speech therapy, and neurology at the large veterans' hospital and got them. They worked for two years with B, at first encouraged by his willingness to try to relearn to speak. Finally, they became discouraged by his regression and growing lack of interest. Repeated tests showed poor prognosis for recovery. However, physicians told S that B was in excellent physical shape and could live until he was 100.

For five years in the city S cared for the supervised her husband at home. Neighbors were extremely supportive and continued to include the couple socially. They were pleased that they could help B recover. One of S's problems was that friends and relatives would not accept B's severe disabilities. The fact B insisted on being immaculately dressed, that he handled his body quite well and walked by himself, and that he remained his quiet, smiling self was deceptive and convinced most people that B's condition was less serious that S claimed it to be. S became irritated and felt a loss of their support when they ignored her stories of B's behavior.

A few of the minor problems included his interest in turning knobs and dials and forgetting that he had done this. Because of the brain injury he turned dials in the wrong direction. He was obsessed with turning on stove knobs, the furnace thermostat to "high" on hot summer days, and water faucets. He also took groceries out of the kitchen cupboards and hid them in remote places such as the attic and then promptly forgot where he had put them. He insisted on trying to drive the car until M had to lock the garage. Finally, S had to sell the house and move to a small apartment because she could no longer afford their home on B's pension.

S became increasingly withdrawn from her social and family contacts. She felt people could not, or refused to, understand the stress of living with B. She felt no hope for having a normal life as a woman. She was unable to leave B alone at home, yet he was not eligible for care in a veterans' hospital or nursing home. B spent his time fishing and practice-shooting one of his six pistols (he had been a marksman in the army) until frightened neighbors wrote complaints. B finally gave up five of his guns (wrapping them in plastic sacks, he had hidden them in various tree hollows) but kept hidden his favorite pistol, refusing to give it up because, as he said casually, "Maybe I'll need it to kill you." Again, friends and relatives paid no heed to such threats, still recalling the stable, kind man that B had been. (Years later the gun was found taped under the bedside stand in their bedroom, with bullets in it.) B became compulsively neat at the apartment; for example, he became extremely upset and angry if any of the pieces of furniture or appliances (such as toaster) were left turned at the slightest angle. Getting along with his obsessions was not easy on S.

Meanwhile M grew up and started a course of studies in another part of the state. S missed M because she had been her sole listener. She understood because she had also lived with her father's changed and erratic behavior. S did speak to her family about a possible separation from B. They, however, maintained the Christian philosophy of the marriage vow, believing that S should remain committed to caring for B until they were parted by death. Relatives sympathized with B, and even S's meek and ailing mother, 73 years of age, insisted that she would care for him herself if S didn't. S's father, her main family supporter, had died a year ago of a heart ailment.

Crisis

The crisis came when M was injured and died. That S had in reality lost her entire family was more than she could bear. That both family members suffered brain damage was ironic and devastating. S reacted with severe anxiety, sleeplessness, and depression. She was unable to resolve her grief or to accept these tragedies as "God's will." Her lonely home life became more frustrating, and thoughts of separation and divorce recurred with extreme guilt feelings. Seeking counseling at a reliable church agency, she was told by an elderly pastor that she couldn't resolve her grief and S became hysterical and ran crying out of the office. (This pastor was "retired" two years later.) She was admitted to a psychiatric unit the following week.

Nursing Intervention

The goal of the intervention was to assist S in recognizing and coping with her feelings of guilt, anger, and low self-esteem. Suppressed feelings about her marriage and ambivalence about divorce were also to be explored.

S adjusted quickly to the psychiatric setting. She believed she could get help there after meeting a concerned psychiatrist. Although she had her own room in the hospital, she did not isolate herself and instead tended to seek out staff, "who could converse intelligently." She tended to be somewhat threatening to staff members and patients because she was extremely perceptive and seemed to enjoy "putting down" others by her astute observations of what they were doing or daying. She astounded the entire staff by her knowledge of psychiatric terminology and understanding of various theoretical concepts. She was amused to cross-examine the nurses on dosages, side effects, and reactions to medications. She obviously enjoyed being surrounded by an interested staff, and she had a quick wit that disguised her lack of confidence and indecisiveness. She like to play bridge, especially with male psychiatrist assistants because they proved to be the best competition she could find on the unit.

During the three-week hospitalization period, S attended group therapy (three times per week). There her psychiatrist, a primary nurse, and approximately ten group members helped her view the present crisis by direct questions and reflection on her verbal and nonverbal behavior. For the first time she felt she was given support and praise for staying with B for six years, attempting to help him recover from his brain damage. Her efforts had been "taken for granted as a wife's duty" by relatives and friends. S heard other patients relate their experiences and talk about similar anxieties and periods of confusion, and she grew in trust. The greatest problem in group work was her tendency to intellectualize. S had an amazing memory for dates and details; she knew exactly what people had said regardless of the number of months or years that had elapsed since the situation had transpired. The words that a physician, relative, or neighbor had said to her were always the same, whenever she repeated them. She never swayed from her original statements. She spoke articulately and with authority. She tended to control or dominate the group by her sophisticated manner and her courage to speak up. Some days, however, she appeared to be quiet and depressed. That she was bitter and cynical about "narrow-minded, self-righteous" people is an understatement.

S continued to intellectualize, calmly listing her problems with alternatives to solutions. Until the third week of hospitalization she was not able to drop her facade and show emotion over the overwhelming loss of her entire family and fear of the future. She was able to talk about her anger at being misunderstood, and at her family's unreasonable expectations.

Another ventilation found helpful almost immediately was writing down her thoughts and feelings on a paper chart daily. Along with her comments were written the nurse's assessment of S's behavior. S found this "open" feedback supporting and believed strongly that she was accepted and cared about. She sought out staff members and engaged them in long conversations. S learned that she could express her anger and found that she could sleep better. She also reacted more often in tears and did not need to repress her religious guilt.

S's creativeness in art was encouraged. She enjoyed going to occupational therapy, where she quickly told the therapists she was bored with their type of art, refusing to work on articles other clients were expected to work on. She preferred to work alone, designing pictures from a variety of materials. The results of her ingenuity and cleverness surprised the therapists, and their reactions were ego boosting for her.

S was still high-strung and vacillated daily between relatively high and low moods. One visitor unknowingly caused a serious regression in S's progress. He was a well-meaning minister, who, after S had confided her fears that her husband might shoot her, agreed with her and described in horrible detail how a former parishioner had been found dead in her bedroom, shot three times through the head by her husband. S reacted hysterically, screaming and frightening the minister out of the room. She was calmed down only by major tranquilizers.

Regardless of S's traumatic interactions with some pastors, she continued to need their intervention. Religion had always played an important part in her life. The one pastor who had supported her during the agonizing hours of deciding to accept M's injury and to have her removed from the respirator continued to be a close friend and confidante. Another extremely helpful minister was a young chaplain on the psychiatric unit who encouraged S to talk about her ambivalent feelings about divorce. He listened. Each day they visited, talking first about any subject she cared to bring up. They discussed the marriage oath, "in sickness or in health," and how S felt guilty because B had cared for her during the years she had had physical problems. They talked about responsibility in marriage, the partnership, the need for involvement by both individuals to maintain its growth, and the view of marriage as a relationship that has expectations for each partner for healthy survival. That B was not the same man that he was before the stroke and that he could no longer bring meaning to their marriage, was discussed. S's depression lifted, and her symptoms of anxiety lessened. She recognized the possibility that the failure of her marriage may not have been because she was not strong enough to stay with B but in the recognition that there was not a meaningful marriage left to sustain. To continue the marriage most likely would result in S's continued need of psychiatric help, which was not seen as healthy. She had a right to choose between her own sanity and staying in an unhealthy marriage.

That S's family approve of her life style was extremely important. Their idea of a psychiatrist's relationship with a client was similar to that of many individuals who do not understand the importance of family involvement and the client's need for support. They thought that they shouldn't talk to the psychiatrist because they feared he would think that they were trying to "tell him his business." The doctor saw their nonparticipation as indifference, a lack of caring about S. During one family session with S, the psychiatrist, the primary nurse, and S's family changed these ideas. The family was able to express their feelings of sympathy for B and his tragedy and began to understand how S felt regarding her future with B. They were able to sympathize with her need to live her own life and to talk about how concerned they were that she should be happy. They had thought "she had known that." The relief S described in her chart that night was overwhelming. She slept well for the first night since she had been hospitalized.

Future Planning

S was granted a dissolution divorce two years later. B moved to another state to live with a single brother and appears to be satisfied and happy. S started an art shop, found new friends, is helping art teachers as a volunteer at the local grade school. She has painted murals for churches and has been in charge of successful adolescent arts and crafts programs. She enjoys working with teenagers immensely: "They remind me of happy times with M."

S has been able to view her painful divorce as a step toward mental health. She is able to be open with new friends about her feelings and is able to accept herself and her need to give to others of the talents she has. She has been able to live with less medication and with fewer physician's visits.

This case study has been included in this chapter to illustrate the traumatic effect that divorce can have on a client. It is apparent that resource people (especially nurses) do have opportunities to intervene and can help clients to have a more productive and serene life when they are aware of the problem and are willing to help solve it.

USING RESOURCES

While listening to people reveal their true feelings and anxieties about divorce, many nurses may realize that they actually don't know much about the problem. The nurse who can recognize her inadequacies as a problem solver in every area of nursing care is an extremely wise nurse. Nurses are not prepared to be experts in every situation. They are not failures because they are unable to deal with every situation with confidence and competence. To make referrals to marriage counselors at family service centers in the area is perhaps the most important help nurses can give since these counselors are experts in the field. Clubs, churches, and community organizations also provide healthy and realistic ongoing support systems (e.g., the group called Parents without Partners). In the hospital other resources may be (1) hospitalized divorced women of the same age to talk with, (2) hospitalized women with similar medical/surgical problems, and (3) women support groups after discharge (e.g., outreach groups).

PREVENTION

In the area of prevention of the stress that accompanies divorce, nurses might do well in planning and becoming involved in teaching high school students in community classes about the psychological aspects of marriage and good parenting. If they are unprepared to do this, they should support such courses in the community. Aguilera and Messick write that the largest proportion of divorces occurs in the early years of marriage among childless couples.[23] The peak period of divorces is in the second year of marriage, after which the rate drops rapidly. A number of factors are precipitating causes of divorce. Among these are early marriages (15 to 19 years of age), short courtships, short engagement, mixed racial or religious marriages, disapproval of friends and relatives, dissimilar backgrounds, and unhappy parental marriages. Since divorce rates are so high and many marriages are centers of friction and unhappiness, something must be lacking in the preparation for marriage. No event in life of equal importance is viewed with so little realism, and marriage seems to come about with little or no preparation.

In summary, with today's increasing divorce rate, nurses need to be aware of the stress that divorce brings to their clients in the hospital and in the community. Nurses should also recognize the need for intervention and the need to improve methods of total patient care that encompass this crisis.

NOTES

1. Sonya J. Herman, "Divorce: A Grief Process," *Perspectives in Psychiatric Care* 12, no. 3, (1974): 108-112.

2. Elisabeth Kübler-Ross, *On Death and Dying* (New York: Macmillan Co., 1969).

3. C. Brisco and J. Smith, "Psychiatric Illness: Marital Units and Divorce," *Journal of Nervous and Mental Disease* 156-157 (1973): 440.

4. Stewart L. Kaplan, "Structural Family Therapy for Children of Divorce: Case Reports," *Family Process* 16 (March 1977): 75.

5. Jack C. Westman et al., "The Role of Child Psychiatry in Divorce," *Archives of General Psychiatry* 23 (November 1970): 414.

6. E. Mavis Hetherington, Martha Cox, and Roger Cox, "Divorced Fathers," *Psychology Today*, April 1977, pp. 42-46.

7. Herman, "Grief Process," p. 108.

8. Westman et al., "Child Psychiatry in Divorce," p. 416.

9. Ruth A. Brandwein, Carol A. Brown, and Elizabeth Maury Fox, "Woman and Children Lost: Divorced Mothers and Their Families," *Nursing Digest*, January-February 1976, p. 39.

10. S. O'Neil, "Divorce and the Professionalization of the Social Scientist," *Journal of Historic Behavioral Science* 2, no. 4 (1966): 291.

11. A. D. G. Gunn, "The Breaking Marriage," *Nursing Times* 66 (1970): 1484-1485.

12. Donna C. Aguilera and Janice M. Messick, *Crisis Intervention*, 2nd ed. (St. Louis: C. V. Mosby Co., 1974), p. 93.

13. Hetherington, Cox, and Cox, "Divorced Fathers," p. 46.

14. Charlotte M. Kaseman, "The Single-Parent Family," *Perspectives in Psychiatric Care* 12, no. 3, (1974): p. 113.

15. Hetherington, Cox, and Cox, "Divorced Fathers," p. 42.

16. Lineley Stafford, "Most Fathers Don't Want Custody of the Children," *Minneapolis Tribune*, May 3, 1977, p. 7A.

17. Kaplan, "Therapy for Children of Divorce," p. 75.

18. Edward Zigler, "The Unmet Needs of America's Children," *Children Today*, May-June 1976, p. 75.

19. Herman, "Grief Process," pp. 109-111.

20. Foster W. Cline, "Generalities Concerning Children and Divorce," *Nurse Practitioner*, March-April 1977, pp. 29-30.

21. Ibid.

22. Kaseman, "Single-Parent Family," p. 115.

23. Aguilera and Messick, *Crisis Intervention*.

17
The Potential Health Care Crisis of Hysterectomy

KAREN STORLIE FINCK

There has always been a consistent pattern of change in the functioning of the female reproductive system. The uterus is the center of the changing process in which the biologic functions of the body are manifested. The actualization of the biologic functions of the female body begins at puberty with the onset of menstruation. For some women the biologic functions are realized with the birth of a child. In the lives of other women, physiology, situation, or choice intercedes and the realization does not occur. When the potential childbearing years end, the biologic functions of the female body terminate in the natural process of menopause.

In recent years this pattern of consistent change has gained the possibility of alteration. With the advancement of medical technology, two surgical procedures that cause the termination of the biologic functions of the female body have been developed and perfected to the extent of increasingly widespread usage. These procedures, hysterectomy and tubal ligation, alter the pattern in such a way that the termination of the childbearing functions no longer necessarily coincides with the natural process of menopause.

Alteration in the pattern of biologic functioning does not in itself constitute a health care crisis. As the surgical procedures themselves are examined, it becomes apparent that one procedure has far-reaching consequences and contains a strong possibility of constituting a health care crisis for women. The other procedure involves a much higher rate of successful adaptation, with generally only very minimal psychological disturbance.

Tubal ligation is a surgical procedure specifically executed for the purpose of terminating the childbearing capacity of a woman. It is well designed, creating only minor alteration in the anatomic structure of the female body and causing only negligible effects on the processes of menstruation and menopause. The decision to perform tubal ligation is based solely on the desire of the woman to alter her pattern of reproductive functioning so that the termination of her childbearing capacity occurs before the onset of menopause. The combination of these factors promotes a response to tubal ligation that is generally very satisfactory and rarely constitutes a health care crisis.

Conversely, hysterectomy is not designed and executed solely for the purpose of terminating the childbearing capacity of a woman. Reasons for the performance of this surgery are varied, and resultant changes in the female anatomic structure are more pronounced. Unlike tubal ligation, hysterectomy involves not only alteration in the pattern of biologic functioning but also removal of an organ from the female body and the concurrent termination of the functions of that organ. Thus, physiologic and psychological effects of hysterectomy are more extensive and provide for wide variations in women's response to the procedure. These variations in response coupled with the incidence of and reasons for performance of the procedure give credence to the view of the hysterectomy experience as a potential health care crisis and provide broad implications in the nursing management of this crisis.

Before examining the components of the hysterectomy experience, it is necessary to clarify terminology and discuss the incidence of the surgery.

TERMINOLOGY OF THE SURGICAL PROCEDURE

The term "hysterectomy" indicates the surgical removal of the uterus. In previous years, only the body of the uterus was removed. This was referred to as a partial or subtotal hysterectomy. More commonly performed at present is a total hysterectomy involving removal of the entire uterus. A radical hysterectomy is the removal of the entire uterus plus lymph nodes and surrounding ligaments.[1]

There are two surgical methods used to remove the uterus. In an abdominal hysterectomy a 4- to 6-inch incision is made in the lower abdomen through which the uterus is removed. In a vaginal hysterectomy, the uterus is removed through the vagina and there is no visible scar. It is generally the method of choice when uterine prolapse, cystoceles, or rectoceles are present.[2]

Although a hysterectomy does not include the removal of the adnexia, in certain conditions these are removed at the same time. This often causes confusion in the terminology for the lay population. In some literature, removal of the uterus and the ovaries is referred to as a panhysterectomy or complete hysterectomy. This is often confused with total hysterectomy, which does not involve removal of the adnexia. This is more readily understood when the adnexia to be removed are specified. Thus, removal of the ovaries is referred to as a bilateral oophorectomy, and removal of the fallopian tubes is known as a salpingectomy. Therefore, a woman who has had her entire uterus, fallopian tubes, and ovaries removed abdominally is referred to as having had a total abdominal hysterectomy and bilateral salpingo-oophorectomy.

There also appears to be another frame of reference for the terminology of hysterectomy. Although it does not appear to be in widespread usage, there is no doubt of its existence. Some medical professionals have referred to hysterectomy as "having the works out" or have told women that "they were rotten inside" or that it was "no good having your tubes tied; your womb would only go bad like a dead tooth without a nerve and you would have to have it out later."[3] This author was told by a young woman that her physician referred to her impending hysterectomy as "taking that old grey bag out." She tearfully stated that this statement made her feel "like an old cow." Further indication of the trauma that this terminology can cause is exemplified in the case of a woman who was told by her physician that she was "all cleaned out" after her hysterectomy because she had been "in a terrible mess and all rotten inside." The woman never felt "clean" again and developed a compulsive need to constantly discuss the surgery.[4] It is clear that this type of terminology is dehumanizing, sexist, and detrimental to the health care recipient and therefore should not be tolerated.

Later, as we investigate the real and imagined effects of changes in female anatomy after hysterectomy on various aspects of women's lives, it will become even more apparent why correct use of terminology is essential.

INCIDENCE OF PERFORMANCE OF HYSTERECTOMY

The surgical removal of the uterus has recently become the most commonly performed major surgery in the United States. Statistics indicate that in 1975 there were 725,000 hysterectomies performed in this country as compared to 658,000 tonsillectomies, the previously most commonly performed major surgery. And it is reported that the trend to perform hysterectomies is increasing. There has been a 25 percent increase in the number of hysterectomies performed in the United States from 1970 to 1975.[5] It is estimated that almost half of all American women over the age of 40 will be advised to have a hysterectomy.[6]

These statistics indicate that alteration in the biologic functioning of the female body by hysterectomy is not only a possibility but, for a vast number of women, a reality.

THEORETICAL FRAMEWORK

The basis for the woman's response to the hysterectomy experience is determined by the woman's concept of her uterine anatomy and physiology. The formulation of this concept includes the woman's knowledge about the actual functions of her uterus and her personal perceptions of uterine anatomy and physiology which are derived from her individual developmental experiences.[7] Realistic and imaginary functions attributed to the uterus intermingle to produce a psychologic response to hysterectomy that is unique to every woman.

However, the literature on hysterectomy reveals frequently held perceptions of various functions attributed to the uterus. These perceptions can be categorized into the related areas of childbearing capacity, menstrual functioning, menopausal process, sexual capacity, and physical condition. Identification of the effects of hysterectomy on each area will assist in delineating the areas in which actual loss is involved, the areas that involve feared loss or change, and the areas that require temporary readjustment. The complex network of relationships among the variables can then be explored and comprehended. The categorization of the areas and the comprehension of the relationships among the variables are key factors that enable a theoretical framework to be devised. This theoretical framework will afford a more comprehensive view of the hysterectomy experience. The structure of the theoretical framework is conceptualized in Figure 17.1.

Indications for Removal of the Uterus

HYSTERECTOMY

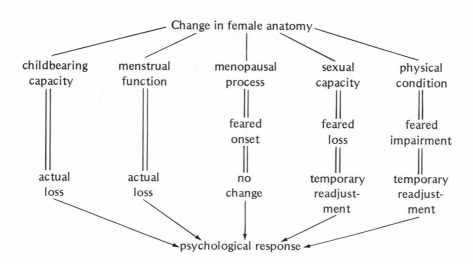

Figure 17.1. Theoretical framework for the relationships among variables and the areas related to hysterectomy.

NURSING INTERVENTIONS

The theoretical framework can be utilized to identify areas in which nursing interventions can be made. The focus of nursing intervention in each area can be derived from the description of the potential hysterectomy crisis along pertinent ego-function parameters. These parameters include affective aspects, defensive aspects, cognitive aspects, reality aspects, and object relations.[8] The three parameters of cognitive aspects, affective aspects, and object relations can be used as the focus of nursing interventions. A description of nursing interventions focused on the three ego-function parameters will enable the nurse to identify nursing interventions in each area and then to individualize the interventions to meet the needs of specific health care recipients.

Nursing Interventions Focusing on Cognitive Aspects

Nursing intervention in this area consists primarily of providing information to health care recipients. Patient teaching has long been recognized as a nursing responsibility. The research of Johnson et al. has revealed the significance of providing information to health care recipients.

Johnson, Morrissey, and Leventhal demonstrated in a study that presenting knowledge to patients affects the patients responses to a given procedure. Patients who were given knowledge about either the technical detail of the procedure or the sensations patients frequently experience during the procedure required less sedation than control patients.[9] Johnson states in further research that "preparatory information may reduce emotional response to procedures which are an unavoidable part of health care, for example, diagnostic examinations, injections, dental procedures, and surgery."[10]

Researchers working in the area of hysterectomy seem to concur with this concept. They suggest that presenting information to a woman undergoing hysterectomy can affect her psychological response to the procedure by reducing the reactions of anxiety, fright, and shock. When concealed anxieties can be brought into the woman's awareness through discussion of the implications of hysterectomy, the postoperative psychiatric complications may be lessened.[11] An explanation of the procedure to be performed can help to prevent fright neurosis, which is often a major factor in the response to hysterectomy.[12] Psychological shock followed by feelings of deprivation and resentment, which occurs in many women after they are told they need a hysterectomy, can be alleviated if information regarding the reasons for and effects of the procedure is provided.[13]

Research reveals to us the importance women who have had hysterectomies place on information. When information is provided, most women find it very helpful and, when information is not given, many women feel it to be a definite unmet need.[14]

Although it is clear that education in this area is of primary importance, it is equally clear when reviewing literature on hysterectomy that education is often not provided. In an attempt to discover what knowledge women possess about the reasons for and effects of hysterectomy, this author examined hysterectomy literature for reported misconceptions and devised a test that measured selected knowledge women had about hysterectomy. The results of this study (referred to as the "Hysterectomy Knowledge Study") are discussed wherever applicable in this chapter. It will provide the nurse with baseline information on what a specific group of women knows about hysterectomy.

Since it deals only with a specific group of women, population characteristics must be discussed. There were 186 women who participated in the study. The age range was equally distributed (except for a smaller percentage of women under 25 and over 65 years old). Women in the study were white (98 percent) and generally Protestant (58 percent) or Catholic (31 percent). They were married (91 percent) and generally had children (88 percent). Almost all of the women completed high school (95 percent), and over half of the women either attended or completed college. About one-half of the women were employed. Twenty percent of the women in the study had had a hysterectomy.

The reader must be cautioned that, although the "Hysterectomy Knowledge Study" will provide useful information about one group of women, this must not be generalized to all women. Williams has demonstrated that there is a strong indication of cultural patterning of the feminine role.[15] This infers that different cultural groups of women possess different knowledge in the area of hysterectomy, as do women of different educational backgrounds. Therefore, the information presented from the "Hysterectomy Knowledge Study" will provide only general guidelines for assessing the knowledge individual women possess about hysterectomy.

Nursing Interventions Focusing on Affective Aspects

Nursing interventions in this area concentrate on accepting, understanding, and providing support for expression of feelings women experience as related to hysterectomy.

Raphael, in a study investigating the perception of the crisis of hysterectomy, found that over half of the study sample perceived the opportunity to discuss their feelings about the surgery as being helpful. None of the women felt that the opportunity to express their feelings was unhelpful. One-third of the women who did not have the opportunity to express their feelings felt that this was an unmet need.[16] Thus it is extremely important in terms of quality health care for women to be afforded the opportunity to express their feelings about hysterectomy.

In order for this to be accomplished in an atmosphere of acceptance, it is necessary for the nurse to comprehend the possible implications of loss of the uterus. If the woman views this loss as significant, the nurse must be prepared to support and encourage expression of the grieving process. As the woman begins a redefinition of her role as a female, the nurse can facilitate the examination of role and identity and provide support and encouragement. With an overall goal of utilizing the individual's strengths to promote healthy long-term adaptation to hysterectomy rather than elimination of psychological pain, the nurse can help the woman to view this time in her life as a redefinition of her role as a woman, similar to that which occurs during menopause.

Nursing Interventions Focusing on Object Relations

Object relations will be confined to those significant persons on whom the health care recipient is emotionally dependent. Nursing interventions will be limited to involvement with those significant persons who can help provide psychological support for the expression of needs by the health care recipient. The focus of interventions in object relations will be on the motivation of significant persons to be accepting and supportive of expression of feelings by the woman as she undergoes the experience of hysterectomy. The nurse can help to motivate significant persons by encouraging direct communication, giving information to them, and accepting the direct expression of their needs and feelings.

A woman tends to develop a diffuse body image and self-concept, which are linked, through dependency, to the evaluation of others. A woman's self-esteem is dependent largely on the expressed feelings of acceptance and appreciation from others.[17] Therefore, as a woman faces hysterectomy, which may be perceived as a threat to her self-esteem, body image, and identity, her needs for acceptance and reassurance of love by significant persons increase greatly. Psychological adjustment to hysterectomy is eased when the response from the woman's environment is not unduly negative.[18] Conversely, rejection by significant others often precipitates posthysterectomy depression.[19] The value of nursing interventions focusing on object relations is further emphasized by a study in which women viewed relationships that encouraged expression of their feelings about hysterectomy as helpful. When these relationships did not exist, women felt this to be an unmet need, an area in which their social network failed them.[20]

INDICATIONS FOR HYSTERECTOMY

Physical Conditions

☐ *Benign uterine disease.* Fibromyomata (commonly referred to as fibroids) constitute the most frequent indication for hysterectomy. Fibroids are benign tumors of the uterus. They are generally slow in growth and painless except when pressure is applied. The presence of fibroids in the uterus is common, occurring in 40 percent of all women over 40 years of age.[21] Often fibroids are asymptomatic and require no treatment. If symptoms appear and are not severe, treatment may be deferred until after the menopause, at which point fibroid tumors tend to regress in size naturally, thus possibly eliminating the need for treatment.

Sarcomatous degeneration of fibroids is rare, malignant change being found in only 0.1 to 0.5 percent of patients operated on for fibromyomata. When symptoms of abnormal uterine bleeding, pelvic pressure, pressure on contiguous organs, and/or abdominal distention occur, treatment may be necessary. Treatment involves myomectomy (removal of the tumors) or hysterectomy.[22]

Adenomyosis is a condition involving enlargement of the uterus caused by the invasion of the hyometrium by the endometrium. Symptoms are acquired dysmenorrhea and menorrhagia. If curettage fails to eliminate the symptoms and if the woman's childbearing needs are over, hysterectomy is recommended.[23]

Dysfunctional uterine bleeding of the menopause is another frequent indication for hysterectomy. Often hysterectomy is chosen as the treatment of choice if there are concurrent changes in the endometrium. The alternative treatment of curettage alleviates the dysfunctional bleeding in 60 percent of the cases the first time it is performed. Curettage performed for the second time alleviates 70 to 75 percent of the dysfunctional bleeding until the menopause supervenes.[24]

☐ *Malignant uterine disease.* Twenty percent of all hysterectomies are performed to alleviate malignancies of the cervix, the body of the uterus, or adjacent organs. The diagnosis is based on the results of the pap smear, dilatation and curettage, or aspiration curettage.[25] Treatment for all types of cancer of the uterus is generally surgical removal of the uterus. In some instances irradiation or chemical therapy is utilized conjunctively with surgery. The presence of precancerous lesions (cell changes that may indicate impending malignancy) may also necessitate hysterectomy.[26]

□ *Removal of the normal uterus.* There are other conditions that may necessitate the removal of the uterus, even if the uterus is not diseased. Established indicators for the removal of the normal uterus are as follows: the presence of ovarian, oviduct, and vaginal cancer; chronic pelvic inflammation; and genital prolapse.

Removal of the normal uterus involves much that is subjective and philosophical; thus, there are differences of opinion as to the necessity of this surgery. This is more clearly indicated in the conditions that have been categorized into the areas of relative indicators for the removal of the normal uterus. These relative indicators include sterilization, mental retardation, ectopic pregnancy, familial history of cancer, pelvic pain, hydatidiform mole, postirradiation of the uterus, benign ovarian disease, pelvic tuberculosis, postpartum hemorrhage, and dysfunctional bleeding.[27]

Psychological Conditions

The uterus is sometimes removed for the psychiatric conditions of phobias (especially cancerophobia) and hypochondriasis. Hysterectomy, in these cases, rarely removes the phobia or lessens hypochondriacal thinking.[28]

On a more general basis, the relationship between the functioning of the female reproductive system and the emotions is close and complex. Psychological factors may influence the development and course of gynecologic disease or symptoms.[29] Or the uterus may become the conversion focus for many psychoemotional ills of women.[30]

The concept that either the emotional status of a woman may precipitate the need for hysterectomy (due to increased gynecologic symptoms) or a woman may displace emotional problems onto her reproductive functioning seems credible, although there have been few studies performed to substantiate this.

Unnecessary Hysterectomies

Research indicates that of all hysterectomies performed, from 32 percent[31] to 39 percent[32] may be unnecessary. These statistics include those cases in which less extensive alternative treatment could have been sufficient and the few cases in which hysterectomy was later determined to be contraindicated.

In general, all physical and psychological conditions, with the exception of malignant disease, may lead to an unnecessary hysterectomy.

Nursing Interventions

Difficulty in understanding and accepting the need for surgery correlates strongly with poor outcome of hysterectomy.[33] This finding provides clear evidence of the importance of satisfactorily explaining the reasons for surgery.

The results of "Hysterectomy Knowledge Study" indicate that 65 percent of the women knew that the most frequent reason for removal of the uterus is the presence of fibroids. However, 19 percent of the women believed that most hysterectomies are performed because the woman has cancer, and 16 percent of the women believed that most hysterectomies are performed unnecessarily.

If the woman believes that most hysterectomies are performed because cancer is present, she probably feels that there is a large possibility of cancer being present in her body. The fear of uterine cancer is experienced by many women,[34] and the fear becomes more pronounced as the woman gets older.[35] This fear of cancer has long been the pretext of proponents of performing hysterectomy for fibroids, by both physicians and patients alike.[36] The magnitude of this fear and the actual percentage of cancerous degeneration of fibroids do not correlate.

The variation in the magnitude of the fear of cancer compared with the rate of cancerous degeneration of fibroids and the percentage of hysterectomies performed for cancer may be a large factor in the woman's decision to have a hysterectomy, regardless of the preoperative diagnosis. Fear of cancer may increase the woman's need for reassurance postoperatively. And the fear of cancer may be a component of preoperative distress.

Recent magazine articles have brought into public awareness the occurrence of unnecessary hysterectomies.[37,38] Women should be aware of their right to obtain a second medical opinion before deciding to have a hysterectomy. Increased efforts in public education may reduce the percentage of unnecessary hysterectomies and help women to make more educated health care decisions. Nursing involvement in public education can help to insure that women are provided information in all areas of the issue.

There are reports in the literature of women who believe that the need for hysterectomy is directly caused by excessive sexual activity.[39,40] There are also reports that hysterectomy is viewed by some women as a punishment for real or imagined "sins," generally sexual in nature (including sexual promiscuity, sexual enjoyment, masturbation, and abortion).[41-43] If these are a woman's perceptions, it is imperative that the beliefs of her sexual partner be assessed to ascertain whether he supports these perceptions. The couple should then be provided with a clear explanation of reproductive functioning and referred for therapy if necessary.

A complete history should be taken on all women before a decision to perform hysterectomy is made. (This is especially necessary for the woman who presents vague, ill-defined complaints.) The history should include physical and emotional components, and present stress-related problems should be explored.[44] If the woman is currently experiencing many stress-related situations, perhaps elective hysterectomy should be postponed. If the stress is severe, psychological therapy may be more appropriate than hysterectomy.

If the woman exhibits an obvious psychiatric disorder, consultation with a psychiatrist or therapist before surgery is recommended. If the hysterectomy is elective, it may be decided against.[45] If the hysterectomy is not elective, the therapist may help the nurse and/or physician to more accurately anticipate postoperative problems.

More nursing research is needed to identify how psychological stress is related to the functioning of the female reproductive system. Increased research in this area could help to insure that women are not treated surgically for psychological problems.

CHANGES IN ANATOMY PRODUCED BY HYSTERECTOMY

The uterus is a hollow, thick-walled, muscular organ shaped somewhat like a pear. In a mature woman, its size at the top measures approximately 2.5 by 2 inches. It narrows to a diameter of about 1 inch at the cervix and is about 3 inches long. The functions of the uterus are those of childbearing and menstruation.[46] Each month the uterine walls become thickened with a lining of blood. If conception has not occurred, the blood exits from the body in the form of a menstrual period. If conception has occurred, the uterus will become the nurturing place of growth for the fetus.

Hysterectomy removes this organ, thus eliminating its functions. When the uterus is removed from the body, fluid and the slight readjustment of other organs displace the resultant gap. The ligaments that held the uterus in place are attached to the vaginal walls.[47] Thus, with the exception of the absence of the uterus, the interior anatomic structure after hysterectomy appears similar to that before hysterectomy. The external anatomic structure appears exactly the same pre- and postsurgically, with the exception of the presence of an abdominal scar if the abdominal surgical technique is utilized.

The two ovaries are almond shaped and measure about 1.25 inches long. Ovaries are connected to the lateral border of the uterus by the ovarian ligament.[48] The functions of the ovaries are the monthly release of ova (eggs) and the production of hormones.[49]

Removal of the uterus may cause a temporary hormonal imbalance. However, the ovaries continue to function and will continue to function normally until the onset of menopause.[50,51]

If an oophorectomy is performed concurrently with hysterectomy, the ovaries are removed and their functions are terminated. Especially if the woman is young, hormonal replacement therapy may be indicated to prevent the onset of surgical menopause.[52]

Nursing Interventions

Many women are ignorant about the anatomy of their sexual and reproductive organs.[53] The functions of the uterus and ovaries are very often confusing to women. When they are asked to identify these functions, general answers like babies, sex, hormones, and regulating are offered.[54] The "Hysterectomy Knowledge Study" results indicate the level of this confusion. Women's responses, when asked to select the functions of the uterus and ovaries, were as follows:

FUNCTIONS OF UTERUS	FUNCTIONS OF OVARIES
Holds menstrual blood, 49%	Hold menstrual blood, 6%
Place where sexual intercourse occurs, 3%	Produce hormones, 54%
Produces hormones, 8%	Release eggs, 92%
Place where a baby grows, 97%	Control a woman's sex drive, 9%
Controls a woman's sex drive, 1%	Place where sexual intercourse occurs, 1%

Only 38 percent of the women answered the question of the functions of the uterus totally correctly, selecting both menstrual and childbearing functions. And only 37 percent of the women indicated that both the release of eggs and production of hormones were the correct responses to the question of ovarian functioning. Thus, it seems well established that more education is needed in the area of the female reproductive system.

As the changes in anatomy after hysterectomy are explored it is discovered that "woman's understanding about what actually happens when they have a hysterectomy is extremely variable and rarely adequate in terms of the degree of understanding they would like to have about what is being done to their bodies."[55] Women often have only a crude understanding of what the surgeon has done to their anatomy,[56] knowing only that their "womb" has been removed.[57] Often women do not even know whether they have had an oophorectomy along with the hysterectomy.[58]

Reports in the literature indicate that some women think they have a hole inside after the uterus is removed.[59] One-fourth of the women in the "Hysterectomy Knowledge Study" thought there would be an empty space where the uterus had originally been. This is an important concept to correct because it leads to speculation and concern by women who wonder if things will pass through the hole or whether something was left behind in surgery to fill the hole.[60]

Women are also confused about the functioning of their ovaries after hysterectomy. Of the women in the "Hysterectomy Knowledge Study," 56 percent knew the ovaries would continue to function, 14 percent thought ovaries functioned at a reduced rate, and 30 percent thought the ovaries no longer functioned at all after hysterectomy.

Obviously education will eliminate many of these misconceptions. Nursing intervention appears to be simple and concise in this area. However, there are factors that complicate the transfer of information from the nurse to the patient. Unformulated personal beliefs about anatomy and physiology of reproductive organs may come into awareness only when the organs are diseased.[61] As one woman stated, "You just don't think about things like your womanly organs until they give you trouble."[62] When the woman is faced with surgery she may have an emotional response that is limiting her awareness. Thus, it may not occur to her to ask questions. Other women may be so confused about the functions of their organs that they have difficulty formulating questions. Some women don't want to show a lack of knowledge or be embarrassed, so they don't ask questions.[63] And other women are not given the opportunity to ask questions.[64]

In providing quality patient care, a nurse cannot afford to wait for the woman to ask questions. The woman may never ask them, or she may ask these questions of people who cannot provide the correct answers.[65]

EFFECTS OF HYSTERECTOMY
ON CHILDBEARING CAPACITY

Hysterectomy affects a woman with total and irreversible loss of childbearing capacity. This loss of the biologic functions of a woman's body is reported by many authors to be of great significance in the emotional response to the surgery.[66–69]

Removal of the uterus and the resultant loss of the ability to bear children have potential psychological consequences for all women.[70] This can be understood only when there is clear differentiation between the ability to bear children and the desire for children. Ability to bear children is the crucial factor, not desire to bear children or desire to bear more children. This concept is evidenced by the findings that wanting more children versus not wanting more children does not correlate with outcome of hysterectomy,[71] nor does having children versus not having children.[72]

The ability to bear children serves a wide variety of needs and functions in the life of a woman. This ability is of significance in the self-image of a woman.[73] The multifaceted relationship between the ability to bear children and the self-image of a woman can be defined in various ways. For many women "the biologic ability to reproduce is intimately connected with the adjustment of women as a feminine figure.[74] For some women childbearing provides a sense of achievement and fulfillment[75] or sense of completeness.[76] For other women it represents a sense of power, with resultant loss of the ability to bear children representing an extreme form of powerlessness.[77]

In the literature, women have defined their sense of self in relation to their ability to have children. Some state that having children is expected of them[78] and is therefore their duty. Other women have defined this in terms of being useful[79] or being a proper women,[80] and yet others have defined the ability to have children as the reason for their existence on earth[81] and even as their total identification as a woman.[82]

The degree to which a woman defines her sense of self in terms of the biologic functions of her body seems to be a crucial factor in the extent of her sense of loss over the cessation of childbearing capacity after hysterectomy. This is probably related in some degree to cultural patterning of the feminine role[83] and the trends of society in general.

In viewing the extensive connections between the self-image of a woman and the ability to bear children, the sense of loss that occurs with the removal of the uterus can be comprehended. However, some women do not appear to experience an extensive sense of loss and perhaps even feel no sense of loss. Many women feel indifferent or delighted about their resultant sterility after hysterectomy.[84] And the relief from fear of pregnancy may be a major factor in the good outcome after hysterectomy for some women.[85] Still other women have hysterectomies for the sole purpose of sterilization. Thus, the response to the loss of childbearing capacity ranges from devastation to delight.

Nursing Interventions

There are isolated reports in the literature which indicate that some women do not know that hysterectomy causes cessation of the childbearing capacity.[86,87] In the "Hysterectomy Knowledge Study" almost 4 percent of the women did not correctly answer the question regarding ability to give birth after hysterectomy. Thus, it cannot be assumed that women know that after a hysterectomy they can no longer give birth to a child.

Comprehension of the meaning of losing the ability to bear children occurs readily when the woman is young, married, and desires to have children. The young woman's sense of loss is easily accepted and even expected by her family, friends, and medical personnel. Although the response of a premenopausal woman with less than two children has been found to be more severe in all gynecologic operations,[88] this does not mean that other women who are not in positions or do not desire to have children will not experience loss. Unless there is a conscious awareness by the nurse that the issue is the ability to bear children (not the feasibility of bearing children), the loss of the unmarried woman, the woman who by choice does not desire children, and the homosexual woman will not be understood.

The inability to differentiate between the ability to have children and the desire to have children may be a factor in the reports of women who express concern and anger that they were not prepared for the sense of loss they felt at the termination of their childbearing capacities after hysterectomy.[89] The "Hysterectomy Knowledge Study" results tend to confirm that women are not aware that the ability to bear children is the crucial issue. Although only 8 percent of the women did not believe that being able to have children is an important part of the way women see themselves, 14 percent believed that, if a woman has all the children she wants, a hysterectomy will have no emotional effect on her. Eleven percent of the women believed that, if a woman is unmarried and does not want children, a hysterectomy will have no emotional effect on her. And 30 percent believed that, after a woman goes through menopause, a hysterectomy will have no emotional effect on her. It can be seen from these data why women are not prepared for the sense of loss.

Even though it would seem likely that the menopausal woman would not be subjected to psychological stress from loss of her childbearing capacity, this is not necessarily the case. Menopause occurs during the climacteric and the climacteric is a time when old doubts and insecurities may emerge, because it is a time of change in a woman's life. Thus, increased psychological stress may occur from hysterectomy at this time.[90] The menopausal process involves the cessation of the ability to bear children, and this carries with it the process of psychological readjustment. When the resolution of psychological components of the climacteric is incomplete, it can be speculated that even the postmenopausal woman may become subject to emotional stress due to reemergence of sense of loss of her childbearing capacity. It can also be speculated that at the age of menopause, if the woman has had children, the children are generally adults. If the children have not fulfilled the mother's expectations by this point, the woman may see herself as having failed in her role of mothering. Menopause and hysterectomy are obvious indications that the woman will have no further chances to reestablish herself in a mothering role. She may express this in excessive concern about her children or bitterness about the way they "turned out."

Women can be encouraged to verbalize their feelings about the significance of their ability to bear children. Older women, women with many children, or women in situations that are not conducive to childbearing may be embarrassed to discuss their feelings about childbearing ability. The nurse can help to minimize embarrassment by helping the woman to verbalize about the basis for her identity. Whether the woman sees herself as primarily a caregiver, a wife, a professional, etc., the nurse can offer support and help the woman to realistically explore changes that hysterectomy may bring to her life. If the loss is felt to be significant to the woman, the nurse, by accepting the woman's expression of feelings, will be assisting her to complete the grieving process.

If the woman wants to be sterilized, this can also be supported by the nurse. However, the performance of hysterectomy solely for sterilization purposes generally should not be supported by the nurse. Tubal ligation is a much more appropriate procedure for sterilization. Standard morbidity of hysterectomy ranges from 42 to 45 percent. Morbidity of tubal ligations ranges from 1.5 to 20 percent.[91] Thus, physical distress from hysterectomy is much greater, as is psychological distress. Tubal ligation has a much higher rate of positive long-term response than does hysterectomy.[92]

Hysterectomies for sterilization purposes only are being labeled more often as unnecessary hysterectomies because of the increased risks of psychological and physical morbidity as compared to the less extensive procedure of tubal ligations. One reason for the performance of hysterectomy for sterilization purposes may be that women do not know of the greater risks hysterectomy entails. The results of the "Hysterectomy Knowledge Study" indicate that almost 30 percent of the women thought that women have the same emotional response to hysterectomy and tubal ligation. Almost half of the women thought that hysterectomies are as medically safe as tubal ligations. These findings indicate that increased efforts should be made in the area of public education.

EFFECTS OF HYSTERECTOMY ON MENSTRUAL FUNCTION

Hysterectomy causes the complete cessation of menstruation. Hormones continue to maintain their cyclic pattern, but the accompanying menstrual bleeding no longer occurs. Thus, a hysterectomy will alleviate dysfunctional bleeding, for example, but will not alleviate symptoms associated with menstruation, such as tension, headaches, water retention, and irritableness.[93]

To understand the potential sense of loss experienced by the woman with the cessation of menstruation, it is necessary to examine how the woman views the experience of menstruation and to identify what functions she attributes to the process of menstruation.

Drellich and Bieber report that the majority of women have positive feelings toward the menstrual function and that many women feel a loss of this valued process when menstrual function is terminated. However, they also report frequent negative attitudes expressed by many women toward the symptoms that accompany menstruation.[94] Thus, it appears that, in order to recognize positive feelings about menstruation, menstruation must be distinguished from the often distressful symptoms that accompany it. The inability to differentiate between the symptoms and the process of menstruation could provide an explanation of the variation in the findings of Drellich and Bieber (in which women viewed the loss of menstruation with sadness) and those of another researcher, who found the vast majority of his study sample to be pleased or unconcerned about the loss of menstrual function after hysterectomy.[95]

The functions women attribute to menstruation also give an indication of their responses to the loss of this process. Some women appear to view menstruation as a cleaning or excretory function. These women seem to associate their menstrual blood with their body wastes. They consider menstruation to be a healthy process that removes "bad blood" and "noxious waste" from the body. Loss of menstrual function causes them to become concerned about what will happen to them if they don't get rid of the waste.[96,97]

Other women view menstruation as a regulatory function. For these women monthly periods provide a predictability to their daily living and serve to regulate their activities. This "rhythm of life" provides a pattern, and some women attribute variations in emotion, strength, and vitality to this pattern.[98]

Menstruation is the outward manifestation of the ability to bear children.[99] With each monthly bleeding comes the reminder that the uterus is capable of nurturing life. When menstruation ceases the woman is faced with evidence that she can no longer bear children. This in turn accentuates an inability that may be vital to the woman's identity.

Nursing Interventions

There are reports in the literature which indicate that not all women know that a hysterectomy causes cessation of menstruation.[100] Thus, a nurse cannot assume that the woman who has had a hysterectomy knows she will no longer menstruate. This is further evidenced by the "Hysterectomy Knowledge Study," in which over five percent of the subjects believed that after hysterectomy the menstrual period either did not stop but became irregular, or continued to occur as it did before the hysterectomy.

Twenty-two percent of the study population in the "Hysterectomy Knowledge Study" believed that hysterectomies would cure premenstrual tension. By increased involvement of nursing in public education programs regarding hysterectomy, the number of hysterectomies performed to alleviate premenstrual tension can be reduced and women who expect that premenstrual tension will disappear with hysterectomy can be spared distress and disappointment.

In responding to a woman who has lost the ability to menstruate, the nurse must remember that feelings about menstruation are dependent on many factors, such as symptoms accompanying menstruation, what the woman believes to be the functions of menstruation, the woman's adolescent experiences involving the onset of menstruation, and cultural attitudes about menstruation. Menstruation is often an emotionally laden process. Some women refer to menstruation as "the curse," and many women feel this terminology is accurate. Other women have positive feelings about this female function and view its termination as a loss. In order to provide an attitude of acceptance of the woman's positive or negative feelings about the cessation of her menstruation after hysterectomy, the nurse may find it necessary to explore her own personal feelings about the menstrual process.

EFFECTS OF HYSTERECTOMY ON
MENOPAUSAL PROCESS

Hysterectomy does not induce menopause, nor does it prevent the process of menopause.[101] There are three aspects of menopause: cessation of the menses, psychological adjustment to the termination of childbearing capacity, and permanent reduction of hormonal (estrogen) level. After hysterectomy the woman experiences cessation of the menses and begins psychological adjustment to the loss of childbearing capacity. However, she does not experience permanent reduction of hormonal levels, and this factor is the qualifying determinant of menopause.

The relation of hysterectomy to menopause becomes increasingly confusing as one examines literature which indicates that, although permanent reduction of hormonal levels does not occur after hysterectomy, a temporary hormonal imbalance often occurs, causing some premenopausal women to experience hot flashes, a symptom commonly associated with menopause.[102] It should be stressed that this condition is temporary, can occur at any age, and generally disappears naturally or can be treated by hormonal replacement.[103]

Therefore, a premenopausal woman who has a hysterectomy may or may not experience some temporary hot flashes after her surgery. Hot flashes in this instance are not indicative of menopause. The woman's ovaries are still functioning and will continue to function until her natural menopause. Masters and Johnson suggest that the only correlation between hysterectomy and menopause is that the young woman who has a hysterectomy may experience menopause a few years sooner than women who have not had hysterectomies.[104]

Hysterectomy with bilateral oophorectomy does induce surgical menopause in the premenopausal woman.[105] In this instance, the woman, again, may or may not experience menopausal symptoms. Although the symptoms of surgical menopause do not appear to be more severe than the symptoms of natural menopause, the suddenness of the surgical menopause can be psychologically distressing. To minimize the distress and lessen the physical discomforts of surgical menopause, generally estrogen therapy replacement is recommended.[106]

Nursing Interventions

The high level of confusion regarding the relationship between hysterectomy and menopause can be seen clearly in the responses of the women who participated in the "Hysterectomy Knowledge Study." Only 52 percent of the women knew that after a hysterectomy menopause would occur when it normally would. Over 36 percent thought that menopause would be brought on by hysterectomy. And just under 12 percent of the women thought menopause could be prevented by hysterectomy.

There are also reports in the literature of women who, not understanding the relationship between hysterectomy and menopause, fear that changes in their physical appearance associated with menopause will occur, such as dry, wrinkled skin, rapid aging, and gray hair or that they will acquire masculine characteristics such as facial hair and a deeper voice.[107-109] Approximately 5 percent of the women in the "Hysterectomy Knowledge Study" believed this to be true. Education can help to alleviate these misconceptions.

The premenopausal woman facing hysterectomy with bilateral oophorectomy should be told she will be experiencing surgical menopause. The menopausal symptoms she may experience should be discussed along with an explanation of estrogen replacement therapy if necessary.

The woman facing hysterectomy may be frightened and most probably will be confused about the relationship between hysterectomy and menopause. She may not ask questions; she may not even be able to formulate questions in her mind about a subject that is extremely confusing to her. The nurse can be most helpful in reducing the stressful fear and confusion the woman may be experiencing by providing information, encouraging the woman to discuss her fears, and accepting the woman's needs for reassurance.

EFFECTS OF HYSTERECTOMY ON SEXUAL CAPACITY

Hysterectomy affects sexual functioning minimally in the areas of sexual ability and libido, generally requiring only a short period of readjustment.

In most cases, sexual intercourse can be cautiously resumed about six weeks after the hysterectomy has been performed. Initial intercourse should be gentle because the woman's abdomen may feel tender. It may take three to four months before normal coital pressure can be comfortable to the woman. This period of adjustment appears to be the same for either vaginal or abdominal hysterectomy.[110]

During this period of readjustment the couple may experience difficulty with intromission, dryness in the vagina, dyspareunia (painful coitus), or bleeding.[111] Frank bleeding and dyspareunia should be brought immediately to the attention of the physician. Dyspareunia generally can be treated and relieved.[112] The majority of women find that sexual intercourse is the same or better after hysterectomy.[113]

The woman's ability to achieve orgasm may diminish for a short time after the surgery due to stress.[114] This is only a temporary condition; there have been only very isolated cases in the literature in which the woman's ability to achieve orgasm was diminished for a great length of time.[115] In general, women retain orgasmic ability.[116]

The woman's desire for sex may decrease for a period of time after hysterectomy.[117] In one study women reported a lack of libido so frequently that the researcher concluded that lack of libido must be considered a normal condition after hysterectomy.[118] Conversely, other studies report that lack of libido is much less frequent[119] or not related to hysterectomy.[120] Although it appears that many women do experience a decrease in desire for sexual activity, it is generally only very temporary. Libido is based on many psychological factors. This is evidenced in the finding that other women report an increase in libido after hysterectomy.[121] This increase may occur because the woman feels relief from the distressing physical symptoms that prompted her hysterectomy or because the woman experiences relief from the fear of pregnancy.

Hysterectomy with oophorectomy does not end a woman's desire for sexual activity. A woman's sex drive often does not diminish even when the ovaries are surgically removed.[122] A woman's desire for sexual intimacy, it appears, is based more extensively on psychological factors than on basic physiology. Thus (regardless of whether an oophorectomy has been performed), the majority of women experience comparable libido and sexual relationships before and after hysterectomy.[123]

Nursing Interventions

Hysterectomy literature abounds with reported fears and misconceptions women have about the effects of hysterectomy on sexual ability and desire. Women fear they will no longer desire sexual intercourse,[124] that sexual intercourse will no longer be a satisfactory experience for their husbands,[125] and that they will no longer be physically able to have sexual intercourse.[126] There are even reports of women and their sexual partners who fear that sexual activity caused the condition that made removal of the uterus necessary and that resumption of sexual intercourse would cause resumption of the disease.[127] There are also reports of men who fear that penile injury will occur if they have coitus with a woman who has had a hysterectomy[128] or that they will contract cancer by having intercourse with a woman who has had her uterus removed because of the presence of cancer.[129] Until recent years, sex was not considered a proper topic of discussion, and it appears that this cultural taboo was also experienced by members of the health care professions.

The "Hysterectomy Knowledge Study" shows a decline in the acceptance of this cultural taboo. Over 99 percent of the women in the study knew that hysterectomy did not end a woman's desire for sex. Just over 96 percent knew that a woman could have sexual intercourse and that it would feel the same to her after hysterectomy. Ninety-three percent felt that a woman could have an orgasm after hysterectomy if she had experienced it before the surgery. Ninety-six percent of the women thought that a woman's desire for six would remain the same or increase after hysterectomy. And 96 percent knew that sexual intercourse would feel the same to the woman's sexual partner after hysterectomy. It appears that articles in women's magazines about sexual functioning after hysterectomy[130,131] along with other media presentations have provided education regarding sexual functioning to the public.

These encouraging statistics, however, do not eliminate the need for informative discussions about the effects of hysterectomy on sexual functioning. It must be remembered that women of various cultural and educational backgrounds will probably display variations of knowledge in this area.

If women are not informed that resumption of sexual intercourse will require a time of readjustment and that they may experience initial difficulties, the experience of sexual intercourse after hysterectomy may be painful, negative, and fear producing. These factors tend to have adverse effects on a woman's libido, thus increasing the possibility of sexual impairment. If women are informed about possible initial difficulties before their first experience with sexual intercourse after hysterectomy, along with methods to alleviate difficulties, the anxiety level can be reduced, which in turn can help make intercourse more pleasurable. If the woman experiences initial dryness in the vagina, the use of water-soluble lubricating jelly can be suggested, or it can be recommended that the couple prolong lovemaking before intercourse. Gentle intercourse will be more pleasurable to the woman. The occurrence of pain during intercourse should be brought to the physician's attention so that treatment can be provided.

The response of the woman's sexual partner is crucial in the sexual adjustment after hysterectomy.[132] He should be included in discussions on sexual functioning and encouraged to ask questions. If he is given information and supported in expressing concerns or fears, he may be better able to support the woman, thus making the sexual adjustment period easier for both of them. This would be true for a homosexual partner as well.

Discussions on sexual functioning are difficult and embarrassing for some people. Many women are uncomfortable asking a male physician questions that are sexual in nature.[133] Such questions as "When will I be healed properly?" are often indicators of a need to discuss when sexual functioning can be resumed.[134] When the nurse is alert to directly and indirectly expressed needs of the health care recipient, more helpful interventions can be made and the quality of health care will improve.

EFFECTS OF HYSTERECTOMY ON PHYSICAL CONDITION

Physical effects of hysterectomy include the mortality rate of the surgery, frequently occurring physical symptoms experienced after the surgery, and the characteristics of the recovery period.

The surgical procedure itself is relatively safe in terms of mortality. In recent years, estimates of mortality range from one death per 1,000 surgeries performed to one death per 4,000 surgeries.[135]

Postoperative urinary tract infections occur frequently, especially after vaginal hysterectomies. In one series of studies, urinary tract infection occurred in approximately 20 to 25 percent of the women.[136]

Headache is another physical symptom that seems to occur frequently after hysterectomy. Richards reports that half of his sample population of women who had hysterectomies complained of headaches postoperatively. (Less than one-sixth of these women complained of headaches preoperatively.)[137]

Weight gain also appears to occur frequently after hysterectomy. Dodds et al. found that approximately one-half of the women in their study sample gained under 10 pounds; the other half gained from 10 to 30 pounds after hysterectomy.[138]

Hot flashes after hysterectomy are experienced by approximately 50 to 60 percent of women.[139,140] These hot flashes occur regardless of the age of the woman and whether or not she has had an oophorectomy along with the hysterectomy. Hot flashes appear to be a temporary symptom, usually subsiding within six months.

Studies dealing with recovery period of hysterectomy report that, for about one-half of the women studied, this period is characterized by extreme fatigue and weakness.[141] Generally most women can resume their normal duties within six weeks to three months after hysterectomy,[142] although there are instances of some women taking up to six months to resume normal duties.[143]

The length of the recovery period from hysterectomy varies. Williams found that the recovery period (time from hospital discharge until the person felt fully recovered) was an average of two months. However, she states that the range was from two weeks to six months and that some women did not feel well at the six-month interview.[144] Richards found the average time for the women in his study to feel fully recovered after hysterectomy was 11.9 months (compared to three months for women in the control group who had other surgeries).[145] The wide variation reported in the length of the recovery time is difficult to understand.

Nursing Interventions

Some women express fears about physical symptoms after hysterectomy that are extreme and occur very rarely, such as permanently losing bowel and bladder control and never being as physically strong or healthy after hysterectomy. The "Hysterectomy Knowledge Study" indicates that these extreme fears about hysterectomy are not as prevalent at present. Under 3 percent of the women in the study thought that a woman would never be as physically strong or healthy after hysterectomy. Only 1 percent thought that many women permanently lost control of bowel and bladder after hysterectomy.

However, results from the "Hysterectomy Knowledge Study" indicate that many women know little about physical symptoms that actually do occur after hysterectomy. Just less than 50 percent of the women knew that temporary urinary problems could occur, that hot flashes were a possible physical symptom, and that weight gain could occur. Less than 20 percent thought headaches were a possible physical symptom.

The nurse can provide women with the information that these symptoms may occur. Women should be told the symptoms of urinary tract infection so that if it does occur it can be treated promptly. Knowing that headaches may occur and that the woman may experience hot flashes can alleviate the possible anxiety that may accompany these symptoms if the woman is not prepared for their possible occurrence. If weight gain after hysterectomy would be distressing to the woman, she can be placed on a moderate diet to prevent this. This information can be presented to the woman in a manner which does not imply that she will experience these symptoms but which indicates that these symptoms are experienced by some women.

In the "Hysterectomy Knowledge Study" most women (97 percent) knew that after hysterectomy women could return to work or household duties six to eight weeks after surgery. Most women (89 percent) thought recovery time was six to twelve weeks after surgery. The remaining 11 percent thought that the recovery time was generally one year or that women never fully recovered.

It appears that when recovery time takes longer than three months (it is often assumed that recovery time for major surgery is one to three months),[146] the woman is probably not prepared for this occurrence. Anxiety may be alleviated if the woman understands in advance that wide variations in the length of recovery time from hysterectomy do occur.

An overview of the goals of nursing interventions in the area of physical effects of hysterectomy include alleviating extreme anxiety about the physical effects of the surgery, bringing into public awareness that hysterectomy contains risks of mortality and physical morbidity, and preparing health care recipients for possible physical symptoms they may experience after hysterectomy.

PSYCHOLOGICAL RESPONSE TO HYSTERECTOMY

The psychological response to hysterectomy has been the focus of many studies. Studies performed to determine the psychological aftermath of hysterectomy, using the criterion of admission to a mental hospital or psychiatric institute, do not prove (either because statistical significance is not established or because of poor study design) that hysterectomy leads to psychiatric disability requiring admission to a psychiatric institute.[147-151] However, studies that use referral to a psychiatrist as the criterion for emotional distress produced by hysterectomy indicate that referral to a psychiatrist after hysterectomy occurs 2.5 times more often than referral after other surgeries.[152] Similarly, studies examining the incidence of psychiatric symptoms after hysterectomy do provide evidence of intense psychological response after hysterectomy.[153-159]

The most common response to hysterectomy is depression. The reported incidence ranges from 4 percent[160] of the women studied to 70 percent,[161] with an average of approximately 30 percent. This depression may or may not be accompanied by agitation.

These studies indicate the level of intensity of the emotional response. Apparently, an adverse response to hysterectomy does not generally necessitate admission to a psychiatric institute. Depression is a common psychological response for which some women may seek treatment from a therapist. Other women may experience depression and not seek treatment.

The identification of women at risk for poor outcome after hysterectomy has also been the focus of studies. Factors that correlate with intense, distressing psychological response have been identified. Poor outcome correlates with women who have a high general anxiety level, are highly neurotic, have a small number of siblings, have a high ordinal position within the family, have a poor relationship with their own mothers, exhibit extensive concern over the effects of the operation on future sexual relationships, and have difficulty understanding and accepting the need for the surgery.[162] Previous history of depression[163] or previous emotional breakdown correlates strongly with poor outcome of hysterectomy.[164] The factor that one researcher found to correlate most significantly with unfavorable outcome was the degree of "unhelpfulness" experienced by the woman from her social network.[165] It has also been discovered that immediate postoperative recovery from anesthesia is indicative of the hospital convalescence.[166]

Nursing Interventions

Previous discussions of nursing interventions have been focused on reducing the possibility of intense psychological distress as a response to hysterectomy. The identification of factors that correlate with poor outcome of hysterectomy can assist the nurse in anticipating and preparing for possible onset of emotional crisis.

The high number of women experiencing posthysterectomy depression is alarming. Some depression (especially as related to the grieving process) may be necessary in order for the woman to make a healthy long-term adaptive response to the loss of her uterus. It is important that the nurse recognize symptoms of depression so that she can direct the woman to treatment if indicated.

Common symptoms of depression include a change in sleeping patterns, a change in eating habits, mood swings, excessive crying, emotional lability, lack of energy, and acquired preoccupation with one's physical condition. This may be accompanied by nervousness and agitation.

FUTURE IMPLICATIONS

The future of hysterectomies is unknown. It is based on another unknown—the future of woman. If females remain dependent and uneducated, it is likely that a large percentage of unnecessary and undesired hysterectomies will continue to be performed. (Hysterectomy performed on a woman who desires hysterectomy, for whatever reason, and makes a conscious decision to have the surgery is not included in the category of unnecessary hysterectomies.) One explanation for the occurrence of undesired, unnecessary hysterectomies lies in the relationship between the physician and the health care recipient. It has been charged that many women unquestioningly surrender their uterus to the whims of the physician—the superior male healer. Hysterectomy, in such instances, is best described as a "socially sanctioned genital trauma performed on a female by a male."[167]

It has further been charged that the physician often "cons" a woman into the surrender of her uterus. In these instances, the physician tells the woman she must have a hysterectomy, either making the decision himself or not providing the woman with enough information so that she can participate in the decision-making process. A partial explanation for this is that a physician can charge more money for a hysterectomy than for a less extensive procedure such as a tubal ligation or dilatation and curettage. It is often women of low socioeconomic backgrounds, generally of the black culture, who are "talked into" hysterectomy when a less extensive procedure[168] would suffice.

These are angry charges, and it is likely that the strength of this anger will help to reduce the number of undesired, unnecessary hysterectomies. The anger is also felt by physicians who are not involved in these practices. Unification of physicians, nurses, and the lay population over this issue may lead to stronger public education programs and increased accountability of physicians to their peers.

Perhaps by having hysterectomies, some women are making statements about the anger they feel about their position in society. The recognition of this anger may be associated with the women's movement. The lives of many women have been ruled by the fruits of their uteri. Childbearing and childrearing are felt to have kept many women in bondage. It can be speculated that increased involvement of fathers in the responsibilities of raising children may decrease the need for women to express their anger by having a part of their body removed.

The high incidence of hysterectomies may also have a partial explanation in the decreased need for biologic functions to be the focus of a woman's identity. With the advent of oral contraceptives, concern with overpopulation, and the number of women working outside the home, women may be less inclined to place a heavy emphasis on retaining their uteri.

Perhaps, in the future, the women's movement will help women to gain a new positiveness about their bodies and their female functioning. This positiveness, if coupled with increased medical management of distressful symptoms of menstruation and menopause, may cause a reduction in the number of hysterectomies performed. Efforts made by nurses through research to identify the effects of stress on the functioning of the female reproductive system may help to reduce the incidence of surgical treatment of a psychoemotional problem.

Notes

1. Marcia Cohen, "Needless Hysterectomies," *Ladies Home Journal* 93, no. 3 (March 1976): 88.
2. Lindsay R. Curtis, *After Hysterectomy What?* (Bristol, Tenn.: Beecham Laboratories, 1975), pp. 14-16.
3. Beverly Raphael, "The Crisis of Hysterectomy," *Australian and New Zealand Journal of Psychiatry* 6 (1972): 114.
4. Beverly Raphael, "Psychiatric Aspects of Hysterectomy, in *Modern Perspectives in the Psychiatric Aspects of Surgery*, ed. John G. Howells (New York: Brunner/Mazel, 1976), p. 438.
5. Associated Press, *Minneapolis Tribune* (May 10, 1977) Section B: 6.
6. Joann Rodgers, "Are This Year's 690,000 Hysterectomies All Necessary?" *Women's Network Directory 1976* (Minneapolis: Women's Network, 1976), p. 136.
7. Marvin G. Drellich and Irving Bieber, "The Psychologic Importance of the Uterus and Its Functions," *Journal of Nervous and Mental Disorders* 126 (1958): 322-336.
8. Raphael, "Crisis of Hysterectomy," pp. 109-111.
9. Jean E. Johnson, John F. Morrissey, and Howard Leventhal, "Psychological Preparation for an Endoscopic Examination," *Gastrointestinal Endoscopy* 19, no. 4 (1973): 190-192.
10. Jean E. Johnson, "Effects of Accurate Expectations About Sensations on the Sensory and Distress Components of Pain," *Journal of Personality and Social Psychology* 27, no. 2 (1973): 273-274.
11. Morris E. Chafetz, "Hysterectomy and Castration: An Emotional Look-Alike," *Medical Insight* 3 (January 1971): 40.
12. M. Steiner and D.R. Aleksandrowicz, "Psychiatric Sequence to Gynecological Operations," *Israel Annals of Psychiatry and Related Disciplines* 8 (1970): 191.
13. Valerie M. Thompson, "Sexual Life After Hysterectomy," (letter to the editor), *British Medical Journal* 3 (July 12, 1975): 97.
14. Raphael, "Crisis of Hysterectomy," p. 113.
15. Margaret A. Williams, "Cultural Patterning of the Feminine Role," *Nursing Forum* 12, no. 4 (1973): 386.
16. Raphael, "Crisis of Hysterectomy," p. 113.
17. Robert L. Green, Jr., "The Emotional Aspects of Hysterectomy," *Southern Medical Journal* 66 (April 1973): 443-444.
18. Ibid.
19. George F. Melody, "Depressive Reactions Following Hysterectomy," *American Journal of Obstetrics and Gynecology* 83, no. 3 (February 1, 1962): 413.
20. Raphael, "Crisis of Hysterectomy," p. 114.
21. Madeline Gray, *The Changing Years: The Menopause without Fear* (New York: Doubleday and Company, 1967), p. 239.
22. S.B. Gusberg, "Indications for Hysterectomy," in *Controversy in Obstetrics and Gynecology*, ed. Duncan Reid and T.C. Barton (Philadelphia: W.B. Saunders Company, 1969), p. 316.

23. Ibid., p. 317.

24. Ibid., pp. 317-318.

25. Cohen, "Needless Hysterectomies," p. 88.

26. Ibid.

27. Henry W. Foster, "Removal of the Normal Uterus," *Southern Medical Journal* 69, no. 1 (January 1976): 13-15.

28. Raphael, "Psychiatric Aspects of Hysterectomy," p. 426.

29. John C. Donovan, "Some Psychosomatic Aspects of Obstetrics and Gynecology," *American Journal of Obstetrics and Gynecology* 75, no. 1 (January 1958): 78.

30. Gusberg, "Indications for Hysterectomy," p. 315.

31. Norman Miller, "Hysterectomy: Therapeutic Necessity or Surgical Racket?" *American Journal of Obstetrics and Gynecology* 51 (1946): 808.

32. James C. Doyle, "Unnecessary Hysterectomies," *Journal of the American Medical Association* 151, no. 5 (January 13, 1953): 364.

33. R. Chynoweth, "Psychological Complications of Hysterectomy," *Australian and New Zealand Journal of Psychiatry* 7 (1973): 103.

34. Raphael, "Psychiatric Aspects of Hysterectomy," p. 425.

35. Waverly R. Payne, "Hysterectomy: A Problem in Public Relations," *American Journal of Obstetrics and Gynecology* 72, no. 6 (December 1956): 1167.

36. Doyle, "Unnecessary Hysterectomies," p. 364.

37. Judith Ramsey, "The Modern Woman's Health Guide to Her Own Body," *Family Circle,* July 1973, pp. 113-120.

38. Cohen, "Needless Hysterectomies," p. 88.

39. Raphael, "Psychiatric Aspects of Hysterectomy," p. 430.

40. Drellich and Bieber, "Psychological Importance of Uterus," p. 326.

41. William S. Kroger, "Hysterectomy: Psychosomatic Factors of the Pre-operative and Post-operative Aspects and Management," *Western Journal of Surgery, Obstetrics and Gynecology* 65 (September-October 1957): 317-323.

42. Raphael, "Psychiatric Aspects of Hysterectomy," p. 430.

43. Drellich and Bieber, "Psychological Importance of Uterus," pp. 330-331.

44. Erich Lindemann, "Observations on Psychiatric Sequelae to Surgical Operations in Women," *American Journal of Psychiatry* 98 (1941): 132.

45. Raphael, "Psychiatric Aspects of Hysterectomy," p. 426.

46. E. Stewart Taylor, *Essentials of Gynecology* (Philadelphia: Lea and Febiger, 1969), p. 35.

47. Ibid., p. 545.

48. Ibid., p. 37.

49. J.C. McClure Browne, *Postgraduate Obstetrics and Gynecology* (London: Butterworths and Co., 1973), p. 38.

50. D.H. Richards, "A Post-hysterectomy Syndrome," *Lancet* (October 26, 1974): 985.

51. T.L.T. Lewis, "The Rationale of Operative Removal of the Ovaries at Hysterectomy," in *The Management of the Menopause*, ed. Stuart Cambell (Baltimore: University Park Press, 1976), pp. 369-370.

52. D.J.S. Hunter, "Oophorectomy and the Surgical Menopause," in *The Menopause*, ed. R.J. Beard, (Baltimore: University Park Press, 1976), pp. 208-209.

53. Barbara Creaturo, "I had a Hysterectomy," *Cosmopolitan*, August 1969, p. 60.

54. Raphael, "Psychiatric Aspects of Hysterectomy," p. 433.

55. Ibid., p. 432.

56. Ralph Patterson, et al., "Social and Medical Characteristics of Hysterectomized and Non-Hysterectomized Psychiatric Patients," *Obstetrics and Gynecology* 15 (1960): 215.

57. Raphael, "Psychiatric Aspects of Hysterectomy," p. 432.

58. Ralph Patterson and James B. Craig, "Misconceptions Concerning the Psychological Effects of Hysterectomy," *American Journal of Obstetrics and Gynecology* 85, no. 1 (January 1, 1963): 107.

59. Raphael, "Psychiatric Aspects of Hysterectomy," p. 432.

60. Ibid.

61. Chaftez, "Hysterectomy and Castration," p. 43.

62. Ibid.

63. Raphael, "Psychiatric Aspects of Hysterectomy," p. 434.

64. Hania W. Ris, "What Do Women Want?" *Journal of American Medical Women's Association* 29, no. 10 (October 1974): 451.

65. Raphael, "Psychiatric Aspects of Hysterectomy," p. 434.

66. Donovan, "Psychosomatic Aspects," p. 78.

67. Marc Hollender, "A Study of Patients Admitted to a Psychiatric Hospital After Pelvic Operations," *American Journal of Obstetrics and Gynecology* 79, no. 3 (March 1960): 500-501.

68. Sanford Wolf, "Emotional Reactions to Hysterectomy," *Postgraduate Medicine* 47 (May 1970): 165-169.

69. R.M. Ellison, "Psychiatric Complications Following Sterilization of Women," *Medical Journal of Australia* 2 (October 17, 1964): 627-628.

70. Prudence Tunnadine, "Gynecological Illness After Sterilization" (letter to the editor) *British Medical Journal* 1 (1972): 748-749.

71. Beverly Raphael, Parameters of Health Outcome Following Hysterectomy," *Bulletin of the Post-Graduate Committee in Medicine, University of Sydney* 30, no. 9 (December 1974): 218.

72. Montagu G. Barker, "Psychiatric Illness After Hysterectomy," *British Medical Journal* 2 (April 13, 1968): 94.

73. Hollender, "Patients After Pelvic Operations," pp. 500-501,

74. Donovan, "Psychosomatic Aspects," p. 78.

75. R.M. Ellison, "Psychiatric Complications Following Sterilization of Women," *Medical Journal of Australia* 2 (October 17, 1964): 627.

76. Drellich and Bieber, "Psychological Importance of Uterus," pp. 323-324.

77. Rollo May, *Power and Innocence: A Search for the Sources of Violence* (New York: Dell Publishing Co., 1972), p. 82.

78. Drellich and Bieber, "Psychological Importance of Uterus," p. 323.

79. Williams, "Cultural Patterning," p. 382.

80. Raphael, "Psychiatric Aspects of Hysterectomy," p. 430.

81. Drellich and Bieber, "Psychological Importance of Uterus," p. 323.

82. Doris Menzer et al., "Patterns of Emotional Recovery from Hysterectomy," *Psychosomatic Medicine* 19, no. 5 (1957): 386.

83. Williams, "Cultural Patterning," p. 386.

84. Patterson et al., "Social and Medical Characteristics," p. 215.

85. Raphael, "Psychiatric Aspects of Hysterectomy," p. 431.

86. Fritz Wengraf, "Psychoneurotic Symptoms Following Hysterectomy," *American Journal of Obstetrics and Gynecology* 52 (1946): 648.

87. Raphael, "Psychiatric Aspects of Hysterectomy," p. 432.

88. Steiner and Aleksandrowicz, "Psychiatric Sequence to Gynecological Operations," pp. 186-192.

89. Rodgers, "Are This Year's Hysterectomies Necessary?" p. 136.

90. Donovan, "Psychosomatic Aspects," pp. 78-79.

91. Russel K. Laros and Bruce A. Work, "Female Sterilization: Vaginal Hysterectomy," *American Journal of Obstetrics and Gynecology* 22, no. 6 (July 15, 1975): 695-697.

92. Peter Barglow et al., "Hysterectomy and Tubal Ligation: A Psychiatric Comparison," *Obstetrics and Gynecology* 25, no. 4 (April 1965): 522-526.

93. Katharina Dalton, "Discussion on the Aftermath of Hysterectomy and Oophorectomy," *Proceedings of the Royal Society of Medicine* 50 (June 1957): 418.

94. Drellich and Bieber, "Psychological Importance of Uterus," p. 324.

95. D.T. Dodds, C.R. Potgieter, and P.J. Turner, "The Physical and Emotional Results of Hysterectomy," *South African Medical Journal* 35, no. 53 (1961): 54.

96. Drellich and Bieber, "Psychological Importance of Uterus," p. 325.

97. Raphael, "Psychiatric Aspects of Hysterectomy," p. 431.

98. Drellich and Bieber "Psychological Importance of Uterus," p. 324.

99. Donovan, "Psychosomatic Aspects," pp. 76-78.

100. Williams, "Cultural Patterning," p. 440.

101. Lewis, "Removal of Ovaries," p. 368.

102. Richards, "Post-hysterectomy Syndrome," p. 985.

103. Margaret Williams, "Easier Convalescence from Hysterectomy," *American Journal of Nursing* 76, no. 3 (March 1976): 440.

104. William H. Masters and Virginia E. Johnson, "What Young Women Should Know About Hysterectomies," *Redbook*, January 1976, pp. 48-50.

105. Gray, *Changing Years*, p. 229.

106. Hunter, "Oophorectomy and Surgical Menopause," pp. 208-209.

107.   Raphael, "Psychiatric Aspects of Hysterectomy," p. 429.

108.   Payne, "Problem in Public Relations," p. 1167.

109.   Drellich and Bieber, "Psychological Importance of Uterus," p. 329.

110.   A.G. Amias, "Sexual Life After Gynaecological Operations. I," *British Medical Journal* 2 (June 14, 1975): 608.

111.   G.A. Craig and P. Jackson, "Sexual Life After Vaginal Hysterectomy" (letter to the editor) *British Medical Journal* 3 (July 12, 1975): 97.

112.   Masters and Johnson, "What Women Should Know," p. 49.

113.   John W. Huffman, "The Effect of Gynecological Surgery on Sexual Reactions," *American Journal of Obstetrics and Gynecology* 59, no. 4 (April 1950): 917.

114.   Gray, *Changing Years*, p. 248.

115.   Tunnadine, "Gynecological Illness After Sterilization," 748-749.

116.   Huffman, "Effect on Sexual Reactions," pp. 915-917.

117.   Gray, *Changing Years*, p. 248.

118.   Dodds, Potgieter, and Turner, "Results of Hysterectomy," p. 54.

119.   Richards, "Post-hysterectomy Syndrome," p. 984.

120.   Patterson and Craig, "Misconceptions," p. 109.

121.   Ibid.

122.   James Leslie McCary, *Human Sexuality* (New York: D. Van Nostrand Company, 1973), p. 259.

123.   Kroger, "Hysterectomy: Psychosomatic Factors," p. 317.

124.   Drellich and Bieber, "Psychological Importance of Uterus," p. 325.

125.   Williams, "Cultural Patterning," p. 382.

126.   Dalton, "Aftermath of Hysterectomy," p. 415.

127.   Drellich and Bieber, "Psychological Importance of Uterus," p. 326.

128.   Melody, "Depressive Reactions Following Hysterectomy," p. 141.

129.   Ibid.

130.   Masters and Johnson, "What Women Should Know," pp. 48-51.

131.   Cohen, "Needless Hysterectomies," p. 88.

132.   Marc H. Hollender, "Hysterectomy and Feelings of Feminity," *Medical Aspects of Human Sexuality* 3 (July 1969): 11.

133.   Raphael "Psychiatric Aspects of Hysterectomy," p. 434.

134.   Ibid.

135.   Cohen, "Needless Hysterectomies," p. 90.

136.   Richards, "Post-hysterectomy Syndrome," pp. 984-985.

137.   Ibid., p. 984.

138.   Dodds, Potgieter, and Turner, "Results of Hysterectomy," p. 54.

139.   London B. Ackner, "Emotional Aspects of Hysterectomy: A Follow-Up Study of Fifty Patients Under the Age of Forty," eds. A. Jores and H. Freyberger, *Advances in Psychosomatic Medicine* (New York: Robert Brunner, Inc., 1960) p. 251.

140.   Richards, "Post-hysterectomy Syndrome," p. 985.

141.   Williams, "Easier Convalescence from Hysterectomy," p. 440.

142.   Dodds, Potgieter, and Turner, "Results of Hysterectomy," p. 53.

143.   Williams, "Easier Convalescence from Hysterectomy," p. 438.

144.   Ibid.

145.   Richards, "Post-hysterectomy Syndrome," pp. 984-985.

146.   Ibid., p. 985.

147.   Robert L. Bragg, "Risk of Admission to a Mental Hospital Following Hysterectomy or Cholecystectomy," *American Journal of Public Health* 55, no. 9 (September 1965): 1403-1410.

148.   Ellison, "Psychiatric Complications," pp. 625-627.

149.   Ralph Patterson et al., "Social and Medical Characteristics," pp. 209-215.

150.   Patterson and Craig, "Misconceptions," pp. 104-111.

151.   Hollender, "Patients After Pelvic Operations," pp. 498-503.

152.   Barker, "Psychiatric Illness After Hysterectomy," p. 94.

153.   Ackner, "Emotional Aspects of Hysterectomy," pp. 248-251.

154.   Dodds, Potgieter, and Turner, "Results of Hysterectomy," pp. 53-55.

155.   Barglow et al., "Hysterectomy and Tubal Ligation," pp. 520-526.

156.   Steiner and Aleksandrowicz, "Psychiatric Sequence to Gynecological Operations," pp. 186-192.

157.   Melody, "Depressive Reactions Following Hysterectomy," pp. 410-413.
158.   Lindeman, "Psychiatric Sequelae," pp. 132-139.
159.   James T. Moore and Dennis H. Tolley, "Depression Following Hysterectomy," *Psychosomatics* 17 (April-May-June 1976): 86-89.
160.   Melody, "Depressive Reactions Following Hysterectomy," p. 411.
161.   Richards, "Post-hysterectomy Syndrome," p. 983.
162.   Chynoweth, "Psychological Complications of Hysterectomy," p. 103.
163.   Melody, "Depressive Reactions Following Hysterectomy," p. 413.
164.   Ackner, "Emotional Aspects of Hysterectomy," p. 250.
165.   Raphael, "Parameters of Health Outcome," pp. 218-219.
166.   Menzer et al., "Patterns of Emotional Recovery," pp. 385-387.
167.   Raphael, "Psychiatric Aspects of Hysterectomy," p. 439.
168.   Rodger, "Are This Year's Hysterectomies Necessary?", p. 138.

18
Menopause

A Closer Look for Nurses

RUTH A. M. DYER

Once menopause was considered one of the most stressful experiences in a woman's life. Although the changes inherent in the menopause event may cause stress, the experience does not necessarily cause distress. Then what is the experience like for women?

Unfortunately, the information available about menopause is inadequate and has too often been inaccurate. Increasing research interest has resulted in the beginning steps of developing accurate knowledge about this event in every woman's life. But women and health professionals must realize the limitations and tentativeness of present information about menopause.

This chapter describes current views of menopause and the surrounding experience and attempts to distinguish commonly held beliefs from those aspects that have research support.

EARLY VIEW OF MENOPAUSE

For years the classic picture of menopause presented a woman in physical and emotional turmoil, exhibiting a multitude of signs and symptoms ranging from a bad taste in the mouth to convulsions and often on the verge of nervous exhaustion. This clinical picture was in keeping with the prevailing view of a woman as a primarily biologic organism whose function was related to attractiveness, childbearing, and child rearing.[1] When menopause took away her capacity to reproduce the human species, it seemed only natural to society that she would have difficulty coping with this impending "uselessness" and "senescence."[2,3] In fact, it seems that women were almost obligated to respond negatively to this period of life: "She realizes vividly that the beautiful past, the loving and beloved womanhood, is now to be left behind forever, and by this an intelligent and sensitive woman cannot fail to be profoundly affected."[4]

While struggling to overcome this "partial death," this "biologic withering," women were expected to experience feelings of hopelessness, sexlessness, purposelessness, and depression. Anxiety, feelings of loss and inferiority, paranoia, urges to have more children, and alterations in sexual desire were common.[5,6] Interestingly, increased sexual desire was believed to be more distressing for women than were decreased sexual feelings. This probably reflected society's expectations that, after menopause, women should quietly fade into sexless oblivion. When experienced by any woman 30 to 60 years old, these feelings and concerns, as well as almost any physical signs and sensations that were not easily explained by other diagnoses, were quickly attributed to approaching menopause. The labels "menopausal syndrome" or "climacteric syndrome" evolved and are still in use today.

The characteristics usually denoted by these labels include the following: vasomotor symptoms of hot flashes, chills, sweats, and palpitations; other somatic symptoms such as rheumatic pains, paresthesias, and dizziness; symptoms often considered psychological or psychosomatic such as weakness and fatigue, headache, nervousness, insomnia, depression, forgetfulness, and melancholia.[7-9]

The idea of a "menopausal syndrome" has become even more firmly established, perhaps in part due to such tools as the Blatt Menopausal Index (BMI). This tool consists of a list of 11 symptoms considered most common in menopausal women. A numerical weight has been assigned to each symptom to reflect its prominence and potential for causing distress in women, as judged by the tool developers. This weight is multiplied by a severity factor when present in a woman, and the sum obtained from all complaints is the Blatt Menopausal Index.[10] Although the BMI was originally devised to measure the effect of various medical therapies on the symptoms listed, the tool has also been erroneously viewed as a method for judging whether a woman is menopausal. This is unfortunate since few of the 11 symptoms have been shown to discriminate between menopause and other times in life, while other signs and symptoms not included in the tool might discriminate more appropriately.[11]

LIMITATIONS OF PRESENT KNOWLEDGE

What is actually known about menopause and the experiences surrounding this event? Quite frankly our knowledge base remains limited. Little research was focused on menopause before 1945. Besides the fact that the life span of only a relatively small proportion of women was expected to exceed the age of menopause, societal taboos made the subject of menopause less than desirable as an area of scientific study. Even when researchers did take an interest, their efforts were often frustrated by the unwillingness of women to share this private aspect of their lives.[12,13]

Current research is limited in both quality and quantity. Most research has been done on women seeking medical care for menopausal complaints. Consequently, we know little about the experience of those women who may not find it necessary to seek medical care. Even the findings based on well women can not be generalized to all women. Also, many other life events and changes commonly take place in the years of menopause, greatly complicating any attempt to define those experiences attributable to menopause rather than the entire middle stage of life.

A focus that has been completely neglected until recently is the study of the individual's subjective response to menopause. In an attempt to obtain "objective" evidence, research has failed to utilize the opportunity to have those women actually experiencing menopause describe this life event in their own words.

Any description of menopause, then, is admittedly sketchy and tentative. However, the information presented here can provide the nurse with some basis for correcting misconceptions and evolving an accurate base of knowledge as new research findings become available.

CURRENT VIEW OF MENOPAUSE

Definitions

Terms such as *menopause, female climacteric,* and *the change of life* have been used interchangeably in both lay and professional literature. Since these terms may refer to a single event or to a continuum of 20 years or more, confusion results. The following definitions are presented to help the nurse be more precise and consistent in discussing menopause and in examining research findings for implications for practice:

Menopause refers to the actual cessation of menstruation and can be said to have occurred after a woman has had no menstrual bleeding for a least one year.[14,15]

Female climacteric refers to the period of life characterized by morphologic and physiologic changes in the body that accompany the decreasing function of the ovaries.[16] The climacteric encompasses the time period and those events leading up to and following the actual cessation of menstruation. The menopause then becomes just one physical event in the entire climacteric experience.

Change of life refers to the time span of the entire climacteric rather than simply the event of menopause.

Middle years refers generally to the same time span as the climacteric.

Premenopausal refers to women whose menstrual pattern is similar to that which they have had in the preceding years.[17-19]

Postmenopausal refers to women who have ceased to menstruate for one full year or more.[20-23] Research studies have also used this term to describe women who have ceased to menstruate for at least three years.[24] The second definition is used in this chapter.

Perimenopausal means around the time of the natural cessation of menstruation. In previous research and in this chapter, the term refers to women who have at some time in the past 12 months had irregularities in menstrual bleeding as compared with their previous pattern or who ceased to menstruate one to three years ago.[25,26]

The overlap of *perimenopausal* and *postmenopausal* when the latter denotes that menstruation has not occurred for one year is acknowledged. Since irregularities in menses may occur two or more years before actual menopause, allowing the term *perimenopausal* to include two or more years after menopause would seem reasonable. Also, the physical changes associated with the postmenopausal period are more likely to become evident two or more years after cessation of menstruation. Further research to clearly define experiences and underlying physiology should lead to more meaningful and consistent definitions.

When Does Menopause Occur?

□ *Age* The precise age at which menstruation will cease for an individual is not predictable. However, 90 percent of women have experienced menopause between the ages of 45 and 54 years. The average age in the United States is 49.5 years.[27] Various factors have been said to affect the age of menopause such as age at menarche, parity, marital status, and geographic location. However, to date these claims have not been adequately substantiated by research. Also, the notion that average age at menopause has been increasing through the years is a misinterpretation of research findings.[28]

☐ *Artificial menopause* When the influence of both ovaries is obliterated by such interventions as bilateral surgical removal or irradiation the woman is said to have experienced an *artificial menopause*. When stimulation of potential cancer is not a contraindication, hormone replacement therapy is often prescribed, especially if the woman is not yet of menopausal age.

☐ *Signs of approaching menopause* The major physical sign of approaching menopause is menstrual irregularity. This can begin several years before complete cessation of periods and may be characterized by lengthening or shortening of cycles, decrease or increase of menstrual flow, or combinations of these characteristics. Often several months pass between menstrual bleedings; occasionally bleeding resumes after a full year's absence, although if this occurs it is wise to investigate for abnormal causes of bleeding. Some women experience menopause without any changes in their usual menstrual pattern before abrupt cessation.

Women have reported that before menstrual pattern changes they experienced alterations of mood and emotional lability that they perceived as signs of approaching menopause. However, a correlation has not yet been supported by research.

Why Does Menopause Occur?

It is often said that menopause occurs because the aging ovaries stop producing estrogen. This oversimplification can lead to misconceptions. In fact, the event of menopause usually occurs long before the ovaries actually stop producing estrogen. It is more accurate to say that the cessation of menstruation occurs because the aging ovary loses its capacity to secrete estrogen and progesterone in the rhythmic pattern necessary for cyclic bleeding to occur.[29] It is, however, accurate to assume that progesterone production from the ovaries ceases.

As a woman enters her 40s, the follicles of the ovary begin to function and mature differently and begin to secrete less and less estrogen. This decrease in estrogen releases the negative feedback inhibition of follicle-stimulating hormone (FSH) and luteinizing hormone (LH) secreted from the pituitary gland. Even in the presence of increased FSH and LH, ovulation often fails to occur, which may be one reason that fertility decreases after age 40. When ovulation does occur, producing a corpus luteum, that structure also functions irregularly, resulting primarily in decreased progesterone secretion. Since these hormones are responsible for the cyclic growth and sloughing of the uterine lining, the usual menstrual pattern is altered.

The frequency of anovulatory cycles increases toward menopause, and a woman is usually considered sterile after menstruation has ceased entirely. However, there is evidence suggesting that, in at least one case, a woman became pregnant 18 months after her final menses.[30] For safety, contraceptive precautions are sometimes advised for a full year following menopause.[31]

By the time a woman ceases to menstruate, the levels of estrogen and progesterone are usually greatly reduced. However, slight amounts of estrogen continue to be secreted by the ovaries, and the adrenal glands also continue to be a source of estrogen.[32] It is important to realize that these hormone levels usually decrease gradually and that there is still some estrogen circulating in the bloodstream even after menopause. This means that the changes most closely associated with estrogen deficiency states (the atrophic changes of external and internal reproductive structures) usually do not become evident for years after the cessation of mentruation.

The increased levels of FSH and LH previously mentioned are currently being examined for their influence, if any, on vasomotor stability. Blood levels of FSH and LH begin to rise a year or more before the last menstrual period and reach a maximum two to three years after menopause, and then FSH continues at higher than premenopausal levels for 20 to 30 years after menopause for 70 percent of women.[33] Further research is needed to shed light on the hypothesis that increased FSH and LH levels increase the vasomotor instability responsible for the hot flashes and sweats experienced by some women perimenopausally.

Physical Signs and Sensations Experienced

☐ *Critical look at the menopausal syndrome* Women report a wide variety of physical signs and sensations perimenopausally, and many of these sensations are included in the symptoms labeled "menopausal syndrome." However, whether such a syndrome actually exists has been questioned.[34-37] In fact, the only characteristics shown to be correlated with the perimenopausal period have been the vasomotor symptoms of hot flashes and episodes of sweating.[38-41] This is not to claim that the other sensations do not occur. However, there is not yet sufficient evidence that women should expect these to occur around menopause. Actually, there is a good chance that many women will experience few if any of the symptoms commonly attributed to menopause, and, if they do, it may be to a very mild degree. A number of studies have found that significant numbers of the women studied, 15 to 40 percent, had no or very few symptoms or complaints perimenopausally.[42-45] As many as 50 percent of those studied viewed menopause as presenting no difficulty even when symptoms occurred,[46] and only about 10 percent considered their symptoms incapacitating.[47] Table 18.1 contains a summary of research findings related to the symptoms labeled "menopausal syndrome."

Among the other physical signs and sensations that have been reported by perimenopausal women but not yet shown to be related to menopause are feeling less coordinated with hands, swollen ankles, soreness in breasts, nausea, pelvic pressure sensations, muscle tightness and tension, decreased perimenstrual discomfort when periods do occur, weight gain, shortness of breath, backache, increased or decreased sexual desire and response, bloatedness, pruritis and foul-smelling vaginal discharge.[71-77]

TABLE 18.1 RESEARCH FINDINGS ON SYMPTOMS LABELED "MENOPAUSAL SYNDROME"

Symptom[48]	Summary of Research
Flushings-hot flashes	Definitely correlated with menopause; 40-75% of women studied experienced to some degree; most prevalent in peri-menopausal group[49-54]
Episodes of perspiration and night sweats	Definitely correlated with menopause; usually but not always associated with hot flashes; 25-40% of women studied experienced to some degree; most prevalent in perimenopausal group[55]
Difficulties sleeping	Has been reported although not clearly related to menopause; seems to be associated with night sweats; one study showed higher incidence in postmenopausal group and suggested this was a geriatric rather than perimenopausal problem[56]
Fatigue	Commonly reported in up to 50% of women studied although not clearly related to menopause[57]
Dizziness, palpitations	Neither clearly related to menopause; possibly an accompaniment of hot flashes; reported in less than 50% of women studied[58,59]
Irritability, nervousness	Not clearly related to menopause; study reports vary from 9 to 90% incindence in perimenopausal women studied[60-63]
Headaches; aches in joints muscles, bones; tingling of extremities	Not clearly related to menopause; usually reported to occur in less than 50% of perimenopausal women studied, although some results suggest higher[64-66]
Depression, feeling blue	Not clearly related to menopause; reported to occur in 17-78% of perimenopausal women studied.[67-70]

☐ *Hot flashes and episodes of sweating* Hot flashes and sweats will be discussed further since they are the only symptoms positively correlated with menopause. Certainly not all women experience these phenomena perimenopausally, but the experience is relatively common. Studies of populations of perimenopausal "well women" rather than populations of women seeking treatment for "menopausal symptoms" have suggested that 40 to 75 percent of women may experience hot flashes, and 25 to 40 percent of women studied have experienced episodes of sweating.[78-83]

Episodes of sweating can occur by themselves, although most commonly the various degrees of sudden perspiration accompany hot flashes.[84] For some women only a slight amount of perspiration appears on the upper lip, forehead, or neck, for example. Other women have described drenching sweats that necessitated changing the bed clothes and linen.[85-87] These sweats are often followed by a chill or cold sensation, which may be explained by the cooling effects of evaporation of perspiration.

The hot flashes, or flushings, have been described by women as sudden warm, clammy warm, hot, very hot, or burning hot sensations of the skin. These are usually felt in the upper body, especially the neck and face, but sometimes include the entire body. For some women the sensation is progressive, beginning at one level of the body and moving up toward the face, whereas others feel the flash first in the neck and face and then the extremities feel warm.[88-91]

The frequency and duration of hot flashes seem to vary greatly, as does the degree of heat sensed. A study reported in 1927 described duration of flushings as momentary to 30 minutes and frequency ranging from twelve or more per day to one or two per week.[92] A more recent descriptive study of one subject reported various measurements recorded for 2 hours on each of four days. The subject experienced two hot flashes during each 2-hour period. The mean duration of the eight flashes was 3.8 minutes; the range was 2.4 to 4.7 minutes.[93] This author obtained subjective reports ranging from "momentary warm feelings occurring three to four times over a span of several months" to "burning, drying heat" lasting 3 to 5 minutes and occuring almost every 15 minutes all day and night.[94] In some women hot flashes may be accompanied by a blush or reddish splotching of some skin area.[95-97]

So far research suggests that the intensity of heat sensation during a flash may be due to the woman's state of mind, which is one of dissatisfaction with her thermal environment, rather than the degree of actual temperature change. Women simply feel much "hotter" than they actually are. Molnar found skin temperature increases of up to 5.5 C on the fingers and toes but increases of only 0.2 to 0.7 C on the cheeks, an area women often describe as feeling the hottest. Internal temperatures and forehead temperatures tended to decrease with the onset of flashes; this was believed to be due to the evaporation of perspiration. It would seem that a hot flash is an explosive activation of certain brain areas. This results in subjective heat distress, vasodilation in extremities, increased heart rate, and stimulation of sweat glands and vasodilators of the face.[98]

As mentioned earlier, the physiologic mechanisms underlying the vasomotor symptoms of hot flashes and sweats are not yet known. Women have reported that conditions of increased environmental temperature or states of increased excitement or stress seem to predispose them to experiencing a hot flash. Stimuli such as a sharp noise, sudden jolt, or a pinprick have at times brought on a flash.[99-101]

Some writers have claimed that the intensity and frequency of vasomotor symptoms are related to the amount or abruptness of estrogen decrease in the bloodstream.[102-104] However, these claims lack research support.

It is known, however, that estrogen replacement can predictably relieve vasomotor symptoms in most cases. Oral estrogen is the medical treatment most often prescribed for those women who find flashes and sweats bothersome enough to consult a doctor. At times tranquilizers or sedatives are given, particularly if estrogen is contraindicated. Women are becoming more aware of potential dangers involved in estrogen therapy, and as a result may increasingly find this form of treatment unacceptable. Currently there is a definite lack of alternatives to help women deal with hot flashes or sweats if they are troublesome. And, as yet, no specific nursing measures have been discussed in the literature.

It should not be assumed that hot flashes and sweats are undesirable experiences. Women have occasionally reported that the sensation of warmth accompanying a hot flash was pleasurable.[105,106]

☐ *Atrophic changes* The physical signs and sensations associated with degenerative changes of the vagina and surrounding structures are frequently included in any discussion of the menopause. As previously pointed out, these atrophic changes usually do not become pronounced until years following menopause, and so associated sensations are more likely to occur in postmenopausal rather than perimenopausal women.

Certain tissues of the urinary tract and the reproductive system are particularly responsive to estrogen and undergo certain changes as this hormone decreases. Atrophy of the urinary meatus may contribute to frequency of, and burning with, urination. The vaginal walls become thinner and less elastic, and secretions become scanty and less acidic. This increases the likelihood of vaginitis developing. Perimenopausally, vaginal changes may result in itching or irritation with intercourse due to decreased lubrication. As the atrophy becomes more evident in the postmenopausal years, cracking of drying, fragile tissue may cause vaginal bleeding and pain for some women. However, these signs are by no means inevitable; there is evidence that as many as 50 percent of women may experience no more than mild vaginal atrophy for many years after menopause.[107]

The gradual loss of subcutaneous fat of the vulva and thinning of pubic hair also usually do not result in marked changes until the late postmenopausal years.

Oral estrogen replacement does predictably relieve atrophic vaginitis.[108] Estrogen-containing vaginal creams can also be helpful. The use of lubricants can help reduce irritation during intercourse, and regular sexual intercourse is considered a prime measure for maintaining lubrication and the vagina's ability to expand.[109] Unfortunately, the alternatives available to women for dealing with atrophic symptoms are still limited.

☐ *Osteoporosis and heart disease* Proponents and lifelong estrogen therapy have claimed that estrogen has the power to slow down the demineralization of bone that occurs with aging and to prevent heart disease.[110] Although some studies do indicate that estrogen can inhibit bone resorption,[111] there is still a lack of conclusive evidence that estrogen replacement will prevent osteoporosis in the minority of postmenopausal women who develop this condition. The relationship between estrogen and the development of coronary artery disease is also inadequately supported.[112] Future research may indicate that estrogen protects women from these conditions. However, nurses should be aware that at present this supposed protection is inadequate reason to advise long-term estrogen therapy. And, in fact, long-term estrogen therapy may be harmful.

Thoughts, Feelings, Concerns: The Woman's Point of View

Nursing's holistic view of humanity dictates that they be concerned with the meaning individuals assign to their total situation; therefore, a focus on the woman's interpretation of her perimenopausal experience seems particularly appropriate for nursing. Unfortunately, the thoughts, feelings, and concerns of women experiencing menopause have received the least research attention. However, the studies reviewed below may provide some additional clues to the nature of the perimenopausal experience and to those aspects that, to be dealt with more effectively, might require a nurse's assistance.

In a study by Neugarten and Kraines, healthy women indicated which of 28 symptoms listed they had experienced. Of the 40 women who reported menstrual irregularities or recent cessation of menstruation, more than 50 percent had experienced being irritable, nervous, excitable, forgetful, or blue and depressed. Less than 50 percent reported being unable to concentrate, having crying spells, feeling suffocated, worrying about body, and feeling fright or panic. Only 12 percent indicated they worried about having a nervous breakdown.[113]

Another group of researchers studied the attitudes and responses to menopause of 51 Israeli women. The analysis of semistructured psychiatric interviews revealed ten major themes that the researchers then judged as either gains or losses. Themes of gain were feelings of (1) freedom from menstruation, (2) freedom from pregnancy, and (3) nonspecific sense of liberation. Themes of loss were feelings of (1) loss of fertility, (2) loss of health as a consequence of cessation of menstruation, (3) loss of femininity, (4) the onset of old age, (5) danger of emotional disturbances, (6) danger of somatic disturbances, (7) generally, menopause had come "too soon."

In this study, gain themes were considered positive expressions of attitude and loss themes were considered negative. A comparison of the number of positive and negative expressions was made to arrive at a measurement of attitude toward menopause. Of the perimenopausal women studied, 29 percent were judged to be more positive than negative toward menopause, 12 percent equally positive and negative, and 59 percent more negative than positive.[114] It is recognized that this method of attitude measurement is crude. Also, it should be noted that many of the women studied were from very traditional cultures that viewed woman's role as that of childbearer.

A survey conducted by the Boston Women's Health Book Cooperative gathered information from 484 women aged 25 to over 60 years. Of those women who considered themselves to be menopausal or postmenopausal, about two-thirds felt neutral or positive about the changes they experienced, and only one-third felt negative. These results differ from those based on Israeli women in Maoz's study. The cooperative's survey also showed that 90 percent of the perimenopausal women polled felt either positive or neutral about the loss of their ability to have a child. Sexual desire was reported as unchanged by approximately 50 percent of the women. The remaining 50 percent were evenly divided between feeling increased or decreased sexual desire. Other feelings and reactions reported included: nervousness and irritation, tearfulness, regret or even rage at aging, feeling "over the hill," a sense of failure, concern over changes in sexual desire, happy that childbearing years are over and can be rid of contraceptive devices, feeling better because of the discovery that fears of going crazy during menopause were unfounded, thoughts that the changes were not drastic or were milder than might have been.[115]

This author carried out a study of perimenopausal unmarried women who were employed. The responses of six women, when asked to describe the thoughts, feelings, and concerns they were experiencing about menopause that were different from their usual experience before the occurrence of menstrual irregularities, varied greatly.

One woman reported no differences in feelings at all. Another woman reported feeling very fortunate that during this menopausal time she felt so good, so healthy, and so unconcerned. She wondered whether depression, hot flashes, or feelings of discouragement would accompany menopause and, if so, whether she had passed the time when those might occur.

All of the remaining four women reported changes in their moods or coping abilities. This is in accordance with other studies that report irritable or emotionally labile states. The following feelings reported were: crabbiness; vulnerability; tendency to react in a magnified way or by crying; feelings of frustration, anger, and nonacceptance of self for crying behavior; and depression and inability to think.

Three of these four women shared thoughts or concerns related to the effect mood changes had on relationships with others; thinking others must be perturbed or angry at moods or behavior, feeling a need to compensate for touchiness or desire to withdraw by making an effort to show caring, and not wanting moods to negatively affect others. Other feelings expressed about relationships included new awareness of needing other people and their understanding, feeling anger at those who failed to be understanding of moods and behavior, increased need to know that family and friends are close, and feeling a greater capacity to have warm feelings toward others.

Two of the women expressed thoughts related to their sexuality, a theme commonly mentioned in other research. Both experienced increased sexual desire or attraction for others and more often wondered what it might have been like to be married and have children. One woman expressed a desire to become more accepting of her own feelings but not to the point that she would dwell on them. The other expressed feelings of guilt and fear at sexual arousal and concern over coping with these feelings in the presence of men. As nuns both women had made early career commitments that precluded marriage and children. This might be one reason sexual feelings at this time were not acceptable to them.

Feelings associated with personal identity were reported by two women: awareness of feeling more capable, and more loving, a sense of being more than the work she produced, and loss of identity due to decreased work productivity.

Other comments were related to the menopause specifically: feeling relief and happiness that menopause is happening, anxious for complete cessation of periods to occur, wondering why others get so upset about menopause and aging, wondering what is still to come with menopause, looking forward to the pace and pressures of life decreasing, and concern over losing sleep at night due to hot flashes and sweats.[116]

Little can be concluded from the studies just discussed. Obviously the thoughts, feelings, and concerns experienced by perimenopausal women vary greatly. Some women find parts of the experience unpleasant or bothersome; however, other women have positive responses to this life event.

What Influences the Perimenopausal Experience?

The influence of a multitude of factors on the nature of the perimenopausal experience has been implied but not adequately supported by research.

☐ *Estrogen* The relation of estrogen to atrophic vaginal changes and vasomotor symptoms of hot flashes and sweats has previously been discussed. The effect of estrogen on other aspects of the perimenopausal experience is still unknown. Claims have been made that estrogen therapy can relieve all the symptoms and distressing feelings associated with a "menopausal syndrome" and increase a woman's general sense of well-being.[117,118] The relief of distressing vasomotor or atrophic symptoms by estrogen could very likely result in an overall increase in peace of mind. However, so far research does not support a clear relationship between estrogen levels and psychological states during menopause.[119-122] Science has only begun to learn of the scope of influence hormones exert over our lives. It is possible that the hormonal imbalance accompanying menopause will be found to physiologically alter emotional lability.

☐ *Emotional stability* At one time if a woman experienced severe physical symptoms or became upset perimenopausally it was considered an indication of limited personality and emotional strength.[123,124] There is some indication that women who experience true depressive reactions and psychoneuroses around menopause are those who have exhibited psychiatric disorders previously.[125,126] However, no correlation has been shown between severity of physical symptoms and emotional stability.[127]

☐ *Marriage and children* Marital status, particularly when associated with the presence or absence of children in the home, is suggested as a factor affecting the perimenopausal experience. A study by the International Health Foundation concluded that the presence of children in the home "buffered" women from experiencing what they labeled "climacteric complaints" as compared with women whose children had left the home.[128] A similar conclusion can be inferred from some findings of Jazsmann et al.[129] A problem arises from responses that may be associated with the departure of the youngest child from the home, sometimes referred to as "the empty nest syndrome."[130] Since most research of menopause has been done with married women who have had children, this is a significant confounding factor. Single women in study populations have had fewer complaints than have married women.[131,132]

☐ *Cultural differences* Research suggests cultural differences in menopausal attitudes and experience, apparently mediated by the prevailing beliefs about women and their role in the family and society.

Dowty et al. compared the response to menopausal changes of 54 Israeli women from three different subcultures. These subcultures represented three points on a hypothetical continuum between traditionalism and modernity. Increased centrality of the childbearing role and a subservient position for women in the family characterized the more traditional subcultures. Diminished importance of the role of wife and mother and increased participation in the labor force were considered characteristics of more modern subcultures.

Those women of the most traditional subculture studied tended to have a negative view of menopause. They had no regrets over the cessation of menstruation but still entertained thoughts of becoming pregnant yet another time, perhaps reflecting the belief that this was their prime function.

The second group of women represented a subculture that was basically traditional but less so than the first group. These women tended to have a more positive view of menopause, feeling great relief that childbearing years were over. They did express concerns over regular menses ceasing since they viewed this as a health-giving phenomenon.

The women of the most modern subculture studied tended to have a negative view of menopause. In contrast with the focus of traditional women on the effects of menopause on childbearing and menstruation, these modern women were more often concerned with changes related to their personality, family, and social environment.[133]

Weideger discussed at length what she considers to be American culture's "menstrual taboo" and commented on the impact this may have on the perimenopausal experience. Not only is menopause considered "unspeakable," "mysterious," and generally of little significance to anyone but women, it is also seen as an ending of womanhood rather than the beginning that menarche represents. She feels that the prevailing negative social attitudes prevent all but the most extraordinary woman from experiencing pleasure rather than discomfort from physical sensations that may occur with menopause.[134]

☐ *Middle years experience* In recent years increased attention has been given to adult developmental processes and the characteristics of the middle years—the 40s through the 60s.[135] Adjustments are demanded by the many events occurring during this time of life. In order to realize the potential for growth presented by these demands, an individual must make an accurate midlife assessment of where she/he is and has been so that she/he can more realistically and meaningfully choose how to spend her/his remaining personal resources which she/he is now beginning to realize may be limited.[136,137] For some individuals this task poses no major difficulty, but for others it constitutes a major crisis.[138]

In her book *Passages*, Sheehy describes some interesting characteristics of this midlife assessment.[139] The individuals she studied most often faced this reassessment between ages 35 and 45. Those who ignored the opportunities for reassessment during this decade were more likely to experience a crisis in their late 40s or 50s. It is interesting to ponder whether the women who accomplish their midlife assessments between the ages of 35 and 45 are better able to cope with the changes of menopause, which usually occur in the late 40s. Could that be a reason few women find menopause a crisis?

MENOPAUSE IN PERSPECTIVE

Any discussion of menopause must finally put that event into proper perspective as but one aspect of the adult woman's growth and development. The influence of events in the middle years on the perimenopausal experience was mentioned, but, more importantly, nurses and women clients as well must realize that the changes occuring perimenopausally are but one portion of the challenge to be faced at this midlife stage of development.

It is hoped that the nurse will use the information presented here to appropriately modify her knowledge base and her interventions with women who will experience menopause. And with increased awareness of the limited knowledge in this area, nurses may be stimulated to increase efforts not only to keep abreast of research findings but also to study the perimenopausal experience themselves, whether as nurse researchers, nurses working with middle-aged female clients, or nurses experiencing menopause firsthand.

NOTES

1. H.J. Osofsky and R. Seidenberg, "Is Female Menopausal Depression Inevitable?" *Obstetrics and Gynecology* 36, no. 4 (October 1970): 611-615.

2. E.H. Kisch, *The Sexual Life of Woman in Its Physiological and Hygienic Aspect* (New York: Allied Book Company, 1916).

3. R.G. Hoskins, "The Psychological Treatment of the Menopause," *Journal of Clinical Endocrinology* 4, (1944): 605-610.

4. Kisch, *Sexual Life of Woman*, p. 344.

5. Ibid.

6. Helene Deutsch, *Psychology of Women*, 2 vols. (New York: Grune and Stratton, 1945), vol. 2.

7. H.S. Kupperman, B.B. Wetchler, and M.H.G. Blatt, "Contemporary Therapy of the Menopausal Syndrome," *Journal of the American Medical Association* 171, no. 12 (November 1959): 1627-1637.

8. B.L. Neugarten and R.J. Kraines, "Menopausal Symptoms in Women of Various Ages," *Psychosomatic Medicine* 27, no. 3 (1965): 266-273.

9. P.S. Timiras and E. Meisami, "Changes in Gonadal Function," in *Developmental Physiology and Aging*, ed. P.S. Timiras (New York: Macmillan Co., 1972).

10. Kupperman, Wetchler, and Blatt, "Contemporary Therapy of Menopausal Syndrome."

11. Neugarten and Kraines, "'Menopausal Symptoms.'"

12. J.H. Hannan, *The Flushings of the Menopause* (London: Bailliere, Tindall & Cox, 1927).

13. G.W. Molnar, "Body Temperatures During Menopausal Hot Flashes," *Journal of Applied Physiology* 38, no. 3 (March 1975): 499-503.

14. Timiras and Meisami, "Changes in Gonadal Function."

15. A.E. Treloar, "Menarche, Menopause, and Intervening Fecundability," *Human Biology* 46, no. 1 (February 1974): 89-107.

16. Timiras and Meisami, "Changes in Gonadal Function."

17. L. Jaszmann, N.D. van Lith, and J.C.A. Zaat, "The Perimenopausal Symptoms," *Medical and Gynaecologic Sociology* 4, no. 10 (1969): 268-277.

18. L. Jaszmann, "Epidemiology of Climacteric and Post-climacteric Complaints," *Frontiers of Hormone Research* 2 (1973): 22-34.

19. P.A. van Keep and J. Kellerhals, "The Aging Woman," *Frontiers of Hormone Research* 2 (1973): 160-173.

20. Jaszmann, van Lith, and Zaat, "Perimenopausal Symptoms."

21. Jaszmann, "Climacteric and Post-climacteric Complaints."

22. van Keep and Kellerhals, "Aging Woman."

23. P.A. van Keep and J. Kellerhals, *The Mature Woman: A First Analysis of a Psychosocial Study of Chronological and Menstrual Ageing* (Geneva: International Health Foundation, 1973).

24. Jaszmann, van Lith, and Zaat, "Perimenopausal Symptoms."

25. Ibid.

26. R.A.M. Dyer, "A Descriptive Study of the Nature of the Subjective Perimenopausal Experience of Single Women" (unpublished paper, University of Minnesota, 1977).

27. Treloar, "Menarche, Menopause."

28. S. McKinlay, M. Jefferys, and B. Thompson, "An Investigation of the Age at Menopause," *Journal of Biosocial Science* 4 (1972): 161-173.

29. Jose Botella-Llusia, *Endocrinology of Woman* (Philadelphia: W. B. Saunders Company, 1973).

30. A. Sharman, "The Menopause," in *The Ovary*, 3 vols. ed. S. Zuckerman (New York: Academic Press, 1962), vol. 1, p. 539.

31. L.R. Curtis, *The Menopause* (Bristol, Tenn.: S.E. Massengill Company, 1969).

32. Timeras and Meisami, "Changes in Gonadal Function."

33. S. Chakravarti et al., "Hormonal Profiles After the Menopause," *British Medical Journal* 2 (October 2, 1976): 784-787.

34. S.M. McKinlay and J.B. McKinlay, "Selected Studies of the Menopause," *Journal of Biosocial Science* 5 (October 1973): 533-555.

35. M.H. Greenhill, "A Psychosomatic Evaluation of the Psychiatric and Endocrinological Factors in the Menopause," *Southern Medical Journal* 39, no. 10 (October 1946): 787-793.

36. M.P. Crawford and D. Hooper, "Menopause, Ageing and Family," *Social Science and Medicine* 7 (1973): 469-482.

37. J.C. Donovan, "The Menopausal Syndrome: A Study of Case Histories," *American Journal of Obstetries and Gynecology* 62, no. 6 (December 1951): 1281-1291.

38. Jaszmann, van Lith, and Zaat, "Perimenopausal Symptoms."

39. J.C. Donovan, "An Investigation of the Menopause in One Thousand Women," *Lancet* 224 (January 14, 1933): 106-108.

40. B. Thompson, S.A. Hart, and D. Durno, "Menopausal Age and Symtomatology in a General Practice," *Journal of Biosocial Science* 5 (1973): 71-82.

41. E. Feeley and H. Pyne, "The Menopause: Facts and Misconceptions," *Nursing Forum* 14, no. 1 (1975): 74-86.

42. Jaszmann, van Lith, and Zaat, "Perimenopausal Symptoms."

43. Crawford and Hooper, "Menopause, Ageing and Family."

44. Donovan, "Investigation of Menopause."

45. Thompson, Hart, and Durno, "Menopausal Age and Symptomatology."

46. Neugarten and Kraines, "'Menopausal Symptoms.'"

47. Donovan, "Investigation of Menopause."

48. Kupperman, Wetchler, and Blatt, "Contemporary Therapy of Menopausal Syndrome."

49. Neugarten and Kraines, "'Menopausal Symptoms.'"

50. Jaszmann, van Lith, and Zaat, "Perimenopausal Symptoms."

51. Donovan, "Investigation of Menopause."

52. Thompson, Hart, and Durno, "Menopausal Age and Symptomatology."

53. Feeley and Pyne, "Facts and Misconceptions."

54. W.H. Utian, "The True Clinical Features of Postmenopause and Oophorectomy, and Their Response to Oestrogen Therapy," *South African Medical Journal* 46 (June 3, 1972): 732-737.

55. Thompson, Hart, and Durno, "Menopausal Age and Symptomatology."
56. Jaszmann, "Climacteric and Post-climacteric Complaints."
57. Jaszmann, van Lith, and Zaat, "Perimenopausal Symptoms."
58. Neugarten and Kraines, "'Menopausal Symptoms.'"
59. Jaszmann, van Lith, and Zaat, "Perimenopausal Symptoms."
60. Neugarten and Kraines, "'Menopausal Symptoms.'"
61. Jaszmann, van Lith, and Zaat, "Perimenopausal Symptoms."
62. Crawford and Hooper, "Menopause, Ageing, and Family."
63. Donovan, "Investigation of Menopause."
64. Neugarten and Kraines, "'Menopausal Symptoms.'"
65. Jaszmann, van Lith, and Zaat, "Perimenopausal Symptoms."
66. Donovan, "Investigation of Menopause."
67. Neugarten and Kraines, "'Menopausal Symptoms.'"
68. Jaszmann, van Lith, and Zaat, "Perimenopausal Symptoms."
69. Crawford and Hooper, "Menopause, Ageing, and Family."
70. Thompson, Hart, and Durno, "Menopausal Age and Symptomatology."
71. Neugarten and Kraines, "'Menopausal Symptoms.'"
72. Jaszmann, van Lith, and Zaat, "Perimenopausal Symptoms."
73. Dyer, "Subjective Perimenopausal Experience."
74. Donovan, "Investigation of Menopause."
75. Thompson, Hart, and Durno, "Menopausal Age and Symptomatology."
76. Feely and Pyne, "Facts and Misconceptions."
77. K. Stern and M. Prados, "Personality Studies in Menopausal Women," *American Journal of Psychiatry* 103, no. 1 (1946): 358-368.
78. Neugarten and Kraines, "'Menopausal Symptoms."
79. Jaszmann, van Lith, and Zaat, "Perimenopausal Symptoms."
80. Donovan, "Investigation of Menopause."
81. Thompson, Hart, and Durno, "Menopausal Age and Symptomatology."
82. Feely and Pyne, "Facts and Misconceptions."
83. P.C. Berger and J. Norsigian, "Menopause," in *Our Bodies, Our Selves,* 2nd. ed., rev. and exp., Boston Women's Health Book Collective (New York: Simon and Schuster, 1976).
84. Thompson, Hart, and Durno, "Menopausal Age and Symptomatology."
85. Dyer, "Subjective Perimenopausal Experience."
86. Miriam Lincoln, *You'll Live Through It: Facts About the Menopause,* new and enl. ed. (New York: Harper and Row, 1961).
87. J. Rogers, "The Menopause," *New England Journal of Medicine* 254, no. 15 (April 12, 1956): 697-704.
88. Hannan, *Flushings of Menopause.*
89. Molnar, "Body Temperatures During Hot Flashes."
90. Dyer, "Subjective Perimenopausal Experience."
91. Rogers, "Menopause."
92. Hannan, *Flushings of Menopause.*
93. Molnar, "Body Temperatures During Hot Flashes."
94. Dyer, "Subjective Perimenopausal Experience."
95. Kisch, *Sexual Life of Women.*
96. Hannan, *Flushings of Menopause.*
97. Rogers, "Menopause."
98. Molnar, "Body Temperatures During Hot Flashes."
99. Ibid.
100. Hannan, *Flushings of Menopause.*
101. Dyer, "Subjective Perimenopausal Experience."
102. Kisch, *Sexual Life of Woman.*
103. Hannan, *Flushings of Menopause.*
104. Paula Weideger, *Menstruation and Menopause: The Physiology and Psychology, the Myth and the Reality* (New York: Alfred A. Knopf, 1976).
105. Hannan, *Flushings of Menopause.*
106. Weideger, *Menstruation and Menopause.*
107. J. Botella-Llusia and P.A. van Keep, "Vaginal Cytology in the Postmenopause: A Study into Some Correlates," *Acta Cytologica* 21, no. 1 (January-February 1977): 18-21.
108. Utian, "Clinical Features."

109. S.E. Dresen, "The Sexually Active Middle Adult," *American Journal of Nursing* 75, no. 6 (June 1975): 1001-1005.

110. J.L. Bakke, "A Teaching Device to Assist Active Therapeutic Intervention in the Menopause," *Western Journal of Surgery, Obstetrics and Gynecology* 71, no. 6 (November-December 1963): 241-245.

111. C. Lauritzen, "The Female Climacteric Syndrome: Significance, Problems, Treatment," *Acta Obstetricia et Gynecologica Scandinavica Supplement* 51 (1976): 47-61.

112. E.A. Graber and H.K. Barber, "The Case for and against Estrogen Therapy" *American Journal of Nursing* 75, no. 10 (October 1975): 1766-1771.

113. Neugarten and Kraines, "'Menopausal Symptoms.'"

114. B. Maoz et al., "Female Attitudes to Menopause," *Social Psychiatry* 5, no. 1 (1970): 35-40.

115. Berger and Norsigian, "Menopause."

116. Dyer, "Subjective Menopausal Experience."

117. Curtis, *Menopause.*

118. K. Achte, "Menopause from the Psychiatrist's Point of View," *Acta Obstetricia et Gynecologica Scandinavica* 49, supplement 1 (1970): 3-17.

119. Greenhill, "Psychosomatic Evaluation."

120. Utian, "Clinical Features."

121. Stern and Prados, "Personality Studies."

122. Rogers, "Menopause."

123. Deutsch, *Psychology of Women.*

124. Achte, "Psychiatrist's Point of View."

125. Greenhill, "Psychosomatic Evaluation."

126. Stern and Prados, "Personality Studies."

127. Ibid.

128. van Keep and Kellerhals, "Ageing Woman."

129. Jaszmann, van Lith, and Zaat, "Perimenopausal Symptoms."

130. M.F. Lowenthal and D. Chiriboga, "Transition to the Empty Nest," *Archives of General Psychiatry* 26 (January 1972): 8-14.

131. Jaszmann, van Lith, and Zaat, "Perimenopausal Symptoms."

132. N. Dowty et al., "Climacterium in Three Cultural Contexts," *Tropical and Geographical Medicine* 22 (1970): 77-86.

133. Weideger, *Menstruation and Menopause.*

134. N. Diekelmann and K. Galloway, "A Time of Change," *American Journal of Nursing* 75, no. 6 (June 1975): 994-996.

135. Gail Sheehy, *Passages* (New York: E. P. Dutton & Co., 1976).

136. L. Greenleigh, "Facing the Challenge of Changes in Middle Age," *Geriatrics* 29, no. 11 (November 1974): 61-68.

137. Sheehy, *Passages.*

138. H. Peplau, "Mid-Life Crises," *American Journal of Nursing,* 75, no. 10 (October 1975): 1761-1765.

139. Sheehy, *Passages.*

19
The Experience of Widowhood

MARIE E. ALBRECHT

Our culture is death denying and, with denial of death, there is denial of free expression of grief. This creates problems for the bereaved. In speaking of this denial of mourning, Gorer commented, "Today it would seem to be believed, quite sincerely, that sensible rational men and women can keep their mourning under complete control by strength of will or character so that it need be given no public expression and indulged, if at all, in private."[1] Overt expression of grieving is thus treated as though it were a weakness instead of a psychological necessity.[2]

The fact that few people are prepared either socially or emotionally to cope with death or to come to the assistance of those touched by death is a serious problem with profound overtones.[3] A widow in our society may not only be unprepared to face or to accept the death of her husband but may also be denied free expression of her grief and supportive assistance from others in coping with and adjusting to her loss.

To further understand what makes becoming a widow a crisis one must look more closely at cultural and sociopsychological factors as well as at the normal grieving process itself. In looking at this process one can recognize the need for preventive intervention in assisting the bereaved to meet their needs during bereavement.

This chapter examines the grieving process and related cultural and sociopsychological factors and then offers an approach to crisis intervention.

FACTORS AFFECTING NORMAL GRIEVING AND ADAPTATION TO LOSS

Cultural Factors

An individual's bereavement is conditioned by his early reaction to loss and biologic adaptive mechanisms as well as by the institutionalized ways that a culture deals with loss.[4]

Most of our losses are assumed to be retrievable, and so we respond accordingly. Also, reproaches against the dead are discouraged, so that expression of guilt, anger, and hostility—all of which are necessary expressions of the urge to recover the lost person—is blocked.[5]

Feifel adds further insight to the problem: "With increasing fragmentation of the family, decline in neighborhood and kinship groups, the growing impersonality of a culture dominated by technology, and the waning of providential faith, death signals . . . man's loneliness and a threat to his pursuit of happiness."[6] Fear leads to a denial that life is limited by time, a denial that conflicts with the nature of reality Thus, when death occurs, it can assume "awesome dimensions."[7]

Some forces, however, are at work to moderate this fear of death in American life. More and more research in the area of death and dying is emerging. Included are the association of psychosomatic symptoms with death anxieties, the knowledge of death's multidimensional meaning for people, the implication that attitudes toward death oscillate within the same individual, and the discovery that the treatment of dying may be conditioned[8] to consideration of wants of the healthy.

Sociologic Factors

All societies must develop some way of containing death's impact because mortality tends to disrupt the ongoing life of social groups and relationships. "Death disrupts the dynamic equilibrium of social life because a number of its actual or potential consequences create problems for a society."[9] One of these is a social vacuum created when a member of society dies. This disruption or gap is more evident for a person in the middle years. Thus, in modern society, where death is more frequent among the old, society rarely interrupts its business. If death occurs mostly among the elderly and the young have severed emotional ties with them, there is little social or psychological need for a vivid community of the dead. Death may simply remind the survivors of the social and psychological debts they owe; so the funeral and memorial may be attempts to compensate for this. Also, disengagement of elderly in modern societies enhances the continuous functioning of social institutions.[10]

A corpse can produce fear, anxiety, and disgust; therefore, the time of exposure is limited. Death, like illness, is generally handled away from the family so that neither dying nor death interferes with the mainstream of life. Even funerals have become relatively unimportant for the life of a large society. Usually only family members and individuals are affected; so bereavement and adaptation become a private responsibility. This can cause serious problems in adjustment. Thus, at a time when death becomes less disruptive in society, its consequences can be more serious for the bereaved individual who experiences grief less frequently but more intensely.[11]

Our youthful orientation, receptivity to innovation, and dynamic social change increase the distance between the dead and the living. The aged become disengaged in present and future status and are left powerless, anonymous, and virtually ignored. As traditional values of the dead and aged lose significance, there is less sense of identity and of belonging with kinship and community. When the threat of death is there but cannot fit into a religious or philosophical context, our society experiences a crisis.[12]

The social changes wrought by death are far more significant than those attending birth, puberty, or marriage. A mourner may be thrown on his own resources with little help in finding a comfortable social status. Consequently, persons who have been widowed at an early age may remain social isolates for the rest of their lives. Having few intimate relationships makes bereavement personally more significant and anxiety producing.[13] Along with this, the nuclear family orientation provides fewer opportunities for people to be bereaved; therefore, there is little if any past experience for guidance.[14]

The role demanded by society wherein grief is suppressed and mourning is inappropriate can lead to unexpected, far-reaching consequences. The period of shock is given social recognition, but tradition generally denies mourning in the period following the funeral.[15]

Two-thirds of all married women are likely to become widows. The increased life expectancy makes it unlikely that one will experience death while young; thus, the loss of a spouse may be the first experience with death in the family. This heightens the effect of the loss of a spouse, which is the loss of an intimate, very meaningful relationship. The problems of bereavement following loss of a spouse may be intensified by the expectation that the marriage relationship compensate for less meaningful relationships elsewhere in society.[16]

Also, the typical American family fails to utilize its opportunities to educate its children for facing death. Social distance is unnecessarily created when adults do not practice their professional beliefs or share with their children their actual beliefs regarding death. There is a need for blending an earlier realism and directness in confronting death with new patterns of socialization involving rationales that have integrity for this age. Personal experience could be melded with contemporary understandings and a renewed sensitivity to people.[17]

Psychological Factors

Because of the cultural and social factors in our country, there are important psychological implications, especially since "the psychological attitudes characteristic of a high civilization are unstable."[18]

A glaring exception to humanity's ability to solve most problems confronting it is its powerlessness to conquer death. Thus, there is the paradox of people today who believe in science and use the scientific method but who resort to magic and irrationality in handling the anxiety of death. The study of death and the defenses against it is extremely important, for it is the consistent experience of psychiatry that "any defense which enables us to persistently escape the perception of any fundamental internal or external reality is psychologically costly."[19]

Death needs to be put in proper perspective. The person who can accept the thought that one day he/she will die can spend time unfettered by fear. Energies bound up by fear can then be released for the constructive aspects of living.[20]

GRIEF

Grieving Process

Grief is a normal adaptive process that enables the bereaved to deal with the psychological disequilibrium caused by loss of a significant other through death. It is sometimes referred to as the work of grieving and it includes (1) making psychologically real an external event that is not desired and for which coping plans may not exist, (2) an emancipation from strong emotional bondage to the deceased, (3) a readjustment to the environment in which the deceased is missing, and (4) forming new relationships and patterns of behavior.[21-23]

Although there are various viewpoints among researchers who have drawn from their experiences in different countries, there seems to be agreement that there are phases of grief. Pentney, a London general practitioner, refers to the three stages of grief as shock, realization, and readjustment.[24] The author accepts this terminology but prefers that suggested by Tyhurst, namely, impact, recoil, and recovery.[25]

Each phase of grief has certain characteristics. The line between impact (with its shock) and recoil (with its awareness) is more distinct than that between recoil and recovery. The author agrees with Bowlby in quoting Shand that the nature of "sorrow is so complex, its effects in different characters so various, that it is rare, if not impossible, for any writer to show an insight into all of them."[26]

Phases

☐ *Impact*. With impact there is numbness—shock. The numbness may be preceded by great distress. Pollock states that the first reaction may be panic with shrieking, wailing, and moaning or perhaps complete collapse with paralysis and motor retardation. The response may vary with the suddenness of death and the degree of preparation preceding death.[27] The bereaved finds herself in disequilibrium, is bewildered, cannot believe what has happened, has a tendency to act as though the lost partner is still present, and may weep or express anger, be accusing or express ingratitude.[28]

Lindemann provides a picture of the physical symptoms, the striking features being a marked tendency toward sighing respiration, lack of strength and exhaustion, digestive symptoms of anorexia, and a feeling of hollowness.[29]

This initial period of shock and disbelief may be followed by a stunned, numbed feeling in which the grief-stricken person does not permit herself any thoughts acknowledging reality. The loss may be accepted intellectually, but the painful character of the loss is denied or muted.[30] This denial may be a defense mechanism, a means to deal with painful feelings.

This period of impact is described by Phyllis Silverman as a time when people restrict their time orientation to the immediate present.[31] It is a time when there is a sense of being lost, of not knowing what to do, of being suspended from life. One is unable to concentrate, is indifferent to needs, and disbelieves the deceased is gone. The feeling that life can never be worth living hinders the ability to plan for ongoing needs.[32]

☐ *Recoil*. The second phase of grief is one of awareness, when there is emergence from the protective fog of numbness. This is a painful period not cushioned by shock. Bowlby describes the period as a state of mental helplessness when the bereaved has conflicting, ambivalent reactions, for example, there is intensified desire for reunion vs. hatred of the deceased and desire for detachment. The bereaved cries for help, yet may reject those who respond. This is a time when there is restlessness, an inability to sit still, a continuous searching for something to do, an inability to initiate and maintain organized patterns of behavior, a feeling of emptiness of self and world, loss of self-esteem, lack of interchange with others, and loss of a significant goal. The feeling that changes in the external world are experienced as changes in the internal world of feeling is not only painful, but alarming.[33]

Psychological loss is felt most acutely at this time; so the bereaved experiences acute loneliness. Silverman's research has shown that loneliness and depression are most difficult six months to a year following the husband's death.[34] Superficially, the widow may appear to carry on, but underneath she is lonely.

Parkes also views loneliness as a major problem. There is a loss of interest in sources of gratification, and the world is viewed as insecure and hostile. The denial continues. There is a marked increase in affect, and insomnia is common. The intense pining, expressed in crying, restlessness, anger, and searching, creates a strong urge to recover the lost person. There is preoccupation with thoughts of the deceased, and attention is directed to the places and objects in the environment associated with him. There may be a sense of presence of the loved one.[35]

Intense psychic pain may be compounded by feelings of guilt. The guilt can be of two types: persecutory or depressive. "In persecutory guilt the main elements are resentment, despair, fear, pain, self-reproaches; its extreme manifestation is melancholia. . . . In depressive guilt the dominant elements are sorrow, concern for the object and the self, nostalgia and responsibility."[36] The latter form of guilt is most frequent during bereavement.

With guilt there may also be resentment against one's self for having exposed one's self to the experience of loss and resentment against the dead person for having taken with him certain parts of one's self. This loss of parts of one's self leads to mourning and loss of identity.[37]

Loss of a widow's identity affects her self-concept, which is the most important factor affecting behavior. Self-concept relates to all the aspects of one's perceptual field. It is the organization of ideas that is more important to its owner than the body in which it exists. The extension of self is observable with respect to other persons or groups; this is the feeling of oneness with those who have special value. This experience is a feeling of identification, which makes us human. In essence, one's self-concept is who one is; its very existence determines what is perceived. Self-concept corroborates the already existing beliefs about one-self and so tends to maintain and reinforce its own existence. Significant others affect self-concept; the feeling that one is loved by someone who matters is positively reinforcing.[38]

It is no wonder that a widow has difficulty accepting the fact that she is a widow: She no longer has an identity; the important aspect of self-concept is gone. This central aspect requires time to change.

☐ *Recovery.* There is no clear-cut transition from the recoil period to that of recovery, but some form of more or less stable organization does begin to develop. Behavior oriented to the lost loved one modifies. The widow continues to miss her husband, but she adjusts to the loss.

Adjustment depends on many factors, some of which are one's ability to accomplish the work of grieving, perception of reality, a viable support system (internal and external), previous coping abilities, life style, and personality.

This is a time when a widow becomes reintegrated into her new situation; she develops a new set of functioning roles.[39] She functions more effectively in the present, can give up the past, and is able to plan for the future. Gerald Caplan states that this period provides the "opportunity for many widows to gain in maturity, to develop psychologically, to be tempered by the fire."[40]

Time Required to Work Through the Grieving Process

There is disagreement over the length of time it takes to pass through the phases of grief. This is not a quick process, for there are many associations to the lost person, and for each association the tie must be dissolved. The breaking of ties and mourning are not only for the lost person, but also for intangibles like missed experiences and relinquished hopes.[41]

Most researchers refer to the length of the total process. This author agrees with Silverman that the impact or shock phase may take one day to six months or more and also that the recoil phase can extend from one month to a year beyond impact phase.[42] In summary, Silverman believes that recovery can occur in three months to two years following death.[43]

Blank thinks similarly, for he believes that the real work of mourning is a prolonged, painful process that begins a week or two following the death of a loved one and continues until the bereaved can accept the loss and direct energies toward the problems and satisfactions of living. Therefore, "if one is to avoid blundering in giving service to the bereaved or avoid making unrealistic demands . . . it would be safe to assume one year to be the minimum duration of mourning, and one to two years the average duration."[44]

APPROACH TO CRISIS INTERVENTION

Crisis

In a crisis there is an upset in a steady state, or disequilibrium. A person is faced with a need to resolve a problem, but the normal repertoire of coping skills does not provide the answer. Where there was equilibrium, there is now disequilibrium and a need to again seek equilibrium. When this happens, there is tension followed by discomfort and a rise in tension.[45] This tension may motivate an individual to either perceive the situation as a challenge and thus initiate action toward solution or perceive the situation as a threat too great to be tackled.[46]

Balancing Factors

Between the perceived effects of a stressful situation and the resolution of the problem are three recognized balancing factors that may determine the state of equilibrium. Aguilera and Messick identify these factors as "perception of the event, available situational supports and coping mechanisms."[47] "Strengths or weaknesses in any one of these factors can be directly related to the onset of crisis or to its resolution."[48] These factors may be utilized in a problem-solving process (assessing, planning, intervening, evaluating) when assisting a widow through the process of grieving.

Assessment of and Needs of Widows

On the basis of personal experience as a widow and limited research with other widows as well as an extensive literature review, this author sees that widows have needs and tasks to perform that can be categorized under the balancing factors presented by Aguilera and Messick in their pattern of crisis intervention.[49] The three balancing factors may be considered when assessing the needs of the widowed person.

Following are some of the questions that a nurse may keep in mind as the widow's needs are assessed. What event has precipitated the widow's stress at this time? How does the widow perceive the event? How realistic is this perception? Does the widow see a relationship between the precipitating event and her stress? What factors in the widow's internal and external environment are influencing her? How is she reacting or coping to the stressors? What is her level and adequacy of functioning in relationship to herself and others? Whom does the widow trust or see as supportive to her? How does she normally react to anxiety? How does the widow feel she can be helped? It is important to remember that the phase of the grieving process that a person is in may influence the reality and breadth of perception.

☐ *Perception of reality*. Before a widow can adequately see and accept herself as a widow, she needs to recognize her loss not only intellectually, but psychologically as well. This takes time. The cushioning effect of shock may initially be a merciful balm, but, as the numbness subsides, the full blast of realization of the loss may hit. The blow is so severe that the widow wants to recoil—hence the appropriateness of the term for this painful second phase of mourning. Because of the degree of anxiety at this time there is a narrowing of perception.

To recognize the reality of loss, Gorer thinks that there is a growing awareness of the need for a bereaved person to see the loved one dead and that this is indeed a necessary prerequisite for carrying out successful grief work.[50]

It is necessary not only to see oneself as a widow, but to accept oneself as such—to accept oneself as a separate individual with an identity, not as a wife, but as a widow and a single person. This acceptance of a change in identity and self-concept takes time, a fact that in itself may be difficult to recognize and accept.

Besides realistically perceiving and accepting oneself as a widow, a widow needs to recognize that grief has ebbs and tides, to perceive grieving as not only normal but indeed necessary, to recognize and accept her feelings, to perceive her strengths and limitations, to recognize that she can change and grow, and to view herself as able.

☐ *Support system*. In order to accomplish the above, a widow needs a support system. An external support system will reinforce the internal support system.

Research by Madison indicates that some widows with high risk of unsatisfactory outcome can be identified shortly after bereavement. One factor of outstanding importance appears to be the widow's perception that the persons in her environment are failing to meet her needs or are actively blocking her expression of affect and her review of her past relationship with her husband.[51] It is therefore important to determine a widow's perception of her support system.

Grief must be released. Although there is a need for a widow to privately release her feelings, there also is a strong need for her to express her thoughts and feelings to others and to talk about the deceased. In recalling the life of and her relationship to the loved one, the widow is recapturing the life that was and also breaking the ties with her spouse so that she can give him up. This is essential to effective grief work.

Matz has summarized the support needs of a bereaved person: acceptance and warm understanding, an opportunity to express feelings and to share them with others, friends who will stay and listen, friends who understand and who can help one know this expression of sorrow is a sign of strength and dignity and will enable one to face the harshness of reality, to recall the life that was lived with its meaning and limitations as well as blessings, to create a framework of meaning for memories so that an enduring image will emerge.[52]

A widow may also feel a need to question or reaffirm her religious beliefs. When religious beliefs and values provide internal support and solace, this can indeed be a balm.

☐ *Coping.* Since the loss of her husband may be the first time that a woman has had to deal with the death of a significant other, she may have no repertoire of coping skills with which to adjust to the loss. Hence, perceiving the loss realistically and having adequate support while achieving this and learning coping skills may be crucial. Gorer believes that the mourner now "is in more need of social support and assistance than at any time since infancy and early childhood."[53]

Realistic perception and support will facilitate the coping abilities of a bereaved person. Fortunately, a widow in stress and crisis may be more amenable to receiving assistance in coping and learning how to cope more effectively. She may need assistance in perceiving reality; in recognizing and accepting her strengths and limitations; in believing she can change and grow; in learning how to make decisions for herself and those dependent on her; in reevaluating her values, goals, and priorities; in adjusting to the role of a single person and perhaps also the role of a single parent; and in learning new skills so that she can be a resourceful, more independent person.

In essence, the widow needs help in recognizing and consciously experiencing her loss, in freeing or emancipating herself from emotional bondage to her husband, in readjusting to the environment in which her spouse is missing, and in forming new relationships and patterns of behavior.[54]

Planning for Intervention and Evaluation

After the needs of a widow are assessed, planning for intervention is done with the widow. There will then be a clearer view as to how to help a widow work through the grieving process or the related problems once the problem areas have been identified, whether they be recognizing or accepting the reality of the situation, needing support, or learning new coping skills. The most pressing concerns can then be more readily ascertained.

Planning with the widow, involving her as much as possible, will help the widow to utilize her strengths in working through her grief. Madison thinks that it is not necessary to direct all approaches at the widow herself, "for in some instances it may be considered that she has the resources to work through her own problems . . . provided certain aspects of the environment can be modified so as to reduce the amount of interference with her . . . coping techniques."[55]

Whether the intervention planning is directed toward the widow or toward modifying her environment, she should, whenever possible, be involved in the planning by determining her goals and how she thinks she can best attain them. Goals should be striven for in realistic steps, small enough so that progress along the way can be recognized and be reinforcing. If behaviors the widow hopes to achieve are identified at this time, these behaviors can, when attained, be indicators of success and goal achievement.

INTERVENTION

Gerald Caplan and others have felt that supportive intervention at a time of crisis is more readily accepted than at other times and can be preventative. Preventive intervention during bereavement could tip the balance between high- or low-level wellness.[56]

Supportiveness seems to be the key to intervention. According to Madison's research as mentioned previously, widows need permissive support to carry out the work of grieving. The intervener who is supportive in accepting the widow, in allowing her to talk about her reaction to her loss and her relationship to her husband, and in providing the opportunity for the widow to express and share her thoughts and feelings may be providing the support opportunity to express and explore feelings that helps the widow to perceive her situation more clearly and arrive at her own solution to her problems.

Widows in the widow-to-widow program in Boston reacted positively to the supportive intervention of aides who were themselves widowed and who understood what the new widow was experiencing. That empathetic support was needed, appreciated, and beneficial. It was found also that support, at least the availability of it, was usually welcomed until the widow was on her way to recovery, but especially during the period of recoil.[57]

Evaluation

If desired terminal behaviors to indicate goal attainment have been identified in planning for intervention, progress can be evaluated in terms of attainment of this change in behavior. Also, one can evaluate progress on the basis of movement through the grieving process; time orientation movement from orientation to present, to past, and finally to future; maintenance of the same level of health as before the loss of spouse; and on accomplishment of the tasks of bereavement as previously listed.

CONCLUSION

This author firmly believes that if a widow can be assisted in realistically perceiving and accepting her loss, has an adequate support system, and either has or develops a successful repertoire of coping skills, she can work through her grieving without falling prey to the physical, mental, or social negative effects of unresolved grief. "Bereavement . . . can lead to bitterness, or it can produce a pearl of great price."[58]

NOTES

1. Geoffrey Gorer, *Death, Grief and Mourning: A Study of Contemporary Society* (Garden City, N.Y.: Anchor Books, 1965), p. 128.

2. Ibid., p. 131.

3. Robert Fulton, "Widow in America: Some Sociological Observations," in *Proceedings of Workshop for Widows and Widowers, April 30, May 1 and 2, 1971* (Boston: Harvard Medical School Laboratory of Community Psychiatry, 1971), p. 8.

4. George R. Krupp and Bernard Kligfeld, "The Bereavement Reaction to a Cross-Cultural Evaluation," *Journal of Religion and Health* 1, no. 3 (April 1962): 227.

5. John Bowlby, "Process of Mourning," *International Journal of Psychoanalysis* 42 (1961): 333-334.

6. Herman Feifel, "The Meaning of Death in American Society: Implications for Education," in *Death Education Preparation for Living*, ed. Betsy Green and Donald Irish (Cambridge, Mass.: Schenkman, 1971), pp. 4-5.

7. Ibid., p. 244.

8. Ibid., pp. 6-7.

9. Robert Blauner, "Death and Social Structure," *Psychiatry* 29 (November 1966): 379.

10. Ibid., pp. 379-383.

11. Ibid., pp. 383-394.

12. Ibid.

13. Krupp and Kligfeld, "Bereavement Reaction," pp. 238-243.

14. Irwin Gerber, "Bereavement and Acceptance of Professional Services," *Community Mental Health Journal* 5, no. 6 (1969): 491.

15. Geoffrey Gorer, *Death, Grief and Mourning*, p. 134.

16. Paul J. Reiss, "Bereavement and the American Family," in *Death and Bereavement*, ed. A.H. Kutscher (Springfield, Ill.: Thomas, 1969), pp. 219-221.

17. Donald Irish, "Death Education Preparation for Living," in *Death Education Preparation for Living*, ed. Betsy Green and Donald Irish, (Cambridge, Mass.: Schenkman, 1971), pp. 45-67.

18. Franz Borkenau, "The Concept of Death," in *Death and Identity*, ed. Robert Fulton (New York: John Wiley & Sons, 1967), p. 47.

19. John P. Brantner, "Death and the Self," in *Death Education Preparation for Living*, ed. B. Green and D. Irish (Cambridge, Mass.: Schenkman, 1971), pp. 17-24.

20. Ibid.

21. Otto F. Thaler, "Grief and Depression," *Nursing Forum* 51, no. 2 (1966): 21.

22. C. Murray Parkes, "The First Year of Bereavement," *Psychiatry* 33 (1970): 445.

23. Irwin Gerber, "Acceptance of Services," p. 489.

24. B.H. Pentney, "Grief," *Nursing Times*, November 13, 1964, pp. 1496-1498.

25. J.S. Tyhurst, cited by L. Rapaport, "The State of Crisis: Some Theoretical Considerations," "Crisis Intervention: Selected Readings," ed. H.J. Parad (New York: Family Service Association of America, 1965), p. 26.

26. John Bowlby, "Process of Mourning," p. 323.

27. G.H. Pollock, "Mourning and Adaptation," *International Journal of Psychoanalysis* 42, no. 4-5 (1961): 346.

28. John Bowlby, "Process of Mourning," pp. 331-338.

29. Erich Lindeman, "Symptomatology and Management of Acute Grief," *American Journal of Psychiatry* 101, no. 2 (September 1944): 144-146.

30. George L. Engle, "Grief and Grieving," *American Journal of Nursing* 60, no. 9 (September 1964): 94-96.

31. Phyllis Silverman, "Services for the Widowed During Period of Bereavement," *Social Work Practice Proceedings* (Conference on Social Welfare, 93rd Annual Meeting) (New York: Columbia University Press, 1966), p. 172.

32. P. Silverman, "Services to the Widowed: First Steps in a Program of Preventive Intervention," *Community Mental Health Journal* 3, no. 1 (1967): 38.

33. Bowlby, "Process of Mourning," pp. 323-336.

34. P. Silverman, "The Widow-to-Widow Program: An Experiment in Preventive Intervention," *Mental Health* 53, no. 3 (July 1969): 336.

35. Parkes, "First Year of Bereavement," pp. 444-467.

36. Leon Grinberg, "Two kinds of Guilt: Their Relations with Normal and Pathological Aspects of Mourning," *International Journal of Psychoanalysis* 35 (April-July 1964): 368.

37. Ibid., pp. 367-368.

38. A.W. Combs, D.L. Avila, and W.W. Purkey, *Helping Relationships: Basic Concepts for the Helping Professions* (Boston: Allyn and Bacon, 1971), pp. 39-46.

39. Silverman, "Services to the Widowed," pp. 41-42.

40. Gerald Caplan, "Foreword," *Proceedings of Workshop for Widows and Widowers, April 30, May 1 and 2, 1971* (Boston: Harvard Medical School Laboratory of Community Psychiatry, 1971), p. v.

41. H. Grayson, "Grief Reactions to the Relinquishing of Unfulfilled Wishes," *American Journal of Psychotherapy* 24 (1970): 287-296.

42. P. Silverman, "Services to the Widowed," p. 38.

43. P. Silverman, "The Widow as a Caregiver in a Program of Preventive Intervention with Other Widows," *Mental Hygiene 54*, no. 4 (October 1971): 541.

44. R.H. Blank, "Mourning," in *Death and Bereavement,* ed. A.H. Kutscher (Springfield, Ill.: Thomas, 1969), pp. 204-206.

45. Gerald Caplan, *Principles of Preventive Psychiatry* (New York: Basic Books, 1964), pp. 38-41.

46. L. Rapoport, "The State of Crisis: Some Theoretical Considerations," in *Crisis Intervention: Selected Readings,* ed. H.J. Parad (New York: Family Service Association of America, 1965), pp. 24-25.

47. D.C. Aguilera and J.M. Messick, *Crisis Intervention Theory and Methodology* (St. Louis: Mosby, 1974), p. 63.

48. Ibid.

49. Ibid., chap. 5.

50. Gorer, *Death, Grief and Mourning,* p. 7.

51. D. Madison, "The Relevance of Conjugal Bereavement for Preventive Psychiatry," *British Journal of Medical Psychology* 40 (1968): 224.

52. M. Matz, "Judaism and Bereavement," *Journal of Religion and Health* 3, no. 4 (July 1964): 350-351.

53. Gorer, *Death, Grief and Mourning,* pp. 134-135.

54. Ibid., p. 489.

55. Madison, "Conjugal Bereavement," p. 231.

56. Caplan, *Preventive Psychiatry,* pp. 41-44.

57. P. Silverman, Comments, "Widow-to-Widow Workshop," Boston, June 30, 1971.

58. N. Autton, "A Study of Bereavement: To Comfort All That Mourn," *Nursing Times,* December 7, 1972, p. 1551.

20

Loss of a Child

Two Case Studies

IDA M. MARTINSON

One of the most stressful situations encountered by a mother is the death of her child. When the death follows a long illness, sometimes years in the case of childhood cancer, the mother not only faces the stress of losing her child but also must cope with the accumulated effects of the ups and downs of treatment, the uncertainty of prognosis, overwhelming physical demands, and often isolation from other family members and friends. During this time of stress a mother must maintain herself and her family throughout the traumatic experience. "A crisis experience may thus be seen as a transitional period, a turning point."[1] As a health professional it would be desirous to make the experience as positive as possible.

SEPARATION OF CHILD AND MOTHER

In our society it is usually the mother who has the most consistent and intimate contact with her child. When a situation arises in a family where a child is dying, the mother most frequently will have the greatest involvement in the care of that child. Health professionals need to know how best they can help a mother who is in the process of caring for a child whose death is imminent. One way this knowledge might be gained is by understanding what a mother experiences during this extended period of stress.

A literature review shows that the child's need for the mother increases during serious illness; hospitalization significantly reduces the child's access to her.[2] Because of the reduced access, the child can reject the parent for not stopping the painful procedures and long hospitalizations. Dependence on hospital staff for relief bypasses the parents and strips them of responsibility and the chance to care for the child.[3] Therefore, parents need the opportunity to participate in this care. A study done at the City of Hope Hospital showed that there was a better adjustment and alleviation of many problems for both parents and child when they could be in constant contact.[4-7]

A great deal of literature has been written on the effects of hospitalization on children.[8-11] For children up to age 5, the worst fear is separation from mother. Involved in this separation is separation from family, home, and belongings. Add to this the introduction to new people, new places and new routines, many of them painful, and hospitalization can be traumatic no matter what the diagnosis is. The child over age five is confronted with the same losses and also fears procedures and mutilation. In regard to the dying child, their questions about death usually express concern for three things:[12,13]

1. Am I safe?,

2. Will there be a trusted person to keep me from feeling helpless and alone to overcome pain?,

3. Will you make me feel all right?

There has been a gradual development of the concept of home care as one segment in the continuum of progressive patient care. The professional health team, hospitals and consumer have shown a growing interest in developing home care services in which a patient and family can receive adequate care at an affordable cost.

HOME CARE AND THE DYING CHILD

For several years the author has been studying the home as an alternate institution to the hospital for nursing care. One aspect of this research is a study of the feasibility and desirability of home care for the dying child.* Since 1972, 66 families who have had a child die from cancer participated in this study. Over three-fourths, or 51, of the children died at home with a parent or both parents having the role of primary care giver to the dying child. Whatever technical procedures that were necessary for the care of the dying child were provided by the parents. The lone exception was the insertion of a Foley catheter. There was sufficient time prior to death of the child to teach procedures to the parents. A home care nurse was also available for help if the parents felt she was needed.

Educational level for the parents in these 66 families ranged from eighth grade to college postgraduate degree. Economic status ranged from a single parent receiving welfare assistance to a family in the upper middle-income level. Family size ranged from zero to nine siblings. Several were single-parent families. Some had large extended families or community resources they were able to utilize. Other families had very little outside resources to call upon for emotional, financial, or physical support. All of the families had the support of a home care nurse they could call at any time, 24 hours a day, 7 days a week. The option of returning to the hospital was always available.

A result of this nursing research study appears to be that the two most important factors necessary for home care for a child dying of cancer are (1) the child's desires to be at home, and (2) the primary care giver's perception of an ability to care for the child at home.

Two case studies are included which describe a situation where a mother has cared for her child at home until death occurred. The two mothers are the first and last of the 66 families the author has worked with over a period of six years. One had no professional nursing experience and the other mother is a registered nurse.

*Supported in part by funds from DHEW, National Cancer Institute, CA 19490.

CASE 1*

> A few months ago I was asked, "What has been your greatest achievement in life?"
>
> "Surviving the illness and death of my son," I replied.
>
> "And your greatest disappointment?"
>
> "Losing Eric."
>
> I did not have to ponder my answer to either question but I had never before thought of how ironic it was that my greatest achievement and disappointment were so closely tied together.
>
> It had been a beautiful July day in the summer of 1970, the kind of day that compensates for long Minnesota winters. "The kids," as we usually referred to them—Eric 7, and Betsy, 4—had been tucked into bed. Del, my husband, and I may not have counted our blessings that evening, but we had many times. After having slept peacefully for several hours, we were awakened by a cry. "I hurt all over," Eric said, as I came to his bedside. Seeming particularly distressed, as we tried to soothe him he asked, "Mommy, am I going to die?" We took him to bed with us.
>
> The next morning, Eric told us, "It felt like a giant worm crawled through my body."
>
> Our pediatrician was not available, so Del carried Eric to another doctor's office without even attempting to make an appointment. The doctor examined Eric, took Del aside, and said, "He must be faking; he doesn't hurt in the right places."
>
> The seed of doubt kept lurking in the background, with denial in the foreground, over the next four weeks, as we continued our search for an answer to Eric's ailments. Eric was finally admitted to the hospital for tests. It was suspected that he had either rheumatic fever or rhematoid arthritis. I was very upset with the doctor's speculations but Del was somewhat relieved. "Thank God," he said, "I thought it was leukemia."
>
> Acute lymphocytic leukemia. The diagnosis was made the next day. I had heard the word, knew it was some awful disease, but that was all that came to my mind. I can remember blasting at my sister, "Of all the rotten, stinking people in the world, why Eric?" And I thought, "Why me? How can I possibly survive without Eric?"
>
> At a conference following diagnosis, the disease was explained and we were told, upon asking, that Eric would probably live 2 to 2½ years. I could remember very little of what was said other than Eric would most likely die and some comments about our lives to come.
>
> As I recall, the physician said, "You have two children, one that is going to live and one that is going to die. The one that is going to live is the most important." His words sounded simple enough at the time, reasonable, good advice to follow. But over the next years of illness, frustration, sometimes despair, we found it was not always an easy task treating our children equally,

much less "the one that is going to live" as the most important. Our youngest, in those so vulnerable years, did not always get the love and attention that she so dearly needed and deserved. Our world began to revolve around Eric as hard as we tried not to make it seem that way. Part or all of one out of four days—over 200 in all—were spent with Eric either being hospitalized or at the outpatient clinic. At gatherings, Eric would be the center of attention and was showered with gifts, some from people we hardly knew. Betsy often seemed relegated to only being Eric's sister, hardly an entity on her own. She loved, admired, and depended on her older brother, but life was very confusing for her at times.

The doctor also said to make the most of the time we had—live life a day at a time. Some parents told him those last years were the best of their lives. Living a day at a time is a good way to live, and we did have some good times, but I am more thankful for the years previous to Eric's illness, as those last ones always had a cloud hovering over. I couldn't forget that our son had been given a death sentence. I grieved—anticipatory grief—and had nightmares of his funeral.

I had been thrown into a situation where the responsibility for my son's health was beyond that customary for a mother. The routines of caring for an ill child had taken a different overtone; the drugs I dispensed were much more potent than anything I had previously dealt with. There were side effects to watch for, symptoms to be aware of, all of which had to be related to the doctor in meaningful context. There were too many times when I didn't know whether physical disturbances were a natural or unnatural part of the disease process or drug reaction. I found that telling a doctor my son's breathing was "short and fast" was much less impressive to him than when I related his respiration was in the 90s.

Six months before Eric died, the leukemia infiltrated the central nervous system for the third time in his illness, leaving him with hemiparesis. He improved some, for a while, and went on another series of chemotherapy, but then he began to go downhill again with more loss of function involving both sides.

Aggressive therapy was discontinued. Eric became bedridden, but we kept him at home.

No matter how many people are around, living with a dying child is in many ways a very lonely life. There are few who can accept the intensity of feelings that a parent goes through or who will acknowledge the fact that a loved one, especially a child, is dying.

When Ida Martinson became part of our life, we were constantly reassured that the care we gave Eric at home was comparable, if not better, than what he would receive in the hospital, and I desperately needed that encouragement. The thought of having Eric die at home wasn't the prime consideration at that point, and it would not have even been given any deliberation had she not gently brought up the possibility.

There were some difficult times, times when we really wondered whether what we were doing was right—keeping Eric at home—but it was what he wanted and we wanted and that made it right in itself.

Eric died November 21, 1972. Del and I had been with him, alternately, through the night. I was sitting on his bed, holding his hand, when Eric found peace.

Eric will always have a special place in my heart, but I have found that I can survive without my beloved son. It hasn't been easy, and there have been times when I really didn't care whether I survived or not. I am very proud to have been his mother, as I am of Betsy, a 12-year-old strawberry blonde, and the light of my life.

CASE 2

Joyce Lindgren, a mother who is also a registered nurse, is from a small city, Olivia, in western Minnesota. Her husband is a Lutheran pastor. Her 18-year-old daughter Brenda died in June 1978 as a result of astrocytoma which had been diagnosed 16 months prior to her death. There are nine other children in the family ranging in age from 19 to 4 years. The six youngest children have been adopted by the family. Three of the children are legally blind.

Joyce responds to a statement made in the manual on implementation of home care services that "occupation, education or religious belief, number of children in the home, martial status, etc., need not be a factor for implementation of home care services."[14]

I think one of the things that annoys me most is when I hear somebody putting labels on others and saying, "She's so busy she can't do that," or "This would never work for them because . . ." or "The reason it worked so well for her is because she was a registered nurse," or "How could they possibly take care of her with all the kids they have?" I really believe that "a desire to have the child home and the perceived ability to care for the child are the two major criteria."[15]

My daughter had a very unrealistic faith in her mother because I am a registered nurse. She placed great emphasis on a lot of the mothering type things that I did at home for her. She felt it was because I am an R.N. that I was "doing it so good." I was quite aware of the fact that the majority of the things I did any mother could do. There really were very few things that I did for Brenda that any mother couldn't do; in fact there weren't any, because mothers can certainly be taught to give shots, too.

I looked at the home care nurse as a professional consultant. I wanted to be the one to make the decisions about my daughter and to give my daughter her shots. I wanted to be the one to talk to the doctors, unless I specifically asked the nurse to make a phone call. A couple of times on a weekend more medications were needed and the clinic doctors, who were familiar with the family and Brenda, were out of town. I did not feel emotionally up to dealing with a doctor that I didn't know very well. I called the nurse and said, "Look, I only have enough meperidine for one shot. Do you think you could get more for me?" And she got it for me.

We bought an intercom because Brenda wanted to stay in her bedroom which was down in the basement. She shared the room with her sister. I would have been in worse shape if it hadn't been for that intercom because I wouldn't have been getting enough sleep. I knew I could call her and she could call me. There were some nights when I had her keep the intercom open so that I could hear her when she turned around and moved. That really eased my mind a lot at night. The last two weeks of her life, I moved her up into the dining room. Her sister was on a canoeing trip, and I didn't want her alone. Brenda was not eager to make the move because she loved that bedroom. We made the dining room into a bedroom. There was a queen-sized hide-a-bed there. Brenda used the dining room table for all the stuff that she was working on. The piano and stereo were in there, and she got so she really enjoyed the room. She did not spend too much time in bed although she began to sleep more and more toward the last.

It was very comforting to me to be able to be the primary care giver for my daughter; to give her her shots, to rub her back and to love her up. I slept with her on the hide-a-bed after she went into the coma. One of the intercoms was then plugged in by me and the other by my husband so that I could call him. This worked out effectively for us.

During this time, I didn't want a lot of people in the house. We live in a parsonage and people are used to coming in. Yet at this point I couldn't bear to share her with anybody. She was ours, and I didn't want people coming in and looking at her. I didn't think Brenda would want that either—I know Brenda would not have wanted that. I stopped at the doctor's office and said, "In the hospital sometimes you put notes up on doors 'No visitors, check at desk' or something. Could you do something like that on our front door?" He said, "I don't see any reason why not." So he wrote a note requesting that nobody come into the house without checking with one of the two doctors or the home care nurse and he put his home phone number on it. We were not bothered with numerous visitors after that. Our neighbor across the street said that many people came up, read the note, turned away and left. This was hard for some people to accept I think, but I felt we had a right to do that. This was our family and we were a family unit. We just locked our front door and used the side door so that we weren't seen going in and out.

The day after Brenda's death was an entirely different thing. I needed support then. There was nothing more that I could do for Brenda and that kind of support was helpful to me.

People were very supportive. They brought in meals for almost a month when she wasn't really all that sick and I could have done it. Actually it was me that was collapsing, not Brenda. It seemed, somehow, that I couldn't muster the energy to make the meals. This help was so appreciated.

One of the heavy burdens for me was the feeling of such major responsibility for meeting the emotional needs of the other children. Having Brenda at home helped immensely because they were able to verbalize with her as well as with me. She was adult enough to handle this. Having her at home seemed to reassure them a lot and seemed to make death a much less frightening thing and heaven more real to them.

We certainly realize that we're really only at the beginning stages of the grieving process. Even though we rejoice with Brenda in her new life, our grief is great. I'm sure there will be many times ahead which will be very rough.

CONCLUSION

As the case studies illustrate, mothers under the stress of a child dying of cancer have demonstrated ability to care for their child at home.

It is important for those who work with mothers of dying children to recognize the strengths women have in time of stress, to help these mothers build on these strengths and to support the decisions they make.

NOTES

1. R.H. Moos and V.D. Tsu, *The Crisis of Physical Illness: An Overview*, Stanford University Medical Center and Veterans' Administration Hospital (Palo Alto, Calif., 1978), p. 7.

2. A.G. Knudson and J.M. Matterson, "Participation of Parents in the Hospital Care of Their Fatally Ill Children," *Pediatrics* 26(1970): 482.

3. André D. Larson, "The Family and the Dying Child," *Medical Times* 97, no. 3 (May 1969).

4. C.M. Binger, et al., "Childhood Leukemia: Emotional Impact on Patient and Family," *New England Journal of Medicine* 280, no. 8 (February 1969): 414-418.

5. S.B. Friedman, et al., "Behavioral Observation on Parents Anticipating the Death of a Child," *Pediatrics* 32 (1963): 610-625.

6. S. Freidman, "Care of the Family of the Child With Cancer," in *Ambulatory Pediatrics*, eds. M. Green and R. Haggerty (Philadelphia: W.B. Saunders Co., 1977).

7. L. Goldfogel, "Working with the Parent of a Dying Child," *American Journal of Nursing* 70, no. 8 (August 1970): 1675-79.

8. G.E. Bloom, "The Reactions of Hospitalized Children to Illness," *Pediatrics* 22 (1958): 509-599.

9. Anna Freund, "The Role of Bodily Illness in The Mental Life of Children," in *The Psychoanalysis Study of the Child*, eds. R.S. Eissler et al. (New York: International University Press, 1952): 69-81.

10. G.H.L. Pearson, "Effect of Operative Procedures on the Emotional Life of the Child," *American Journal Diseases of Children* 62 (1941); 716-729.

11. D.G. Prugh, "Investigations Dealing with the Reactions of Children and Families to Hospitalization and Illness." *Emotional Problems of Early Childhood*, ed. G. Caplon (Basic Books, 1955), pp. 307-311.

12. Morris Green, "Care of the Dying Child," *Pediatrics* 40, no. 3, part 2, (September 1967).

13. Eugenia H. Waechter, "Children's Awareness of Fatal Illness," *American Journal of Nursing*, 71 (June 1971): 1168-1172.

14. I.M. Martinson, et al., *Home Care: A Manual for Implementation of Home Care For Children Dying of Cancer* (School of Nursing, University of Minnesota, 1978), p. 6 (Mimeographed)

15. Ibid.

Index

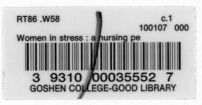